UCLA Symposia on Molecular and Cellular Biology, New Series

Series Editor
C. Fred Fox

UCLA Symposia Published Previously

(Numbers refer to the publishers listed below.)

1972
Membrane Research (2)

1973
Membranes (1)
Virus Research (2)

1974
Molecular Mechanisms for the Repair of
    DNA (4)
Membranes (1)
Assembly Mechanisms (1)
The Immune System: Genes, Receptors,
    Signals (2)
Mechanisms of Virus Disease (3)

1975
Energy Transducing Mechanisms (1)
Cell Surface Receptors (1)
Developmental Biology (3)
DNA Synthesis and Its Regulation (3)

1976
Cellular Neurobiology (1)
Cell Shape and Surface Architecture (1)
Animal Virology (2)
Molecular Mechanisms in the Control of Gene
    Expression (2)

1977
Cell Surface Carbohydrates and Biological
    Recognition (1)
Molecular Approaches to Eucaryotic Genetic
    Systems (2)
Molecular Human Cytogenetics (2)
Molecular Aspects of Membrane Transport (1)
Immune System: Genetics and Regulation (2)

1978
DNA Repair Mechanisms (2)
Transmembrane Signaling (1)
Hematopoietic Cell Differentiation (2)
Normal and Abnormal Red Cell
    Membranes (1)

Persistent Viruses (2)
Cell Reproduction: Daniel Mazia Dedicatory
    Volume (2)

1979
Covalent and Non-Covalent Modulation of
    Protein Function *(2)*
Eucaryotic Gene Regulation (2)
Biological Recognition and Assembly (1)
Extrachromosomal DNA (2)
Tumor Cell Surfaces and Malignancy (1)
T and B Lymphocytes: Recognition and
    Function (2)

1980
Biology of Bone Marrow Transplantation (2)
Membrane Transport and Neuroreceptors (1)
Control of Cellular Division and
    Development (1)
Animal Virus Genetics (2)
Mechanistic Studies of DNA Replication and
    Genetic Recombination (2)

1981
Immunoglobulin Idiotypes (2)
Initiation of DNA Replication (2)
Genetic Variation Among Influenza Viruses (2)
Developmental Biology Using Purified
    Genes (2)
Differentiation and Function of Hematopoietic
    Cell Surfaces (1)
Mechanisms of Chemical Carcinogenesis (1)
Cellular Recognition (1)

1982
B and T Cell Tumors (2)
Interferon (2)
Rational Basis for Chemotherapy (1)
Gene Regulation (2)
Tumor Viruses and Differentiation (1)
Evolution of Hormone-Receptor Systems (1)

Publishers

(1) Alan R. Liss, Inc.
     41 E. 11th Street
     New York, NY 10003

(2) Academic Press, Inc.
     111 Fifth Avenue
     New York, NY 10003

(3) W.A. Benjamin, Inc.
     2725 Sand Hill Road
     Menlo Park, CA 94025

(4) Plenum Publishing Corp.
     227 W. 17th Street
     New York, NY 10011

MONOCLONAL ANTIBODIES AND CANCER THERAPY

MONOCLONAL ANTIBODIES AND CANCER THERAPY

Proceedings of the Roche–UCLA Symposium
Held in Park City, Utah
January 26 – February 2, 1985

Editors

Ralph A. Reisfeld
Department of Immunology
Scripps Clinic and
Research Foundation
La Jolla, California

Stewart Sell
Department of Pathology
and Laboratory Medicine
University of Texas Medical School
Houston, Texas

Alan R. Liss, Inc. • New York

Address all Inquiries to the Publisher
Alan R. Liss, Inc., 41 East 11th Street, New York, NY 10003

Library of Congress Cataloging-in-Publication Data
Main entry under title:

Monoclonal antibodies and cancer therapy.

    Comprised of a series of papers presented at the Roche-UCLA Symposium on "Monoclonal Antibodies and Cancer Therapy."
    Includes index.
    1. Cancer—Immunological aspects—Congresses.
2. Antibodies, Monoclonal—Therapeutic use—Congresses.
3. Immunotherapy—Congresses. I. Reisfeld, Ralph A.
II. Sell, Stewart, 1935-   . III. Hoffmann-LaRoche,
Inc. IV. University of California, Los Angeles.
V. Roche-UCLA Symposium on "Monoclonal Antibodies and
Cancer Therapy" (1985 : Park City, Utah)
[DNLM: 1. Antibodies, Monoclonal—therapeutic use—
congresses. 2. Neoplasms—drug therapy—congresses.
W3 UN17N new ser. v. 27 / QZ 267 M738 1985]
RC271.I45M66 1985   616.99′4061   85-19829
ISBN 0-8451-2626-1

Contents

Contributors

P.G. Abrams, NeoRx Corp. Inc., 410 West Harrison Street, Seattle, WA 98119 **[233]**

Anthony C. Allison, Institute of Biological Sciences, Syntex Research, Palo Alto, CA 94304 **[397]**

Kenneth C. Anderson, Department of Tumor Immunology, Dana-Farber Cancer Institute, Boston, MA 02115 **[113]**

N. Armitage, Department of Surgery, University Hospital, University of Nottingham, NG7 2RD, UK **[215]**

Ruth Arnon, Department of Chemical Immunology, The Weizmann Institute of Science, Rehovot, Israel **[243]**

Cliff Astley, Regional Primate Research Center, University of Washington, Seattle, WA 98195 **[121]**

Robert W. Baldwin, Cancer Research Campaign Laboratories, University Hospital, University of Nottingham, NG7 2RD, UK **[215]**

K. Ballantyne, Department of Surgery, University Hospital, University of Nottingham, NG7 2RD, UK **[215]**

Jacques Barbet, Laboratory of Mathematical Biology, NCI, National Institutes of Health, Bethesda, MD 20205 **[473]**

Robert C. Bast, Jr., Duke University Medical Center, Durham, NC 27710 **[37]**

Lydia Bator, Department of Pathology, Tufts New England Medical Center, 171 Harrison Ave., Boston, MA **[565]**

Jacquelyn Beauregard, University of California San Diego School of Medicine and Cancer Center, and Veterans Administration Medical Center, San Diego, CA 92161 **[133]**

Christopher D.V. Black, Laboratory of Mathematical Biology, NCI, National Institutes of Health, Bethesda, MD 20205 **[473]**

Hildur E. Blythman, Department of Immunology, Centre de Recherche Clin Midy (Groupe Sanofi), 34082 Montpellier Cedex, France **[263]**

Joseph Bolen, Pediatric Branch, Carcinogenesis Branch, National Institutes of Health, Bethesda MD 20205 **[551]**

Michael B. Bolger, School of Pharmacy, University of Southern California, Health Science Campus, Los Angeles, CA 90033 **[289]**

Michael J. Borowitz, Department of Pathology, Duke University Medical Center, Durham, NC 27710 **[63]**

Bernard J.P. Bourrié, Department of Immunology, Centre de Recherche Clin Midy (Groupe Sanofi), 34082 Montpellier Cedex, France **[263]**

Vera Brankovan, ONCOGEN, 3005 First Avenue, Seattle, WA 98121 **[149]**

Joan S. Brugge, Department of Microbiology, State University of New York, Stony Brook, NY 11794 **[551]**

Thomas F. Bumol, Department of Immunology, Lilly Research Laboratories, Lilly Corporate Center, Indianapolis, IN 46285 **[257]**

The number in brackets is the opening page number of the contributor's article.

X. Canat, Department of Immunology, Centre de Recherche Clin Midy (Groupe Sanofi), 34082 Montpellier Cedex, France **[263]**

Walter P. Carney, Biomedical Products Department, E.I. DuPont deNemours, 331 Treble Cove Rd., North Billerica, MA 01862 **[565]**

Jorge Carrasquillo, BRMP, NCI, Frederick, MD 21701, and Nuclear Medicine Department, Clinical Center, National Institutes of Health, Bethesda, MD 20205 **[233,473]**

Dominique Carrière, Department of Immunology, Centre de Recherche Clin Midy (Groupe Sanofi), 34082 Montpellier Cedex, France **[263]**

Ann M. Carroll, Department of Pathology, Harvard Medical School and Department of Medicine, Tufts New England Medical Center, Boston, MA **[359]**

A. Caruso, Laboratory of Tumor Immunology and Biology, NCI, National Institutes of Health, Bethesda, MD 20205 **[23]**

Pierre Casellas, Department of Immunology, Centre de Recherche Clin Midy (Groupe Sanofi), 34082 Montpellier Cedex, France **[263]**

Jerome Charles, Department of Pathology, University of Michigan Medical School, Ann Arbor, MI 48109 **[327]**

David A. Cheresh, Scripps Clinic and Research Foundation, La Jolla, CA 92037 **[173,193]**

W.L. Cleveland, Department of Microbiology, Columbia University and the Cancer Center, New York, NY 10032 **[345]**

Maureen Clutter, University of California San Diego School of Medicine and Cancer Center, and Veterans Administration Medical Center, San Diego, CA 92161 **[133]**

Man Sung Co, Department of Pathology, Harvard Medical School, and Department of Medicine, Tufts University Medical School, Boston, MA 02111 **[367]**

S.P.C. Cole, Department of Microbiology and Immunology, Queen's University, Kingston, Ontario, Canada K7L 3N6; presently at: The Ontario Cancer Treatment & Research Foundation, Kingston Regional Centre, King Street West, Kingston, Ontario, Canada K7L 2V7 **[77]**

P.J. Conlon, Immunex Corporation, 51 University St., Seattle, WA 98101 **[413]**

Geoffrey M. Cooper, Department of Pathology, Dana Farber Cancer Institute, 44 Binney St., Boston, MA **[565]**

David G. Covell, Laboratory of Mathematical Biology, NCI, National Institutes of Health, Bethesda, MD 20205 **[473]**

Yogeshwar Dayal, Department of Pathology, Tufts New England Medical Center, 171 Harrison Ave., Boston, MA **[565]**

Ronald DeLellis, Department of Pathology, Tufts New England Medical Center, 171 Harrison Ave., Boston, MA **[565]**

Robert O. Dillman, Department of Medicine, Division of Hematology/Oncology, San Diego VAMC-V111E, San Diego, CA 92161 **[133]**

Steven K. Dower, Immunex Corporation, 51 University St., Seattle, WA 98101 **[383]**

Lindy Durrant, Cancer Research Campaign Laboratories, University Hospital, University of Nottingham, NG7 2RD, UK **[215]**

M.J. Embleton, Cancer Research Campaign Laboratories, University Hospital, University of Nottingham, NG7 2RD, UK **[215]**

B.F. Erlanger, Department of Microbiology, Columbia University and the Cancer Center, New York, NY 10032 **[345]**

Nadir R. Farid, Thyroid Research Laboratory, Health Sciences Centre, St. John's, Newfoundland, Canada A1B 3V6 **[299]**

M.F. Fer, Hematology-Oncology, University of Kentucky Medical Center, Lexington, KY 04536-0084 **[233]**

Isaiah J. Fidler, Department of Cell Biology, The University of Texas, M.D. Anderson Hospital and Tumor Institute, 6723 Bertner Ave., Houston, TX 77030 **[573]**

Olivera J. Finn, Department of Microbiology and Immunology, Duke University Medical Center, Durham, NC 27710 **[63]**

K.A. Foon, Biological Response Modifiers Program, NCI, Frederick, MD 21701 **[233]**

S.A. Gaffar, U.C. San Diego Cancer Center, T-011, Department of Medicine, University of California, San Diego, CA 92103 **[97]**

M. Garnett, Cancer Research Campaign Laboratories, University Hospital, University of Nottingham, NG7 2RD, UK **[215]**

Glen N. Gaulton, Department of Pathology, Harvard Medical School, and Department of Medicine, Tufts University Medical School, Boston, MA 02111 **[367]**

Raffaella Giavazzi, Department of Cell Biology, The University of Texas, M.D. Anderson Hospital and Tumor Institute, 6723 Bertner Ave., Houston, TX 77030 **[573]**

Steven Gillis, Immunex Corporation, 51 University St., Seattle, WA 98101 **[383]**

Albert Giorgio, Naval Blood Research Laboratory, Boston University School of Medicine, Boston, MA 02118 **[121]**

Mark C. Glassy, U.C. San Diego Cancer Center, T-011, Department of Medicine, University of California, San Diego, CA 92103 **[97]**

Gary E. Goodman, Tumor Institute, Swedish Hospital Medical Center, Seattle, WA 98104 **[149]**

Mark I. Greene, Department of Pathology, Harvard Medical School, and Department of Medicine, Tufts University Medical School, Boston, MA 02111 **[359,367]**

Samuel E. Halpern, University of California San Diego School of Medicine and Cancer Center, and Veterans Administration Medical Center, San Diego, CA 92161 **[133]**

Peter Hamer, Biomedical Products Department, E.I. DuPont deNemours, 331 Treble Cove Road, North Billerica, MA 01862 **[565]**

P. Horan Hand, Laboratory of Tumor Immunology and Biology, NCI, National Institutes of Health, Bethesda, MD 20205 **[23]**

Michael G. Hanna, Jr., Litton Institute of Applied Biotechnology, 1330 Piccard Drive, Rockville, MD 20850-4373 **[505]**

John A. Hansen, Fred Hutchinson Cancer Research Center, Seattle, WA 98104; Department of Medicine, University of Washington, Seattle, WA 98195; and Puget Sound Blood Center, Seattle, WA 98104 **[121]**

J.D. Hardcastle, Department of Surgery, University Hospital, University of Nottingham, NG7 2RD, UK **[215]**

Martin V. Haspel, Litton Institute of Applied Biotechnology, 1330 Piccard Drive, Rockville, MD 20850-4373 **[505]**

Ingegerd Hellström, Department of Microbiology and Immunology, University of Washington, Seattle, WA 98195; presently at: ONCOGEN, 3005 First Avenue, Seattle, WA 98121 **[149]**

Karl Erik Hellström, Department of Pathology, University of Washington, Seattle, WA 98195; presently at: ONCOGEN, 3005 First Avenue, Seattle, WA 98121 **[149]**

Christopher S. Henney, Immunex Corporation, 51 University St., Seattle, WA 98101 **[383]**

Ronald B. Herberman, Biological Therapeutics Branch, Biological Response Modifiers Program, DCT, National Cancer Institute, Frederick, MD 21701 **[193]**

Dorothee Herlyn, The Wistar Institute of Anatomy and Biology, Philadelphia, PA 19104 **[165]**

B.L. Hill, Department of Microbiology, Columbia University and the Cancer Center, New York, NY 10032 **[345]**

Thomas Hoffman, Division of Blood and Blood Products, and Division of Bacterial Products, Food and Drug Administration, Bethesda, MD 20205 **[431]**

Oscar D. Holton, III, Laboratory of Mathematical Biology, NCI, National Institutes of Health, Bethesda, MD 20205 **[473]**

Herbert C. Hoover, Jr., Division of Surgical Oncology, Health Sciences Center, State University of New York, Stony Brook, NY 11794 **[505]**

T. Hopp, Immunex Corporation, 51 University St., Seattle, WA 98101 **[413]**

L.L. Houston, Department of Biochemistry, University of Kansas, Lawrence, KS 66045; presently at: Cetus Corp., 1400 53rd St., Emeryville, CA 94608 **[275]**

Pei-Ling Hsu, Department of Pathology and Laboratory Medicine, University of Texas, Houston, TX 77030 **[53]**

Su-Ming Hsu, Department of Pathology and Laboratory of Medicine, University of Texas, Houston, TX 77030 **[53]**

Martin J. Humphries, Howard University Medical School, Cancer Center and Department of Oncology, Washington, DC 20060, and Membrane Biochemistry Section, Laboratory of Molecular Biology, NCI, National Institutes of Health, Bethesda, MD 20205 **[443]**

Ashraf Imam, Department of Microbiology, University of Southern California School of Medicine, Los Angeles, CA 90033 **[523]**

Mark Israel, Pediatric Branch, Carcinogenesis Branch, National Institutes of Health, Bethesda, MD 20205 **[551]**

F.K. Jansen, Department of Immunology, Centre de Recherche Clin Midy (Groupe Sanofi), 34082 Montpellier Cedex, France [263]

June Kan-Mitchell, Department of Microbiology, University of Southern California School of Medicine, Los Angeles, CA 90033 [523]

Andrew Keenan, Nuclear Medicine Department, Clinical Center, National Institutes of Health, Bethesda, MD 20205 [473]

Raymond A. Kempf, Department of Internal Medicine, University of Southern California School of Medicine, Los Angeles, CA 90033 [523]

James Kenimer, Division of Blood and Blood Products, and Division of Bacterial Products, Food and Drug Administration, Bethesda, MD 20205 [431]

Robert C. Knapp, Dana-Farber Cancer Institute, Boston, MA 02115 [37]

Hilary Koprowski, The Wistar Institute of Anatomy and Biology, Philadelphia, PA 19104 [165]

D. Kozbor, Department of Microbiology and Immunology, Queen's University, Kingston, Ontario, Canada K7L 3N6; presently at: The Wistar Institute of Anatomy & Biology, Thirty-Seventh Street at Spruce, Philadelphia, PA 90026 [77]

H.H. Ku, Department of Microbiology, Columbia University and the Cancer Center, New York, NY 10032 [345]

Michael S. Lan, Department of Microbiology and Immunology, Duke University Medical Center, Durham, NC 27710 [63]

Steven M. Larson, Nuclear Medicine Department, Clinical Center, National Institutes of Health, Bethesda, MD 20205 [473]

Guy Laurent, Department of Immunology, Centre de Recherche Clin Midy (Groupe Sanofi), 34082 Montpellier Cedex, France [263]

D. Scott Linthicum, Department of Pathology, University of Texas Health Science Center, Houston, TX 77025 [289]

Leah Lipsich, Department of Microbiology, State University of New York, Stony Brook, NY 11794 [551]

Philip O. Livingston, Department of Medicine, Sloan-Kettering Institute, 1275 York Ave., New York, NY 10021 [537]

Michael Lubeck, The Wistar Institute of Anatomy and Biology, Philadelphia, PA 19104 [165]

H. Luk, Immunex Corporation, 51 University St., Seattle, WA 98101 [413]

Richard G. Lynch, Departments of Pathology and Microbiology, University of Iowa College of Medicine, Iowa City, IA 52242 [317]

David M. Mahvi, Department of Surgery, Duke University Medical Center, Durham, NC 27710 [63]

Wayne A. Marasco, Department of Pathology, University of Michigan Medical School, Ann Arbor, MI 48109 [327]

Maurie Markman, University of California San Diego School of Medicine and Cancer Center, and Veterans Administration Medical Center, San Diego, CA 92161 [133]

Paul J. Martin, Fred Hutchinson Cancer Research Center, Seattle, WA 98104, and Department of Medicine, University of Washington, Seattle, WA 98195 [121]

Richard P. McCabe, Litton Institute of Applied Biotechnology, 1330 Piccard Drive, Rockville, MD 20850-4373 [505]

Richard S. Metzgar, Department of Microbiology and Immunology, Duke University Medical Center, Durham, NC 27710 **[63]**

William C. Meyers, Department of Surgery, Duke University Medical Center, Durham, NC 27710 **[63]**

Malcolm S. Mitchell, Departments of Medicine and Microbiology, University of Southern California School of Medicine, and Comprehensive Cancer Center, Los Angeles, CA 90033 **[495,523]**

Alton C. Morgan, Jr., Biological Response Modifiers Program, DCT, NCI, Frederick, MD 21701; presently at: NeoRx Corp., 410 W. Harrison Street, Seattle, WA 98119 **[193,233,237]**

R. Muraro, Laboratory of Tumor Immunology and Biology, NCI, National Institutes of Health, Bethesda, MD 20205 **[23]**

Lee M. Nadler, Department of Tumor Immunology, Dana-Farber Cancer Institute, Boston, MA 02115 **[113]**

H.F. Oettgen, Sloan-Kettering Institute, 1275 York Ave., New York, NY 10021 **[537]**

L.J. Old, Sloan-Kettering Institute, 1275 York Ave., New York, NY 10021 **[537]**

Kenneth Olden, Howard University Medical School, Cancer Center and Department of Oncology, Washington, DC 20060, and Membrane Biochemistry Section, Laboratory of Molecular Biology, NCI, National Institutes of Health, Bethesda, MD 20205 **[443]**

R.K. Oldham, Biological Therapy Institute, Riverside Drive, Franklin, TN 37064 **[233]**

John R. Ortaldo, Biological Therapeutics Branch, Biological Response Modifiers Program, DCT, NCI, Frederick, MD 21701 **[193]**

L. Park, Immunex Corporation, 51 University St., Seattle, WA 98101 **[413]**

Robert J. Parker, Office of the Director, Division of Cancer Etiology, NCI, National Institute of Health, Bethesda, MD 20205 **[473]**

Gowsala Pavanasasivam, Biological Response Modifiers Program, DCT, NCI, Frederick, MD 21701; presently at NeoRx Corp., 410 W. Harrison Street, Seattle, WA 98119 **[237]**

John W. Pearson, Biological Response Modifiers Program, DCT, NCI, Frederick, MD 21701 **[237]**

A.S. Penn, Department of Neurology, Columbia University, New York, NY 10032 **[345]**

Mark D. Pescovitz, Immunology Branch, NCI, Bethesda, MD 20205 **[53]**

Robert E. Peters, U.C. San Diego Cancer Center, T-011, Department of Medicine, University of California, San Diego, CA 92103 **[97]**

Debra Petit, Biomedical Products Department, E.I. Dupont deNemours, 331 Treble Cove Rd., North Billerica, MA 01862 **[565]**

Michael D. Pierschbacher, Cancer Research Center, La Jolla Cancer Research Foundation, 10901 North Torrey Pines Road, La Jolla, CA 92037 **[489]**

M.V. Pimm, Cancer Research Campaign Laboratories, University Hospital, University of Nottingham, NG7 2RD, UK **[215]**

Nicholas Pomato, Litton Institute of Applied Biotechnology, 1330 Piccard Drive, Rockville, MD 20850-4373 **[505]**

Harvey Rabin, Biomedical Products Department, E.I. DuPont deNemours, 331 Treble Cove Rd., North Billerica, MA 01862 **[565]**

S. Ramakrishnan, Department of Biochemistry, University of Kansas, Lawrence, KS 66045; presently at Cetus Corp., 1400 53rd Street, Emeryville, CA 94608 **[275]**

Ralph A. Reisfeld, Department of Immunology, Scripps Clinic and Research Foundation, La Jolla, CA 92037 **[xxi,173,193,207,523]**

Jerome Ritz, Department of Tumor Immunology, Dana-Farber Cancer Institute, Boston, MA 02115 **[113]**

R.A. Robins, Cancer Research Campaign Laboratories, University Hospital, University of Nottingham, NG7 2RD, UK **[215]**

J.C. Roder, Department of Microbiology and Immunology, Queen's University, Kingston, Ontario, Canada K7L 3N6; presently at: Mount Sinai Research Institute, Mount Sinai Hospital, 600 University Ave, Toronto, Ontario, Canada M5G 1X5 **[77]**

Ivor Royston, U.C. San Diego Cancer Center, T-011, Department of Medicine, University of California, San Diego, CA 92103 **[97]**

Kevin P. Ryan, University of California San Diego School of Medicine and Cancer Center, and Veterans Administration Medical Center, San Diego, CA 92161 **[133]**

R. Sarangarajan, Department of Microbiology, Columbia University and the Cancer Center, New York, NY 10032 **[345]**

Bilha Schechter, Department of Chemical Immunology, The Weizmann Institute of Science, Rehovot, Israel **[243]**

J. Schlom, Laboratory of Tumor Immunology and Biology, NCI, National Institutes of Health, Bethesda, MD 20205 **[23]**

Alain B. Schreiber, Institute of Biological Sciences, Syntex Research, Palo Alto, CA 94304 **[397]**

Robert W. Schroff, Biological Response Modifiers Program, DCT, NCI, Frederick, MD 21701; presently at NeoRx Corp., 410 W. Harrison Street, Seattle, WA 98112 **[233,237]**

Gregor Schulz, Scripps Clinic and Research Foundation, La Jolla, CA 92037 **[173]**

H.F. Seigler, Department of Surgery, Duke University Medical Center, Durham, NC 27710 **[63]**

Stewart Sell, Department of Pathology and Laboratory Medicine, University of Texas Health Science Center at Houston, Houston, TX 77025 **[xxi,3]**

Daniel L. Shawler, University of California San Diego School of Medicine and Cancer Center, and Veterans Administration Medical Center, San Diego, CA 92161 **[133]**

Susan M. Sieber, Office of the Director, Division of Cancer Etiology, NCI, National Institutes of Health, Bethesda, MD 20205 **[473]**

Kathryn E. Stein, Division of Blood and Blood Products, and Division of Bacterial Products, Food and Drug Administration, Bethesda, MD 20205 **[431]**

Zenon Steplewski, The Wistar Institute of Anatomy and Biology, Philadelphia, PA 19104 **[165]**

H.C. Stevenson, Biological Response Modifiers Program, NCI, Frederick, MD 21701 **[233]**

Tak Takvorian, Department of Medical Oncology, Dana-Farber Cancer Institute, Boston, MA 02115 **[113]**

A. Thor, Laboratory of Tumor Immunology and Biology, NCI, National Institutes of Health, Bethesda, MD 20205 **[23]**

Arthur S. Tischler, Department of Pathology, Tufts New England Medical Center, 171 Harrison Ave., Boston, MA **[565]**

F.M. Uckun, Department of Therapeutic Radiology, University of Minnesota, Minneapolis, MN 55455 **[275]**

David L. Urdal, Immunex Corporation, 51 University St., Seattle, WA 98101 **[383,413]**

C. Robert Valeri, Naval Blood Research Laboratory, Boston University School of Medicine, Boston, MA 02118 **[121]**

Nissi M. Varki, Department of Immunology, Scripps Clinic and Research Foundation, La Jolla, CA 92037 **[207]**

V. Vilasi, Laboratory of Tumor Immunology and Biology, NCI, National Institutes of Health, Bethesda, MD 20205 **[23]**

Leslie E. Walker, Department of Immunology, Scripps Clinic and Research Foundation, La Jolla, CA 92037 **[207]**

Peter A. Ward, Department of Pathology, University of Michigan Medical School, Ann Arbor, MI 48109 **[327]**

N.H. Wasserman, Department of Microbiology, Columbia University and the Cancer Center, New York, NY 10032 **[345]**

M.O. Weeks, Laboratory of Tumor Immunology and Biology, NCI, National Institutes of Health, Bethesda, MD 20205 **[23]**

Barbara Weiblen, Naval Blood Research Laboratory, Boston University School of Medicine, Boston, MA 02118 **[121]**

John N. Weinstein, Laboratory of Mathematical Biology, NCI, National Institutes of Health, Bethesda, MD 20205 **[473]**

Sandra L. White, Howard University Medical School, Cancer Center and Department of Oncology, and Department of Microbiology, Washington, DC 20060 **[443]**

Meir Wilchek, Department of Biophysics, The Weizmann Institute of Science, Rehovot, Israel **[243]**

Hubert J. Wolfe, Department of Pathology, Tufts New England Medical Center, 171 Harrison Ave, Boston, MA **[565]**

C.S. Woodhouse, NeoRx Corp. Inc., 410 West Harrison Street, Seattle, WA 98119 **[233]**

D. Wunderlich, Laboratory of Tumor Immunology and Biology, NCI, National Institutes of Health, Bethesda, MD 20205 **[23]**

Wes Yonemoto, Department of Microbiology, State University of New York, Stony Brook, NY 11794 **[551]**

Vincent R. Zurawski, Jr., Centocor, Malvern, PA 19355 **[37]**

Preface

This volume is comprised of a series of papers presented at the Roche-UCLA Symposium on "Monoclonal Antibodies and Cancer Therapy", held in Park City, Utah, January 26 – February 2, 1985. This meeting was attended by scientists from around the world and was the first meeting on this topic sponsored by the UCLA Symposia on Molecular and Cellular Biology.

Judging from comments and discussions during and after the meeting, it was a big success. The science was excellent and led to many useful exchanges of information among the participants. This certainly was evident from the lengthy and thought-provoking discussions that followed every session, even after the evening programs that often lasted well after eleven o'clock. Most presentations were very well attended, although many people were exhausted by the intensity of the program and the afternoons spent skiing. The extensive and lively discussions during the plenary sessions and workshops were a tribute to the generally excellent presentations of the speakers.

Following a stimulating keynote address by Hilary Koprowski of the Wistar Institute, that defined the theme for the meeting, subjects covered dealt with many of the current issues in cancer diagnosis and therapy with monoclonal antibodies. These included the following topics: monoclonal antibodies to human cancer, human-human hybridomas, antibody therapy for leukemia and lymphoma, modulation of effector cells by monoclonal antibodies to cell surface receptors, monoclonal antibodies to lymphokines, antibody radionuclide conjugates, cancer vaccines, and monoclonal antibodies to oncogene products. Five workshop/poster sessions dealt with such topics as status of blood tests, monoclonal antibodies to premalignant cells, to conjugates with drugs or toxins, to glycolipids, and to extracellular matrix and cytoskeletal components.

A timely and thoughtful special lecture on monoclonal antibodies and cancer metastasis by I.J. Fidler, University of Texas, was the piece de resistance at the close of the meeting.

Not all the lectures and workshop presentations of the meeting are summarized in this volume since contributions herein were made voluntarily. It is nevertheless a tribute to the speakers at the symposia that more than eighty percent of them contributed a paper to this volume which is arranged according to the organization of the meeting.

It is evident that no meeting can be successful without dedicated administrative and financial support. We would like to acknowledge the excellent assistance received from Robin Yeaton, Betty Handy and Robert Harwood and their associates in the UCLA Symposia office. We would like to express our thanks and appreciation to Hoffman–LaRoche, Inc. for its generous sponsorship of this meeting. We also would like to thank the following for their financial support: Monsanto Corporation Research Laboratories; Meloy Laboratories; Bristol-Myers Co., Pharmaceutical Research & Development Division; Damon Biotech, Inc.; E.I. duPont de Nemours & Company; Lilly Research Laboratories, Eli Lilly and Company; Boehringer-Mannheim GmbH; Pel-Freez Clinical Systems; Merck, Sharp and Dohme Research Laboratories; American Hoechst Corp; Hybritech, Inc., and Cutter Laboratories, Division of Miles Laboratories. Needless to say, without these generous contributions, the 1985 Roche-UCLA Symposium on Monoclonal Antibodies and Cancer Therapy would not have been possible.

Ralph Reisfeld, Ph.D.
Department of Immunology
Scripps Clinic & Research
    Foundation
La Jolla, CA 92037

Stewart Sell, M.D.
Department of Pathology and
    Laboratory Medicine
University of Texas Medical
    School
P.O. Box 20708
Houston, TX 77025

I. MONOCLONAL ANTIBODIES TO HUMAN CANCER

Monoclonal Antibodies and Cancer Therapy, pages 3–21
© **1985 Alan R. Liss, Inc.**

CANCER MARKERS: PAST, PRESENT AND FUTURE

Stewart Sell

Department of Pathology and laboratory Medicine
University of Texas Health Science Center at Houston
Houston, Texas 77025

ABSTRACT Cancer markers include secreted proteins,
cell surface molecules, hormones, enzymes and isozymes,
cytoplasmic constituents and chomosomal changes. The
most useful markers are monoclonal immunoglobulins,
alphafetoprotein, and carcinoembryonic antigen.
Although the clinical applications of AFP and CEA have
not fulfilled all the optimistic expectations that
many predicted, they have achieved a place in cancer
diagnosis and management. Many other markers have not
been nearly as useful and the verdict has not yet been
returned on several now being studied. Claims of a
universal cancer marker have been made repeatedly, but
have gone unsubstantiated. Identification of cancer
markers by monoclonal antibodies offers an exciting
opportunity not available with previous approaches.
It is also possible that molecular probes for human
oncogenes or gene rearrangements might become a
diagnostic approach in the future. A continued search
for new tumor markers is more than justified by the
tremendous potential for clinical applications.

INTRODUCTION

The ultimate goal of cancer research is to understand
the etiology and progression of cancer in order to prevent
cancer. However, given the present state of the art the
practical application of our knowledge of cancer must be
primarily directed not to prevention, but to treatment.
The key to the successful treatment of cancer lies in detecting cancer early while it may be treated effectively,

primarily by surgery or in a more limited extent by other modalites.

The primary diagnosis of malignancy depends upon the identification by a pathologist of structural features of cancer tissue that differentiates it from normal or non-cancerous tissue. Pathologists recognize cancer tissue to be " less differentiated" than normal tissue. Until recently analysis of body fluids chemically or immunologi-cally added little useful information for diagnosis. However, if such fluids contained malignant cells the diagnosis of cancer could be made by morphologic examina-tion of these cells.

During the last 20 years there has been a growing appreciation that the morphologic resemblence of cancer cells to embryonic or fetal cells is also reflected in the production of cellular macromolecules by cancer cells that are more typical of embryonic or fetal cells than of adult tissue (1,2).

Examples of different types of cancer markers are listed in Table 1.

TABLE 1
TYPES OF CANCER MARKERS

TYPE	EXAMPLE
Exposure of backbone or blood group markers	ABH
Cell surface glycoproteins	Carcinoembryonic antigen
Secreted proteins	Alphafetoprotein
Enzyme Alterations	Glycosyltransferases
Isozymes	Alkaline phosphatase
Ectopic hormone	Human chorionic gonadotropin
Antigens identified by monoclonal antibodies	Melanoma proteins
Cytoskeletal elements	Prekeratin
Immunoglobulin gene rearrangements	B Cell tumors
Gene translocations	Philadelphia (Chomosome)
Fragile siles	Leukemia

Many of these macromolecules are not only present in the cell or on the cell surface, but are also secreted into the body fluids. Measurement of these "oncodevelopmental markers" (3) by the clinical laboratory has become increasingly important in the diagnosis of cancer. In addition, antibodies to cancer markers are being used to determine pronosis, monitor therapy by serial determinations, label tissue by immunohistology, localize in vivo by radioimmunoscintigraphy and treat cancer by therapy using isolated antibody or drug antibody conjugates.

The production of oncodevelopmental markers is closely related to the tissue of origin that normally produce them during development (Table 2).

TABLE 2
"LEVELS" OF EXPRESSION OF ONCODEVELOPMENTAL MARKERS

PRODUCTION BY TUMORS

EXAMPLE	NORMAL PRODUCING TISSUE	EMBRYOGENICALLY CLOSELY RELATED	DISTANTLY RELATED	DIFFERENT
carcino-embryonic antigen	colon	stomach, pancreas liver	lung breast	lymphoma
alphafeto-protein	liver yolk sac	colon, stomach pancreas	lung	
serotonin	"Entero-endocrine" carcinoid	adrenal	oat cell lung	epidermal lung
chorionic gonado-tropin	placenta	germinal tumors	liver	epidermal lung
monoclonal immuno-globulin	plasma cell	B cell tumors	T Cell tumors	monocytic tumors

CANCER ANTIGENS

Changes in cancer "antigens" have been recognized as either a loss of normal or a gain of "new"cellular macromolecules. Cancer antigens are not necessarily immunogenic in the host of origin (Autochlonous), and in fact are usually identified by immune products of a different stain or species. Thus human carcinoembyonic antigen is not antigenic in humans, and is identified by antisera made in goats or rabbits. Most "cancer antigens" are identified by serologic activity (i.e. by immunoglobulin antibody) but some animal cancer antigens are recoynized by in vitro reactivity with immune cells or by transplantation rejection. These latter antigens are called tumor specific transplantation antigens when the rejection is specific for one tumor. Such "tumor specific" antigens have not been convincingly demonstrated in human tumors.

HISTORY OF CANCER MARKERS

YEAR	AUTHOR	MARKER
1846	H. Bence-Jones	Bence-Jones Protein
1928	W.H. Brown	Ectopic hormone syndrome
1930	B. Zondex	HCG
1932	H. Cushiny	ACTH
1938	Gutman and Gutman	Prostatic Acid Phosphatase
1949	K. Oh-Uti	Deletion of Blood Group Antigens
1959	C. Markert	Isozymes
1960	P. Nowell	Philadelphia Chromosome
1963	G.I. Abelev	Alphafetoprotein
1965	Gold and Freeman	Carcinoembryonic
1969	Heubner and Todaro	Oncoyenes
1975	Kohler and Milstein	Monoclonal antibodies
1980	Cooper, Weinberg, Bishop	Oncoyene probes and transfection
1981	J. Yunis	Fragile sites

MYELOMA PROTEINS

The first cancer marker identified was almost certainly Bence-Jones protein (4). In a series of lectures delivered to the Royal College of Physicians in London in 1846, Dr. H. Bence Jones, M.D., F.R.S., described studies on a urine sample referred to him by another physician, a Dr. McIntire, who wrote "Dear Dr. Jones: The tube contains urine of a very high specific gravity. When boiled it become slightly opaque---". The urinary precipate was found in a patient with "mollities ossium", a bone disease now known as multiple myloma. One hundred years later Bence-Jones proteins were identified as being immunoglobulin light chains associated with the presence of monoclonal immunoglobulins in the serum. With application of immunoassays or quantitative electro-phoresis, the amount of Bence-Jones protein found in urine or the amount of myeloma immunoglobulin in the serum may be used to follow the effects of therapy; the amount of these proteins closely reflects the amount of myeloma tumor mass. This general principle also applies to other secreted tumor markers.

HORMONES AND ECTOPIC HORMONE PRODUCTION

A number of clinical syndromes are caused by the increased production of hormones by tumors (6). When the hormone is produced by a tissue that does not normally produce the hormone, it is termed ectopic (7,8) (Table 3). A given hormone may be produced by many different tumors. For instance, the production of human growth hormone by teratocarcinomas has been shown to be particularly useful, but elevations are also found with other tumors including hepatocellular (21%), pancreatic (33%), gastric (23%) colonic (12%), breast (11%) and renal cell (6%) carcinoma. These markers may be extremely useful for a small number of individuals but have had little impact on the diagnosis of cancer in general.

TABLE 3
SOME PARAENDOCRINE SYNDROMES ASSOCIATED WITH
ECTOPIC HORMONE PRODUCTION

Aberration	Hormone	Source
Hypercalcemia	PTH,*	Bronchogenic, pancreatic and breast CA
Hypokalemia	ACTH	APUDomas
Diarrhea	VIP	Pancreatic CA, APUDomas
Gynecomastia, precocious puberty	HCG	Pancreatic, gastic, liver CA
Erthrocytosis	ERP	Lung CA, Ranal CA
Achromegaly	GH	Breast, lung, stomach CA

PTH, parathyroid hormone; ACTH, adrenocorticotrophic hormone; VIP vasoactive intestinal polypeptide; HCG, human chorionic gonadotropin; ERP; erythryopoietin; GH, growth hormone.

APUDomas. Certain cells, recognized at first only as clear cells found in relatively small numbers in the GI tract, pancreas, bile ducts and bronchi, came to be iden- tified in over 24 different tissues by the ability of these cells to synthesize and store neurotransmitter biogenic amines, such as serotonin (9). APUD cells share properties of both neural and endocrine tissues and are referred to as neuroendocrine cells. The important point for our con- sideration is that these neuro-endocrine tissues synthesize a number of polypeptide hormones including, ACTH, calcito- nin, insulin, melanocyte stimulating hormone (MSH), gluco- gon, gastrin, secretin, GIP, VIP etc. Cancers of these cells often secrete the hormone of the tissue of origin, but APUDomas may also secrete hormones of other tissues in the APUD system. The frequency of production of a given hormone appears to correlate with the degree of embryologic relationship of the cancer of origin to other tissues in the APUD system (8). One effect of the production of dif- ferent hormones by cells in different tissue sites is that one cannot necessarily locate the site of an APUDoma by the hormone produced. Thus the finding of excess ACTH produc- tion that does not respond to physiologic control does not necessarily indicate a pituitary adenoma (although that must be the first site considered), but could be caused by APUDomas at other sites.

ENZYMES AND ISOZYMES

There are two basic abnormalities of expression of enzymes in cancer: expression of "fetal" forms of an enzyme, and "ectopic" production of enzymes. Of particular interest are isozymes, i.e. forms of enzymes that migrate differently under electrophoresis than does the normal dominant form (10,11). Unfortunately,these changes occur mainly within tumor tissue, and are expressed in the circulation only when the tumor is very large, or widespread metastases have occurred. For instance, pancreatic amylase is elevated in fewer patients with pancreatic cancer than in those with pancreatitis. An exception is prostate acid phosphatase (PAP) first described as a marker for prostatic cancer in 1938 (11).

An example of the complexity of isoenzyme analysis in cancer is that of alkaline phosphatase (13). Different electrophoretic mobilities are noted for alkaline phosphatases from bone, liver, intestine and placenta. In view of the incomplete separation of alkaline phosphatases by electrophoresis, selective heat inactivation (time for inactivation at different pH's and temperatures) is the best method for identifying these isozymes. An increase in liver alkaline phosphatase occurs frequently with malignant infiltration of the liver and in bone alkaline phosphatse with secondary malignant growth in bone and with Paget's disease. Successful treatment may be followed by a decrease in these enzymes, but the initial decrease in liver alkaline phosphatase may be masked by a concomitant healing response of bone and an increase in bone phosphatase if total activity alone is measured. Elevations of placental alkaline phosphatase occur with a variety of cancers including trophoblastic and G.I. cancers.

An isozyme of enolase, neuron specific enolase (NSE) normally found in brain tissue has been associated in large amounts with all forms of neuroendocrine tumors and with up to 70% of patients with small-cell carcinoma of the lung, a particularly difficult cancer to diagnose at a time when therapy is still effective (14). In addition elevations may be used to determine the response to therapy. Further results on this marker are awaited with interest.

BLOOD GROUP ANTIGENS

The accumulation of precursor blood group core glycolipid structures in colonic carcinomas, first identified biochemically, has been shown to be caused by a decreased activity of glycosyltransferases in certain tumors (14).

The expression of the various carbohydrate moieties of the blood group substances has been shown to be aberrant in a variety of epithelial cancers: Of particular interest is the correlation of expression with the biologic behavior of bladder cancers. Urothelial (bladder) cells normally possess A,B, and H antigens which are identical to the blood group antigens. In patients with bladder carcinomas, those which have lost blood group antigens show a much greater tendency to invade than those which do not. It has been proposed that the expression of blood group antigens on bladder cancer be used as a guide to therapy; more radical surgery being applied to tumors which lack blood group antigens (16). Thus, limited resection of a non-invasive blood group antigen positive tumor may permit preservation of a functional bladder without risk of later development of an invasive carcinoma.

A monosialoganglioside blood group precursor "antigen" in human colonic cancer has been identified by a monoclonal antibody (17). This monoclonal antibody is being studied as a possible therapeutic agent and has served as a prototype for other glycolipid antigens identified by monoclonal antibodies (18).

ALPHAFETOPROTEIN

The modern era of cancer markers began with the discovery of alphafetoprotein by G.I. Abelev of the Soviet Union in 1963 (19,20). He identified this protein in the sera of normal fetal mice and in the sera of adult mice with hepatocellular carcinoma, but not in normal adult mice! Alphafetoprotein is an antigenically distinct serum protein with properties similar to albumin. It is found in high concentrations (up to 10 mg/ml) in fetal serum and in the serum of patients with hepatocellular or teratocarcinomas but is low (<10 ng/ml) in sera of adults (21). Elevations up to 500 ng/ml occur frequently in association with a variety of non-malignant diseases, but elevations above this are essentially diagnostic of an AFP producing tumor. Approximately half of the patients with hepatocellular car-

cinoma may be diagnosed by such an elevation. Serial
determinations of AFP may be used clinically to determine
the effectiveness of therapy (Figure 1). Failure of elevated serum AFP to return to normal after surgery is an
indication that the tumor has not been completely removed
or that metastases are present. These patterns essentially
hold true for other cancer markers found in the serum.

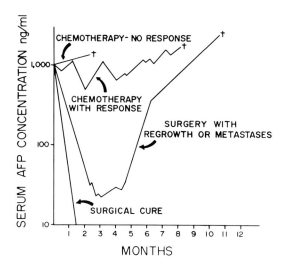

REPRESENTATIVE RESPONSES OF SERUM AFP
TO THERAPY

MONTHS

The amount of carbohydrate on AFP depends upon the level of glycosylase in fetal and tumor tissue (20). The amount of glycosalation of AFP differs among normal liver, yolk sac and hepatocellular carcinomas (23,24). Differences in glycosylation of AFP can be measured by binding of AFP to the lectins Concanavalin A (Con A) and lens culinaris lectin (LCA) (25). Completely glycosylated AFP binds to Con A at a low percentage and to LCA at a high percentage. Ratios of the percent of binding of AFP to Con A to the percent binding to LCA below 0.2 are usually found in cord serum and in patients with AFP elevations associated with benign liver disease (completely glycosylated), whereas in hepatocellular carcinomas Con A/LCA binding ratios are above 0.2 (incompletely glycosylated).

In animals exposed to chemical carcinogens, serum AFP elevations occur many months before cancer develops. The implication of this experimental observation in regard to detecting precancerous exposure of humans to chemical hepatocarcinogens remains undetermined (26).

CARCINOEMBRYONIC ANTIGEN

Carcinoembryonic antigen is a cell surface glycoprotein that is normally produced by colonic epithelium and secreted in the intestine (27). In colonic and other cancers, alterations in the polarity of cells are associated with release of CEA in elevated levels into the blood. During development, CEA is produced by the fetal gastrointestinal tract; elevations of CEA associated with cancers in the adult reflect the developmental relationship to gastrointestinal tissue. CEA elevations also occur in association with non-malignant diseases so that elevated serum CEA can only be used as an adjunct to other diagnostic procedures (28). In patients with colo-rectal cancer who have elevated serum CEA the serum levels may be used to determine the effectiveness of therapy. Unfortunately, re-elevation CEA has not proven useful as an indication for "second-look" surgery. CEA levels in breast cancer became elevated with metastatses and serial determinations are useful for determining effectiveness of chemotherapy, for determining prognosis, and to measure progression of the disease.

Radiolabeled antibodies to AFP and CEA have been used to localize clandestine tumors by radioimmunescintigraphy (29,30). Accuracy of diagnosis has been improved by application of computer analysis to photoscans. Primary cancers have been localized in 83% of colo-rectal cancer and in 22% of patients cancer sites were located that no other method had been able to detect. An interesting finding with AFP is that in experimental systems, AFP is taken up by some non-AFP containing cancers in mice, and that localization of selected tumors using radiolabelled AFP and scintigraphy is possible even when the tumor does not produce AFP (31). Extension of this system to humans is proposed.

Antibodies to CEA and AFP have also been used to treat tumors producing these markers in animals. So far the results, even when drugs such as daunomycin have been attached to the antibodies, have been equivocal. Trials in humans now underway with drug conjugated horse anti-AFP, are not yet interpretible (32).

MIXED MARKERS

Since some tumors may produce more than one marker, the simultaneous measurement of more than one marker often provides informatin leading to a more precise diagnosis or prognosis than one marker alone (33). For instance, differentation of germ cell tumor types can be accomplished on the basis of elevation of serum AFP or HCG:

	HCG	AFP
SEMINOMA	-	-
EMBRYONAL	+	+
CHORIOCARCINOMA	+	-
YOLK SAC	-	+
TERATOMA	-	-

Similarly the significance presence of the presence of other mixtures of tumor markers, for instance CEA, AFP and/or ectopic hormones is being analyzed at several centers.

Combined use of serum prostate specific antisera and prostatic acid phosphatase measurement give the following positive results in patients with prostate cancer. Stages A or B, 58%; Stage C 68%; Stage D 92% (34).

OTHER TUMOR MARKERS

A number of other human tumor markers detected by heteroantisera are listed in Table 4 (35). Many of these have been tested and found lacking in their ability to diagnose or determine prognosis of cancer. Others such as melanoma associated antigen have been chemically characterized and analyzed by monoclonal antibodies (36). Pancreatic oncofetal antigen has shown promising preliminary evidence of being useful diagnostically and prognostically (37).

TABLE 4
SOME SEROLOGICALLY DEFINED HUMAN TUMOR MARKERS

Name	Tumor Tissue	Fetal Tissue
Beta Oncofetal Antigen	Many types	Epithelial, placenta
Carcinofetal Ferritin	Many	Liver
Gamma-Fetoprotein	Many	Serum and some tissues
Fetal Gut Antigen	GI CA (32%)	GI
Fetal Sulphoglyco-protein	CI Ca	GI
Melanoma Associated Antigen	Melanoma (240K), Carcinoma(95K)	Melanocytes
Melanoma Fetal Antigen	Melanomas	Skin, brain
Pancreatic Cancer Associated Antigen	Pancreas,stomach, others	Pancreas,stomach
Pancreatic Oncofetal Antigen	Pancreas, others	Pancreas, others
Pregnancy Specific Protein 1	Trophoblastic germ cell	Pregnancy sera, etc.
Prostate Antigen	Prostate CA	? Prostate (BPH)
Tissue Polypeptide Antigen	Various	Placenta growing cells

MONOCLONAL ANTIBODIES TO CANCER MARKERS

We have recently entered the third era of cancer markers. The selectivity of hybridoma techniques for producing monoclonal antibodies to tumor antigens could revolutionize the field of cancer markers in the next year.

Monoclonal antibodies to melanoma, neuroblastoma, glioma, colorectal (CEA), liver (AFP), prostate (prostate specific antigen), lung, breast and lymphoid tissue are being used to localize the respective antigen in tumor tissue by immunoperoxidase procedures. A monoclonal antibody to the major antigenic protein of melanomas is now being tested in therapeutic trials as is a monoclonal antibody to T cells for selected T cell tumors (see below). The result of this approach will be presented by a number of authors at this meeting.

Lymphoid Tumors

The application of monoclonal antibodies to lymphocyte differentiation antigens is changing the classification of lymphoid tumors (39,40). Using conventional markers, it has been shown that the survival of patients with histologically similar tumors is markedly different if B, T, and "null" cell tumors are classified separately.

The critical finding in lymphoid cancers is that the normal mixture of cells with different markers is replaced by a homogenous population of cells with limited marker expression. A normal lymph node contains B cell zones (follicules) with a mixture of cells containing different immunoglobulin light chains and Ig classes although any individual B cell only expresses one light chain and usually one heavy chain, normal mixtures of B cells contain some cells that express one light chain and one Ig class and other cells that express the other light chain and another Ig class in fairly predictable ratios. Tumors of B cells result in replacement of this mixed population so that each cell of the cancer expresses the same light chain and the same Ig class. Similarily mixtures of different T cell populations are seen in the normal lymph node cortex. In T cell tumors this is replaced by a diffuse infiltration of a homogeneous population of T cells, with each cell bearing only one set of the same T cell markers.

Extensive analysis of lymphoid tumor cells using monoclonal antibodies have failed to identify a tumor specific leukemia or lymphoma antigen. Thus, like hormone and enzyme expression in epithelial cancers, lymphoid tumors express normal markers in abnormal proportion and distribution. The so-called common acute lymphocytic leukemia associated antigen (CALLA) detected by xenogeneic antisera raised against acute leukemic cells detects antigens on lymphoblasts of most cases of non-T, non-B ALL. It is also present on some cells in fetal regenerating bone marrow.

The use of monoclonal antibodies to T cells for passive immunotherapy of T cell tumors (ie Sezary Syndrome) has resulted in providing anecdotal case reports of success (41), but application of monoclonal antibody therapy to a controlled series of patients has not been reported.

Cytoskeletal Elements

Monoclonal antibodies to cytoskeletal elements (intermediate filiments, 42,43) have been used to identify the cellular origin of cancers by immunohistology. Glial fibrillary acidic protein (GFAP) is a major component of the intermediate filiments of astrocytes (42) and appears to be useful for diagnosis of astrocytic neoplasms and mixed glial tumors as if not found in epidermial tumors, menningiomas or other non-Astrocytic brain tumors (43). Prekeratin in the form of intermediate sized filaments is found exclusively in cells of epidermial origin (44) and may be used immunohistologically to identify cancer cells of epithelial origin (45). Neurofiliments are found in neuroblastomas and pheochromocytomas; vimentin in sarcomas and lymphomas.

CANCER MARKERS OF THE FUTURE - CHROMOSOMAL TRANSLOCATIONS

In 1960 Nowell and Hungerford described the classic finding of a translocation of one arm of chromosome 22 to chromosome 9 (or 6), in the cells of patients with chronic granulocytic leukemia (46). The smaller chromosome 22 become known as the Philadelphia chromosome (Ph') and may be used as a marker for CGL cells. Acute blastic crisis may be predicted by an increase in the number of marrow cells containing Ph'. In Burkitts" lymphoma a portion of chromosome 8 containing the myc oncogene is translocated to chromosome 14 (or less often to 2 or 22). There are other tumors associated with detectable translocations (47) and some investigators feel, with justification, that all tumors would contain some chromosomal abnormalities if we had the appropriate methodology to detect them.

IMMUNOGLOBULIN GENE REARRANGEMENTS

The presence of immunoglobulin gene arrangements in lymphomas may give evidence of B cell lineage even if the tumor cells do not produce cytoplasmic or surface monoclonal Ig (48). Immunoglobulin gene rearrangements that result in splicing out of intervening DNA sequence has been associated with maturation of B cells and the ability to produce Ig. However, some gene rearrangements are not associated with the capacity to synthesize ig, but are still believed to be characteristic of B cells. Some non-Ig producing null cell lymphomas will demonstrate gene rearrangement whereas others will not. The finding of gene rearrangements in a null cell tumor indicates 1) that the cell line is monoclonal and therefore probably neoplastic and 2) that the tumor is most likely of B cell origin. Studies on rearrangement of Ig genes and T cells receptor genes in T cell lymphomas is now underway.

FRAGILE SITES

Many cells from human cancers when cultured in vitro in folic acid deficient mediam will show "breaks" in chromosomes when examined by high resolution banding techniques (49). The location of these "fragile sites" appears to correlate with the type of malignancy. Although breaks are also found in normal chromosomes, these occur in a scattered fashion and in a smaller number of cells, whereas most cancer cells will have a consistant site of breakage.
Preliminary evidence suggests that cancer associated fragile sites may also be found in normal cells of patients with cancer. An hypothesis now being tested is that "cancer prone" individuals may also have such fragile sites.

ONCOGENES

The confirmation of the prediction made in 1969 by Heubner and todaro (50) that genetic structures associated

with cancer in animals (oncogenes) are also present in at
least some human cancers raises the possibility of applying
this property of cancer cell to diagnosis. Although there
is evidence already that expression of oncogenes or gene
rearrangements (which are well documented in leukemias) are
not uniformily found in all cancers, the observations so
far are promising (51,52). In the future, probes for oncogenes, the ability of DNA from cancer cells to transform
tissue culture cell in vitro, or restriction endonuclease
analysis of transforming sequences activated in neoplastic
cells might be applied to DNA derived from human tumors as
diagnostic procedures.

REFERENCES

1. Sell, S. (Ed.) (1980) Cancer Markers: Diagnostic and
    Developmental Significance. The Humana Press. Crescent
    manor, Clifton, New Jersey.
2 . Sell, S. and Wahren, B. (Eds) (1982). Human Cancer
    Markers. The Humana Press, Crescent Manor, Clifton,
    N.J.
3. Fishman, W.H. and Sell, S. (1976) Oncodevelopmental
    Gene Expression. Academic Press, New York.
4. Sell, S. (1978) Tumor Immunity: Relevance of animal
    models to man. Human Pathology 9:63.
5. Bence-Jones, H. (1847). Papers on Chemical Pathology,
    Lecture III. Lancet 2:269-274.
6. Gritting, G. and Vaitukaitis, J.L. (1980) Hormone
    Secreting Tumors in Ref. p. 169.
7. Brown, W.H. (1928). A case of pluriglaudular syndrome.
    Lancet 17:1022.
8. Baylin, S.B. (1975). Ectopic production of hormones and
    other protein by tumors. Hospital Practice 10:117.
9. Pearse, A.G.E. (1969). The cytochemistry and
    ultrastructure of polypeptide hormone producing cells
    of the APUD series and the embryologic, physiologic and
    pathologic implications of the concept. J. Histochem
    Cytochem. 17:303.
10. Balinsky, D. (1980. Enzymes and isozymes in cancer in
    (Ref. 1). p.191.
11. Schapira, R. (1981). Resurgence of fetal isozymes in
    cancer: Study of aldolase, pyruvatekinase, lactic
    dehydrogenase and B- hexasosaminidase. Current topics
    in Biol and Med. Res. 5:27.

12. Gutman, A.B. and Gutman, E.B. (1938). An "acid" phosphatase occuring in the serum of patients with metastasizing carcinoma of the prostate gland. Am. J. Cancer 28:485.

13. Moss, D.W. (1982). Alkaline phosphatase isoenzymes. Clin. Chem. 28:2007-2016.

14. Carvey, D.N., et al (1982) Serum neuron-specific enolase: A marker for disease extent and response to therapy of small-cell lung cancer. lancet 1:583.

15. Kuhn, W.J. and Schoentag, R. (1981). Carcinoma related alterations of glycosyltransferase in human tissues. Cancer Res. 41:2767.

16. Alroy, J. Teramura, K., Miller, B. et al (1978). Isoantigens A, B and H in Urinary Bladder Carcinomas Following Radiotherapy. Cancer 41:1739.

17. Magnani, J.L., Brockhaus, M., Smith, D.F. et al (1981). A monosialoganglioside is a monoclonal antibody defined antigen of colon carcinoma. Science 212:55.

18. Koprowski, H. and Steplewski, Z. (1982). Recognition of human tumor antigens by monoclonal antibodies in Genes and Tumor Genes (Eds E. Winnacker and H.H. Schoene) Raven press, new york. 101.

19. Abelev, G.I., Perova, S.D., Khramkova, N.I. et al (1963. Production of embryonal β -globulin by transplantable mouse hepatomas. Transplantation 1:174.

20. Abelev, F. (1971) Alpha-fetoprotein in oncogenesis and its association with malignant tumors. Adv. Cancer Res. 14:295-358.

21. Sell, S, Becker, F.F. (1978). Alphofetoprotein Cancer Res. 60:19.

22. Zimmerman, E.F., Bowen, D., Wilson, J.R. and Madappally, M.M. (1976). Developmental microheterogeneity of mouse α -fetoproteins: Purification and partial characterization. Biochemistry. 15:5534.

23. Smith, C.J., Morris, H.P. and Kelleher, P.C. (1977). Concanavalin A affinity molecular variants of α fetoprotein in neonatal rat serum and in the serum of rats bearing hepatomas. Cancer Res. 37:2651.

24. Ruoslahti, E., Engvall, E. Pekkala, A. and Seppala, M. (1978). Developmental changes in carbohydrate moiety of human alphafetoprotein. Int. J. Cancer 22:515.

25. Smith, C.J., Adjukiewicz, A. and Kelleher, P.C. (1983). Concanavalin A - affinity molecular heterogentic of human hepatomas AFP and cord-serum AFP. Ann. N.Y. Acad. Sci. 417:69.

26. Sell, S, Leffert, H.L. (1982). An evaluation of cellular lineager in the pathogenesis of experimental lhepatocellular carcinoma. Hepatol. 2:77.

27. Gold, P. and Freedman, D.O. (1965). Demonstration of tumor specific antigens in human colonic carcinomata by immunological tolerance and absorption techniques. J. Exp. Med. 121:439.

28. Go. V. 1976). Carcinoembryonic antigen. Cancer.37:562.

29. Goldenberg, D.M., Deland, F. Kim, E. et al (1978). Use of radiolabeled antibodies to carcinoembryonic antigen for the detection and localization of disease cancers by external photo scanning. N. Eng. J. Med. 298:1384.

30. Mach, J.-P., Buchecyer, F., Forni, M. et al (1981). Use of radiolabeled monoclonal anti-CEA antibodies for the detection of human carcinomas by external photo scanning and tonoscintigraphy. Immunol. Today 2:239, 1981.

31. Uriel, J. Villacampa, M-J, Moro, R. et al (1983) Selective uptake of radiolabelled alphafetoprotein by spontaneous mammary carcinoma in the mouse. C.R. Adad. Sci. Paris 297:589.

32. Koji, T, Ishii, N., Munehisa, T. et al (1880). Localization of radioiodinated antibody to α-fetoprotein antibody treatment of a hepatoma patient. Cancer Res. 40:3013.

33. McIntire, K.R. (1984). Tumor Markers: How useful are they? Hospital Practice 19:55.

34. Kuriyama, M., Wang, M.C., Lee, C.L. et al (1982).

35. Sell, S. (1978). The biologic and diagnostic significance of oncodevelopmental gene kproducts in the Handbook of Cancer Immunology, Vol. 3 (H. Waters, Ed) Garland STPM, press New York pl.

36. Reisfeld, R. (1985) Monoclonal antibodies a probes for the molecular structure and biological function of memanoma associated antigen in Monoclonal Antibodies in Cancer. Humana Press, Clifton, New Jersey. p.205.

37. Hobbs, J.R. (1982) Pancreatic Tumor Markers in Ref 1a p.165.

38. Sell, S. and Reisfeld, R. (1985). Monoclonal antibodies in Cancer. Humana Press. Clifton, N.J.

39. Foon, K.A., Schroff, R.W. and Gale, R.P. (1982). Surface markers in leukemia and lymphoma cells: Recent Advances Blood 60:1.

40. Hsu, S-M., Zhang, H.-Z. and Jaffe, E.S. (1983). Utility of monoclonal antibodies directed against B and T lymphocytes and monocytes in paraffin - embedded sections. Am. J. Clin. Path. 80:415.
41. Levy, R. and Miller, R.A. Tumor therapy with monoclonal antibodies. Fed. Proc. 42:2651-2656, 1983.
42. Lazarides, E., Dorsett, B., Ioachim. H.L. (1981). Identification of prekeratin by immunofluoresence staining in the differential diagnosis of tumors. Hum. Pathol. 12:452.
43 Tascos, N.T., Parr, J. and Gonatas, N.K. (1982). Immunocytochemical study of the glial fibrillary acidic protein in human neoplasma of the central nervous system. Hum. Pathol. 13:454.
44. Franke, W.W., Scharid, E., Osborn, M. and Weber, K. (1978). Different intermediate sized filaments distinguished by immunofluorenscence microscopy. Proc. Nat'l Acad. Sci. 75:5034.
45. Sienski, W., Dorsett, B., Ioachim. H.L. (1981). Identification of prekeratin by immunofluoresence staining in the differential diagnosis of tumors. Hum. Pathol. 12:452.
46. Nowell. P., and Hungerford, D.A. (1960). A minute chomosome in human chronic granulocytic leukemic. Science 132:1497.
47. Gilbert, F. (1983). Chromosomes, Genes, and Cancer: A classification of chomosome abnormalities in cancer. J. Nat'l Cancer Invest. 71:1107.
48. Korsmeyer, S.J. and Waldmann, T.A. (1984). Immunoglobulin genes: Rearrangement and translocation in human lymphoid malignancy. J. Clin. Investig. 4:1.
49. Yunis, J.J. (1983). The chomosomal basis of human neoplasia. Science 221:227.
50. Huebner, R.J. and Todaro, G.J. (1968) Oncogenes of RNA tumor viruses as determinants of cancer Proc. Nat'l Acad. Sci. 64:1087.
51. Cooper, G.M. Cellular transforming genes. Science 217:801-806, 1982.
52. Cline, M.J., Slamon, D.J., Lipsick, J.S. (1984) Oncogenes: Implications for the diagnosis and treatment of cancer. Am. Int. Med. 101:223.

Monoclonal Antibodies and Cancer Therapy, pages 23–36
© 1985 Alan R. Liss, Inc.

COMPARISONS OF QUALITATIVE AND QUANTITATIVE IMMUNOASSAYS
FOR ras p21

P. Horan Hand, A. Thor, A. Caruso, D. Wunderlich, R. Muraro,
M.O. Weeks, V. Vilasi, and J. Schlom

Laboratory of Tumor Immunology and Biology, National Cancer
Institute, National Institutes of Health, Bldg. 10, Rm 8B07,
Bethesda, Maryland 20205.

ABSTRACT   Monoclonal antibodies RAP 1-5 (RA, ras; P,
peptide), generated by using a synthetic peptide
reflecting amino acid positions 10-17 of the Hu-ras^{T24}
gene product as immunogen, have previously been shown to
react with the ras gene product, p21 (1,2). Using the
avidin-biotin complex immunoperoxidase method and
formalin-fixed tissue sections, monoclonal RAP-5 IgG
reacted with the majority of human colon and mammary
carcinomas. The majority of all abnormal ducts and
lobules from fibroadenoma and fibrocystic disease
patients were negative, as were benign colon tumors and
inflammatory colon lesions. Antigenic heterogeneity of
expression of ras p21 was observed among mammary and
colon carcinomas, as well as among different tumor cell
populations of a given tumor mass. Variable levels of
the ras gene product were also observed among metastatic
colon carcinomas indicating that continuous expression of
p21 in all tumor cells may not be required of ras for
maintenance of the transformed phenotype.
    A quantitative liquid phase competition radio-
immunoassay for ras p21 capable of detecting as little
as 0.001fM p21 per ng of cellular protein has been
developed. This immunoassay which uses monoclonal
antibody YA6-259 (3) directed against native p21 and
the 568 H-transformed NIH-3T3 cell line as source of
p21 antigen, is capable of detecting and quantitating
both the point mutated and proto- ras p21 in E. coli
vectors and mammalian cell lines. The immunoassays
described here now provide the means for the quantitative and qualitative evaluation of the role of ras p21
expression in the initiation, promotion, and progression
of carcinomas.

INTRODUCTION

Transforming genes, activated in neoplasias from a variety of species including humans have been identified by several investigators by transfection of cellular DNAs (4). One group of transforming genes thus identified are related to the ras genes of Harvey and Kirsten sarcoma viruses. Members of the human ras gene family (H-ras, K-ras, and N-ras) have been identified in cell lines or biopsy material from a variety of malignant disease states including carcinomas, lymphomas, sarcomas, and leukemias.

Several studies have shown that activation of the ras genes either by a point mutation causing a change in one amino acid of the 21,000d (p21) ras gene product or by enhanced expression of the proto- ras gene product mediates transformation of NIH-3T3 mouse fibroblast cells (5-7). This methodology has shown that none of many human breast tumors contain point mutated ras and that only approximately 10-15% of human colon cancers contain this altered gene; this latter figure is probably an overestimate since many negative results tend not to be reported in the literature. Radioimmunoassays (RIAs) and immunohistochemical studies using monoclonal antibodies (MAbs) would provide alternative methodologies in an attempt to determine if correlates exist between increased expression of ras p21 and a specific malig-nant disease state. Immunohistochemical methodologies would make possible localization of ras p21 in specific cell popu-lations, while RIAs would provide quantitation of ras p21.

We have reported (1,2) the production of MAbs designated RAP (ras peptide) 1-5, which were developed using as immuno-gen a synthetic peptide of position 10-17 of the Hu-ras protein of T24 human bladder carcinoma cells coupled to thyroglobulin (1,2,8-11). The RAP MAbs have previously been shown by solid phase RIAs to react with both the T24 Hu-ras and the Hu-ras[Ha] peptides (which differ in a single amino acid at position 12, Val to Gly, respectively). Consistent with the prediction that amino acids at positions 10-17 are located within the tertiary structure of the ras p21, detection of the ras gene product was enhanced using formalin or glutar-aldehyde denatured cell extracts or tissue sections. Using the immunoperoxidase method on formalin-fixed tissue sections and tissue culture supernatant containing RAP MAbs, we have demonstrated the expression of ras p21 in human colon and mammary carcinomas (1,2).

We report here the range and pattern of expression of
ras p21, as detected by purified IgG of MAb RAP-5, in human
mammary and colon carcinomas, benign disease states and
normal tissues as well as both primary and metastatic colon
lesions from each of several patients. We also describe
here the development of a quantitative liquid competition
RIA for ras p21 using MAb YA6-259 (3), and the use of this
RIA in the quantitation of ras p21 in E. coli and mammalian
cells containing the ras gene product.

RESULTS

Expression of ras p21 in Human Colon Carcinomas. To
determine the expression of ras p21 within individual cell
types in a spectrum of colonic disease states, purified (12)
RAP-5 IgG was reacted, using the immunoperoxidase method
(13,14), with formalin-fixed tissue sections of 29 colon
adenocarcinomas, 9 benign colon tumors, 16 inflammatory colon
lesions and 5 normal colon tissues from non-cancer patients.
An isotype-identical primary antibody (UPC-10) (15) was used
as a negative control in all immunoperoxidase experiments.
Cytoplasmic ras p21 was detected in 27 of 29(93%) of the
colon carcinomas (Figs. 1A, 2A), with 16 of the 29(55%) containing $\geq$ 20% of tumor cells positive for ras p21 expression.
The malignant epithelium is the cell type expressing ras in
these sections (Fig. 1A). Smooth muscle and stroma of the
colon do not express detectable levels of the ras gene
product. Normal colonic epithelium in the same section as
carcinoma cells was either negative or contained <1% of
epithelial cells reactive with MAb RAP-5. In contrast to
the reactivity observed with the colon carcinomas, only 1 of
5 normal colon tissues from 5 different non-cancer patients
contained cells expressing ras p21; this specimen contained
<1% positive cells with the remainder negative (Fig. 2C). A
variety of benign colon tumors and inflammatory colon
lesions were also assayed for ras p21 (Figs. 1B, 2B). The
vast majority of these tissues (24 of 25, 92%) were either
negative for ras p21 or contained $\leq$5% of cells scoring positive for the ras p21 (Fig. 2B).

In most primary colon carcinomas, a heterogeneity of
expression of ras p21 was observed. This heterogeneity was
manifested by a variation in the number of ras p21 positive
tumor cells within a given tumor as well as by a variation
in the level of p21 expression among individual cells in
the "positive" population. Primary colon carcinomas,
regional lymph node metastases and distal metastases from

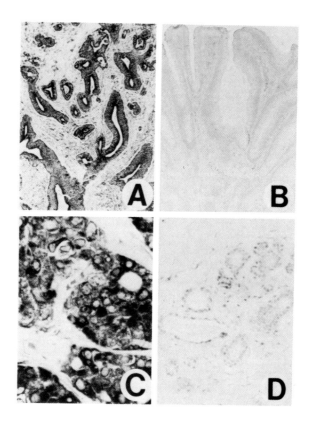

Figure 1.   Immunoperoxidase staining of paraffin-embedded
formalin-fixed tissue sections with MAb RAP-5.   (A) adenocarcinoma of the colon, invasive component.   The darkly
stained areas represent the reaction of the diaminobenzidine
substrate and therefore MAb RAP-5 binding to cytoplasmic
ras p21 in carcinoma cells.   The lighter region is the
hematoxylin counter stain, showing no antibody reactivity
(x34).   (B) Tubulovillous adenoma.   Dysplastic colonic
epithelium, stroma and a mixed inflammatory mononuclear
cell infiltrate are negative (x27).   (C) Human mammary
infiltrating ductal carcinoma positive for cytoplasmic
reactivity with MAb RAP-5 (x270).   (D) Fibrocystic disease
with epithelial hyperplasia negative for reactivity with
MAb RAP-5 (x110).

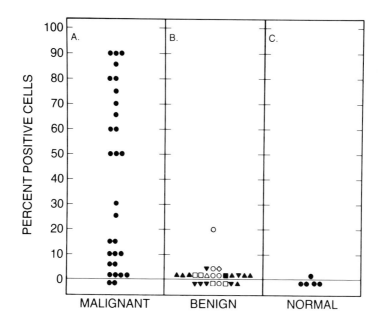

<u>Figure 2</u>.   Reactivity of MAb RAP-5 with several colonic
disease states. Using the immunoperoxidase method, MAb RAP-5
was reacted with formalin-fixed tissue sections of colonic
adenocarcinomas (A, closed circles); benign tumors including
tubular adenomas (B, closed triangles), tubulovillous
adenomas (B, inverted triangle), villous adenoma with <u>in situ</u>
carcinoma (B, closed squares), hamartomatous polyp (B,
diamond); inflammatory bowel diseases including diverticulitis
(B, open circles), ulcerative colitis (B, open squares),
Crohn's disease (B, open triangle); and normal colon (C,
circles).   Each symbol represents a tumor or tissue from a
different patient. The percent positive cells denotes the
number of tumor cells positive for <u>ras</u> p21 divided by the
total number of tumor cells x 100 in carcinomas and benign
tumors (A,B) and denotes the total number of epithelial cells
positive for <u>ras</u> p21 divided by the total number of epithelial
cells x 100 in inflammatory bowel disease and normal colon
(B,C).

each of 4 patients were studied for ras p21 expression using
the immunoperoxidase method and MAb RAP-5 IgG. As seen in
Fig. 3, all the primary colon carcinomas and metastatic
lesions scored positive for ras p21. Heterogeneity of ras
p21 expression was observed for the primary colon carcinomas,
with a range of 80-90% of tumor cells positive for ras p21.
The regional lymph node metastases and distal metastases
also showed antigenic heterogeneity with 70-100% and 25-95%
of ras p21 positive tumor cells, respectively.

Expression of ras p21 in Human Mammary Carcinomas.
Twenty-one formalin-fixed infiltrating ductal carcinomas
(IDCs) from 21 patients were examined for ras gene activation with purified IgG of MAb RAP-5. Nineteen of the 21
IDCs (90%) were positive for ras p21 (Figs. 1C, 4). Using
the criterion of >20% of tumor cells expressing detectable
levels of ras p21 as a positive reaction, 18 of 21 IDCs
(86%) versus 2 of 21 benign breast lesions (0 of 11 fibrocystic disese and 2 of 10 fibroadenomas) scored positive
(Figs. 1D, 4). The vast majority of all abnormal ducts and
lobules from fibrocystic disease patients (Fig 1D) and
fibroadenomas were negative. Normal lobules and ducts from
both benign breast disease patient groups were also routinely negative for ras p21.

Heterogeneity of expression of ras p21 was also observed
in the majority of mammary carcinomas (Figs. 1C, 4). This
heterogeneity included a variation in the number of tumor
cells within a given tumor expressing ras p21, as well as the
amount of ras p21 expressed among tumor cells within a given
tumor section.

Liquid Competition RIA for ras p21. To determine the
presence and quantity of the ras p21 antigenic determinant
detected by MAb YA6-259 (3), a liquid phase competition RIA
was developed. In this assay, MAb YA6-259 is incubated in
liquid phase with dilutions of competitor antigen. Unbound
MAb is detected by further incubation of the antibody antigen
mixture with a protein extract of the H-transformed NIH-3T3
cell line (568) dried to polyvinyl chloride microtiter wells;
the wells are then washed and incubated with rabbit anti-rat
IgG, and subsequently with ^{125}I-Protein A. The wells are
counted and percent bound determined by dividing the counts
bound in the presence of competitor antigen by the counts
bound in the absence of competitor antigen.

To determine the specificity of the RIA, ras p21 puri-
fied from E. coli containing the point mutated (T24) human
H-ras gene product (16) was used as competitor antigen.
Binding of MAb YA6-259 to the H-transformed 3T3 detection

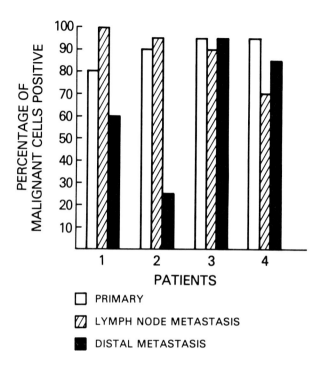

Figure 3.   Reactivity of MAb RAP-5 with primary colonic adenocarcinomas and metastases from four different patients.   MAb
RAP-5 was reacted with each of four primary colonic adenocarcinomas (open bar) and metastases of the primary carcinoma
to the lymph node (hatched bar) and to sites distal to the
primary lesion (closed bar) from four different patients.   The
percent positive cells denotes the number of tumor cells
positive for ras p21 divided by the total number of tumor
cells x 100.

antigen could be inhibited completely by approximately 7 ng
of the purified ras p21 (95% pure), with less than 0.3 ng
required to demonstrate competition (20%).   Lysates of E.
coli containing the T24 and proto-forms of the human H-ras
gene product (16) were also used as competitors in the RIA.
Approximately 100 ng of the T24 and 250 ng of the proto-

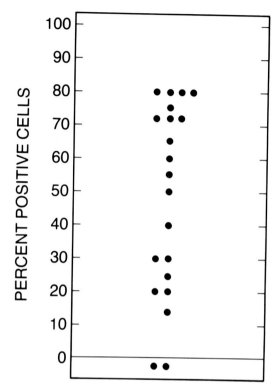

Figure 4.   Reactivity of MAb RAP-5 with infiltrating ductal
carcinomas of the breast.   Using the immunoperoxidase method,
MAb RAP-5 was reacted with formalin-fixed sections of primary
mammary carcinomas.   Each symbol represents a tumor from a
different patient.   The percent positive cells denotes the
number of tumor cells positive for ras p21 divided by the
total number of tumor cells x 100.

ras p21 E. coli lysates were required for 100% competition.
The similar slopes and complete competition demonstrated by
the 95% pure ras p21 and both E. coli lysates strongly suggest that the identical antigenic determinant is being detected in each of these preparations.   This RIA therefore
detects an antigenic determinant shared by the proto- and
point mutated ras gene products.   The displacement observed
between the E. coli lysates containing the proto- and point
mutated H-ras p21s is probably due to their relative efficiency of production using the E. coli expression vector

system. The specificity of the ras p21 RIA was further
demonstrated since no competition was observed when as much
as 10^5 ng of E. coli lysate was used as competitor antigen.

The presence of ras p21 was then demonstrated in a
variety of mammalian cell lines using the ras p21 liquid
competition RIA. Protein extracts of both the H-transformed (568) and K-transformed (DT) NIH-3T3 murine cell
lines competed completely. More than 100- to 200-fold less
p21 was detected in the 568 and DT protein extracts, respectively than in the E. coli lysate containing the H-ras p21.
Approximately two-fold more input protein was required of
the DT K-transformed cell line to achieve the same level of
competition as the 568 H-transformed NIH-3T3 cell protein
extract. This RIA may therefore be termed group-specific
since it detects both the H-ras and K-ras gene products as
well as interspecies since it detects both rodent and human
ras. The murine fibroblast cell line, NIH-3T3, contains the
proto- ras gene product. A protein extract of this cell
line competed completely at input concentrations of 10^5 ng.
Five- to 10-fold more protein was required for the NIH-3T3
cell protein extract to achieve levels of competition identical to those of the 568 H-transformed cells. Competition of
the NIH-3T3 cells in the ras p21 RIA therefore confirms the
ability of this assay to detect both the proto- and point
mutated ras p21.

Protein extracts of two transfected mammalian cell
lines were also assayed for ras p21. Both the viral H-ras
transfected NIH-3T3 and the activated Hu ras^{T24} transfected
NIH-3T3 cell lines competed completely at levels of protein
comparable to those of the K-transformed NIH-3T3 cell line.
Approximately 1.4-fold less protein was required for competition of the viral H-ras transfected NIH-3T3 cell line than
the activated Hu-ras^{T24} transfected NIH-3T3 cell line. H-ras
p21 was also detected in the T24 human bladder carcinoma
cell line with approximately 4- to 8-fold more protein extract required than that of the H-transformed NIH-3T3 cell
line to achieve equivalent levels of competition.

Based on the reactivity observed with purified ras p21
in the liquid competition RIA, it is possible to quantitate
the amount of p21 in this sample and in protein extracts
used as competitors. The purified ras p21 was therefore
determined to contain 45.1 fM p21 per ng total protein,
while the proto- and point mutated H-ras p21 E. coli lysates
contained 0.73 and 0.87 fM p21 per ng protein, respectively.
In contrast, less than 0.0003 fM p21 was detected per ng of
the E. coli lysate.

Protein extracts of the H- and K-transformed NIH-3T3 cell lines have 0.006 and 0.004 fM p21 per ng protein, respectively, while the NIH-3T3 cells contain approximately 0.001 fM p21 per ng. The H-transfected NIH-3T3 cells and the Hu-H^{T24} transfected NIH-3T3 cells were determined to contain 0.004 and 0.003 fM p21 per ng protein extract, respectively.

DISCUSSION

A higher percent of colon carcinoma cells positive for ras p21 expression was detected using the RAP-MAbs in the immunohistochemical studies detailed here than that reported in DNA transfection studies. Furthermore, since DNA transfection experiments designed to detect activated ras gene expression in human mammary carcinomas have thus far been unsuccessful, the number of mammary carcinomas expressing ras p21 as detected by the RAP MAbs was surprising. One possible explanation for these discrepancies is that the NIH-3T3 transfection system may not be a sensitive indicator model for the ras gene present in these carcinomas. Alternatively, enhanced expression of the proto- ras gene may be responsible for ras activation in some colon or mammary carcinomas, perhaps at times, by means of a promotor sequence regulated by a hormone. The only two benign breast lesions that scored with percentage of tumor cells positive similar to those of mammary carcinomas were from patients with multiple fibroadenomas (a total of 7 tumors removed from the two patients prior to 24 years of age). Hormonal factors may be involved in the development of these benign lesions (17).

Some colon carcinomas may evolve from benign disease states or inflammatory bowel diseases such as adenomas, familial adenopolyposis or ulcerative colitis (18-20). If carcinogenesis is a multistep event, it would be interesting to determine if ras p21 expression is related to a specific stage in this process. We have observed the reactivity of RAP MAbs in a specimen of invasive carcinoma in a pseudo-polyp from a patient with ulcerative colitis (2). Weak reactivity of the RAP MAb was observed to the hyperplastic epithelial cells of the pseudopolyp, while the invasive carcinoma cells and adjacent hyperplastic epithelia contained higher levels of ras p21. ras activation may therefore be a late event in the process of transformation (21-23).

The RAP MAbs were generated using as immunogen a syn-

thetic peptide representing an amino acid sequence thought
to be located internally in the molecule. The studies
reported here confirm our earlier findings and provide
additional evidence that alteration of ras p21 with an
agent such as formalin permits the binding of the RAP MAbs
to their antigenic determinants. This is opportune since
formalin-fixed tissue sections provide better histologic
detail and are more easily available than frozen tissue
sections. In contrast, using formalin-fixed tissue sections
we have been unsuccessful in detecting the determinant recognized by MAb YA6-259 (prepared against native ras p21 (3)).

We have demonstrated heterogeneity of expression of ras
p21 in both human colon and mammary carcinomas. Antigenic
heterogeneity was observed (1) among carcinomas from different
patients, (2) among cells within a given tumor specimen, and
(3) among primary carcinomas, lymph node metastases, and
distal metastases from the same patient. There was also a
variation in the level of expression of ras p21 within the
population of cells positive for the ras gene product. Therefore, if ras activation is involved in the transformation of
colon or mammary epithelium or in the progression of carcinomas, uniform and constant expression does not appear to be
required for the maintenance of the transformed phenotype.
Several factors may be involved in the initiation and maintenance of ras p21 expression in carcinoma cells including
cell cycle, as demonstrated for other tumor-associated antigens (24), and ras p21 (25). The possibility also exists
that activation of the ras gene may be required solely for
initiation and/or promotion and not for maintenance of the
transformed phenotype.

We have developed a highly sensitive and specific
quantitative liquid competition RIA for ras p21. This
immunoassay as well as the quantitative solid phase RIAs
which utilize the RAP-MAbs (1) are termed "group-specific"
since they identify antigenic determinants shared by
members of the ras gene family. The antigenic determinant
detected in the liquid competition RIA is shared by the
proto-oncogenic as well as the activated ras p21. This
is demonstrated by the identical slopes of the competition
curves generated by extracts of the E. coli and mammalian
cells containing either ras gene translational product.
The development of additional MAbs that recognize "class-
specific" and "type-specific" antigenic determinants
representing the more variable regions of this gene family
will eventually be utilized to determine which member of
the Hu-ras gene family is being expressed in a given cell.

It is important to note that the liquid competition RIA allows for the first time the direct measurement of ras p21 concentration within cells. The RIA has been used here to detect ras p21 in E. coli or mammalian cells containing the proto- and point mutated form of p21. Based on the reactivity observed with the purified ras p21, we have determined that approximately 1.5% of the total proteins of the E. coli ras p21 samples is p21 while the amount of p21 detected in mammalian cell lines ranged from 0.013% for the Ha-transformed NIH-3T3 to as little as 0.003% for the NIH-3T3 cell lines. Due to its high degree of sensitivity, this RIA may be valuable in determining the relationship between ras gene expression and a specific malignant disease state.

The quantitative liquid competition RIA described here as well as the quantitative solid phase RIAs using the RAP-MAbs (1) now make possible determination of levels of ras p21 in biopsy material and mammalian cell lines, while immunohistochemical studies using formalin-fixed tissues permit the identification of specific cell types expressing ras p21. These immunoassays now provide the technology for the evaluation of the role of ras gene translation products in the processes of initiation and maintenance of carcinomas.

REFERENCES

1. Horan Hand P, Thor A, Wunderlich D, Muraro R, Caruso A, Schlom J (1984). Monoclonal antibodies of predefined specificity detect activated ras gene expression in human mammary and colon carcinomas. Proc Natl Acad Sci USA 81: 5227.
2. Thor A, Horan Hand P, Wunderlich D, Caruso A, Muraro R, Schlom J (1984). Monoclonal antibodies define differential ras gene expression in malignant and benign colonic diseases. Nature 311:562.
3. Furth ME, Davis LJ, Fleurdelys B, Scolnick EM (1982). Monoclonal antibodies to the p21 products of the transforming gene of Harvey murine sarcoma virus and of the cellular ras gene family. J. Virol. 43:294.
4. Cooper GM (1982). Cellular transforming genes. Science 217:801.
5. Ellis RW, DeFeo D, Shih TY, Gonda MA, Young HA, Tsuchida N, Lowy DR, Scolnick EM (1981). The p21 src gene of Harvey and Kirsten sarcoma viruses originate from divergent members of a family of normal vertebrate genes. Nature (London) 292:506.

6. Tabin CJ, Bradley SM, Bargmann CI, Weinberg RA, Papageorge AG, Scolnick EM, Dhar R, Lowy DR, Chang EH (1982). Mechanism of activation of a human oncogene. Nature (London) 300: 143.

7. Schwab M, Alitalo K, Varmus HE, Bishop JM (1983). A cellular oncogene (c-Ki-ras) is amplified, overexpressed and located within karyotypic abnormalities in mouse adrenocortical tumor cells. Nature (London) 303:497.

8. Audibert F, Jolivet M, Chedid L, Arnon R, Sela M (1982). Successful immunization with a totally synthetic diphtheria vaccine. Proc Natl Acad Sci USA 79:5042.

9. Kohler G, Howe SC, Milstein C (1976). Fusion between immunoglobulin-secreting and nonsecreting myeloma cell lines. Eur J Immunol 6:292.

10. Herzenberg LA, Herzenberg LA, Milstein C (1978). Cell hybrids of myelomas with antibody forming cells and T lymphocytes with T cells. In Weir DM (ed.): "Handbook of Experimental Immunology," London: Blackwell Scientific Publications, p. 25.1.

11. Colcher D, Horan Hand P, Teramoto YA, Wunderlich D, Schlom J (1981). Use of monoclonal antibodies to define the diversity of mammary tumor viral gene products in virions and mammary tumors of the genus Mus. Cancer Res 41:1451.

12. Colcher D, Zalutsky M, Kaplan W, Kufe D, Austin F, Schlom J (1983). Radiolocalization of human mammary tumors in athymic mice by a monoclonal antibody. Cancer Res 43:736.

13. Hsu SM, Raine L, Fanger H (1981). Use of avidin-biotin-peroxidase complex (ABC) in immunoperoxidase techniques: a comparison between ABC and unlabelled antibody (PA) procedures. J Histochem Cytochem 29:577.

14. Nuti M, Teramoto YA, Mariani-Costantini R, Horan Hand P, Colcher D, Schlom J (1982). A monoclonal antibody (B72.3) defines patterns of distribution of a novel tumor-associated antigen in human mammary carcinoma cell populations. Int J Cancer 29:539.

15. Potter M (1972). Immunoglobulin-producing tumors and myeloma proteins of mice. Physiol Rev 52:631.

16. Feramisco JR, Gross M, Kamata T, Rosenberg M, Sweet R (1984). Microinjection of the oncogene form of the human H-ras (T24) protein results in rapid proliferation of quiescent cells. Cell 38:109.

17. Robbins SL, Cotran SR (1979). "Pathologic Basis of Disease," Philadelphia: Saunders, p. 1317.

18. DeVita VT, Hellman S, Rosenberg SA (1982). "Cancer: Principles and Practice of Oncology," Philadelphia:

Lippincott, p. 674.

19. Edwards FC, Truelove SC (1964). The course and prognosis of ulcerative colitis. Gut 5:15.

20. Bussey HJR (1975). "Familial Polyposis Coli," Baltimore: Johns Hopkins University Press.

21. Land H, Parada LF, Weinberg RA (1983). Cellular oncogenes and multiple carcinogenesis. Science 222:771.

22. Land H, Parada LF, Weinberg RA (1983). Tumorigenic conversion of primary embryo fibroblasts requires at least two cooperating oncogenes. Nature 304:596.

23. Needleman SW, Yuasa Y, Srivastava S, Aaronson SA (1983). Normal cells of patients with high cancer risk syndromes lack transforming activity in the NIH-3T3 transfection assay. Science 222:173.

24. Kufe DW, Nadler L, Sargent L, Shapiro H, Horan Hand P, Austin F, Colcher D, Schlom J (1983). Cell surface binding properties of monoclonal antibodies reactive with human mammary carcinoma cells. Cancer Res 43:851.

25. Campisi J, Gray HE, Pardee AB, Dean M, Soneshein GE (1984). Cell cycle control of c-myc but not c-ras expression is lost following chemical transformation. Cell 36:241.

Monoclonal Antibodies and Cancer Therapy, pages 37–51
© **1985 Alan R. Liss. Inc.**

CLINICAL APPLICATION OF MONOCLONAL ANTIBODIES
REACTIVE WITH EPITHELIAL OVARIAN CANCER

Robert C. Bast, Jr., Vincent R. Zurawski, Jr., and
Robert C. Knapp

Duke University Medical Center,
Durham, North Carolina 27710
Centocor,
Malvern, Pennsylvania 19355
Dana-Farber Cancer Institute
Boston, Massachusetts 02115

ABSTRACT   Several monoclonal reagents have been
prepared in different laboratories which react
with epithelial ovarian carcinomas. The murine
IgG1 immunoglobulin OC125 reacts with CA125
determinants expressed by more than 80% of non-
mucinous epithelial ovarian carcinomas. Traces of
CA125 can be detected in amnion and in fetal
tissues derived from the coelomic epithelium, but
CA125 is not found in fetal or adult ovary. Using
a radioimmunometric sandwich assay, CA125 levels
have been found in sera from more than 80% of
patients with surgically demonstrable ovarian
cancer (1). Doubling or halving of abnormal
antigen levels has correlated with increasing or
decreasing tumor burden in greater than 90% of
instances studied. Elevation of CA125 preceded
clinical recurrence of disease by 1-14 (median=3)
months in 94% of 35 patients (2). In one patient
for whom serial blood samples had been frozen,
CA125 levels were elevated 10-12 months prior to
the primary diagnosis of ovarian cancer (3).
Among 988 non-pregnant patients with benign
gynecologic disease, CA125 levels were comparably

elevated in 1% on a single determination and in 0.5% on two determinations (4). In patients undergoing diagnostic laparotomy for pelvic masses, CA125 was elevated in 13 of 14 with frankly malignant gynecologic tumors, but in only one of 78 with benign disease (5). CA125 deserves further evaluation as a test for early detection of ovarian neoplasms.

INTRODUCTION

Ovarian carcinoma exhibits an unusual pattern of spread. The tumor can metastasize through lymphatics and blood borne metastases are sometimes encountered, but by far the most frequent pattern of spread is over the peritoneal surface. Small tumor nodules stud the serosal surfaces of abdominal viscera and block diaphragmatic lymphatics. Outflow of lymph is impeded and ascites fluid accumulates. Once a surgeon removes the bulk of the ovarian tumor during a total abdominal hysterectomy and bilateral salpingo-oophorectomy, the only disease remaining often consists of small tumor nodules, which cannot be detected on careful physical examination or by the most sophisticated radiographic procedures. As this is one of the tumors that can respond to combination chemotherapy, the oncologist must often treat patients for a period of months without knowing whether the treatment is benefitting the patient. Consequently, a good deal of effort has been invested in defining serum markers for tumor burden in patients undergoing treatment for epithelial ovarian carcinoma.

CA125: A LINEAGE ASSOCIATED DETERMINANT

Some five years ago we had applied the technique of Kohler and Milstein (6) to the production of monoclonal antibodies reactive with human ovarian cancer. In collaboration with Dr. Herbert Lazarus, cell lines

had been established from epithelial ovarian carcinomas. B lymphocyte lines had also been established
from the tumor cell donors by Epstein-Barr virus
transformation of peripheral blood lymphocytes. Mice
were immunized with epithelial ovarian carcinomas and
hybridomas were prepared with the P3-NS1 cell line.
Clones were screened for the production of antibodies
that would bind to the immunizing ovarian tumor cell
line, but not to autologous B lymphocytes or to enzymatically dissociated allogeneic normal ovarian cells.
One of the most promising reagents isolated in our
early studies was designated OC125 (7), an IgG1 immunoglobulin which recognized a determinant associated with
a high molecular weight glycoprotein. Multiple CA125
determinants are associated with each glycoprotein molecule. Using a biotin-avidin immunoperoxidase technique, CA125 determinants are found in coelomic epithelium during embryonic differentiation (8). CA125 can
be found in the fetal pleura, pericardium, peritoneum,
Müllerian duct and amnion. Traces of the antigen can
also be detected adult structures derived from the
coelomic epithelium, but importantly are not found in
ovary, either in the fetus or in the adult. CA125 is
expressed by approximately 80% of non-mucinous
epithelial ovarian carcinomas (9).

CA125 IN MONITORING RESPONSE TO TREATMENT

In collaboration with Tom Klug an immunoradiometric assay has been developed to detect CA125 antigen
in serum and body fluids (1, 9). As there are multiple
CA125 determinants on each glycoprotein molecule, a
sandwich immunoradiometric assay could be constructed.
In this assay, antigen in 100 ul of serum is bound to a
solid phase immunoabsorbent containing non-labeled
OC125. Bound antigen can then be detected using ^{125}I
labeled OC125 as a probe. Antigen in serum or a body
fluid is compared to an arbitrary standard. Using this
assay, it is possible to measure from 1.4 to more than
20,000 units of antigen activity per milliliter of

serum. As the day-to-day coefficient of variation of the assay is 12-15%, a two-fold increase or halving of antigen level has been considered significant.

In our early studies, using 35 U/ml as a cutoff, elevated CA125 levels were found in 1% of apparently healthy controls, 6% of patients with non-malignant disease, 28% of patients with non-gynecologic malignancy and more than 80% of patients with some amount of surgically demonstrable epithelial ovarian cancer (1). Subsequent studies in England, France, Germany and the People's Republic of China, have confirmed the presence of elevated CA125 in 79% of sera from 437 patients studied (Table 1). A subsequent report has also demonstrated elevated levels of CA125 in sera from the majority of patients with adenocarcinomas of the fallopian tube, endometrium and endocervix (17). Squamous cell tumors of the cervix, vulva and vagina have generally not been associated with elevated CA125 levels. In a retrospective analysis of serum samples from the cryobank at the Dana-Farber Cancer Institute and the Brigham and Women's Hospital, increases or decreases in antigen levels correlated with progression or regression of tumor in 42 of 45 instances studied (1).

Subsequent studies have better defined the limitations of this assay in judging residual tumor prior to second or third-look surgical surveillance procedures (2). Among 56 patients with elevated CA125 levels, CA125 returned to less than 35 U/ml prior to a surgical surveillance procedure in 36 cases. In 14 of those 36 patients (39%) no tumor was found on multiple biopsies or washings. In 22 of the 36 patients, small amounts of tumor were detected. In no case did the largest tumor nodule exceed 1 cm in diameter. Conversely, in 20 of 56 patients, CA125 levels remained elevated, despite the lack of conclusive evidence for persistent disease by non-invasive evaluation. In some cases, it was possible to detect nodules as small as 0.4 cm in diameter. In two cases, no tumor was found at second-look procedure, but recurrent carcinoma was detected within 3 months. Consequently, a return of

CA125 to normal levels cannot be taken as evidence that the patient is disease free. A persistently elevated or rising level of CA125, however, has generally been associated with persistent tumor. In 35 patients who have responded to therapy, a persistent elevation of CA125 preceded disease recurrence in 33 cases (19). The interval between the first elevation of CA125 and the clinical appearance of recurrent disease by non-invasive techniques was from 1 to 14 months with a median of 3 months. From these early studies, it appeared that elevated levels of CA125 could be detected in sera from more than 80% of the patients with surgically demonstrable epithelial ovarian carcinomas. Antigen levels correlated with clinical course in 93% of instances. If these studies are confirmed, CA125 may prove to be the first generally useful marker for monitoring patients with epithelial ovarian carcinoma.

POTENTIAL OF CA125 FOR
EARLY DETECTION OF EPITHELIAL OVARIAN CANCER

From a clinician's perspective, the problem in epithelial ovarian carcinoma is not only monitoring the disease course more accurately, but also detecting the disease at a time when it could be treated effectively with conventional surgery and radiation therapy. In approximately two thirds of the ovarian cancer patients, tumor has spread outside of the pelvis to the abdominal cavity or beyond the diaphragm at the time the tumor is diagnosed. This may, however, be one of the tumors that lends itself to early detection with a blood test. Knauf and Urbach (20) had developed a radioimmunoassay for OCA, a tumor marker defined by polyclonal heteroantiserum. OCA levels were elevated in 60-70% of patients with stage I or stage II epithelial ovarian cancer. Elevated antigen levels were also found in approximately 10% of apparently healthy individuals, precluding the use of this assay for screening large populations. These data did, however, suggest that shed tumor products could be found in the circulation at an early stage of tumor development.

In one fortuitous case, it has been possible to study CA125 levels prior to the diagnosis of ovarian cancer (2). Serum samples from a patient with acquired hypogammaglobulinemia had been saved for several years prior to the presentation of a stage III serous cyst-adenocarcinoma. In retrospect, CA125 was greater than 35 U/ml 12 months prior to clinical presentation and greater than 100 U/ml 10 months prior to diagnosis of the malignancy. This case raises the question of whether CA125 would provide a useful marker for early detection of epithelial ovarian cancer.

If one wants to utilize an assay for early detection of a malignancy, there can be few false positive values among healthy individuals or patients with benign disease. Consequently, we have studied CA125 levels in 1,020 patients with benign gynecologic disease seen at a clinic in Boston. If a cutoff of 65 units is chosen, 1.8% of patients had elevated antigen levels. When pregnant patients were excluded, the false positive rate dropped to approximately 1%. When a second blood sample was obtained, only 0.5% had elevated CA125 on two occasions. More than 70% of patients with advanced ovarian carcinoma have greater than 65 U/ml of antigen. In our own experience, 8 of 11 patients with stage I or stage II disease also had elevated CA125 prior to exploration. In collaboration with Dr. Nina Einhorn at the Karolinska Institute, we have measured CA125 levels in 100 patients undergoing laparotomy for diagnosis of a pelvic mass (5). Among patients with benign disease at laparotomy only 1 of 78 had had more than 65 units of antigen per milliliter of serum. Conversely, 9 of 11 patients with frankly malignant non-mucinous epithelial ovarian cancer had elevated antigen levels. Several patients had gynecological tumors arising from other sites. Overall, 13 of 14 patients with a pelvic mass and an elevated CA125, had some form of gynecologic malignancy. The assay failed to detect mucinous tumors and borderline neoplasms. If these results can be confirmed, it may be possible to identify patients preoperatively who should be referred for cytoreductive surgery.

OTHER MONOCLONAL ANTIBODIES REACTIVE WITH EPITHELIAL OVARIAN CANCER

Following the development of OC125, several different groups have obtained a number of monoclonal reagents by immunizing mice with ovarian tumor cell lines, ovarian tumor tissues or cyst fluid (Table 2). Some of these reagents react solely with mucinous ovarian tumors and others with both serous and mucinous neoplasms. Monoclonal antibodies reactive with ovarian carcinoma have also been developed by immunizing mice with tumor cells which had arisen from other tissues, including the endometrium, colon, pancreas, breast and bone. In most cases these reagents react with the epithelial components of tumors. Most antibodies react with tumors from more than one primary site. Reagents react with at least one normal tissue with the possible exception of the 632 reagent of Fleuren and the OV-TL-3 reagent of Poels. Although no antibody appears absolutely specific, the binding of two reagents to tumor cells or to shed tumor products might provide a more specific or more sensitive test for this ovarian tumor.

CA19-9 has reacted with approximately 40% of epithelial ovarian cancers in tissue section (33). Shed antigen was detected in only 17% of serum samples from 105 patients with some amount of persistent epithelial ovarian carcinoma. Given the excellent correlation observed between disease course and levels of CA125, a combination of CA19-9, carcinoembryonic antigen and CA125, was no more effective than CA125 alone for monitoring the course of patients. A remarkable parallel was, however, observed between levels of CA125 and levels of CA19-9 when a single patient was monitored at weekly intervals over a 5 month period (34). Among samples from different patients, no correlation was found between CA125 and CA19-9 levels. Moreover, anti-19-9 did not compete for binding of CA125 in the double determinant immunoassay and OC125 did not affect binding of CA 19-9 to anti-19-9. Consequently, the two epitopes appeared antigenically distinct. When antigen was purified from culture supernatants of tumor cells that bore both epitopes, OC125 bound to two distinct glycoproteins of greater than 300,000 daltons. Anti-19-9 bound to a single band which co-migrated with the higher molecular weight moiety to which OC125 had bound. CEA was not detected in either band. This suggested that a single high molecular weight species might express both epitopes. When sera and ascites fluid from patients with elevated CA125 levels were analyzed, approximately 40% contained molecules which bound both antibodies (35).

CA125 and CA19-9 are co-expressed in two normal tissues, the endocervix and fallopian tube. To construct an assay which would discriminate between malignant and benign disease, antibodies which had completely complementary expression in normal tissue might be of value. In this setting, normal cells should not be capable of synthesizing a molecule which bears both epitopes and levels of doubly positive molecules should not be detectable in serum. To obtain such reagents, CA125 mucin has been isolated from ovarian tumor cell culture supernatants using antibody affinity techniques. Mice have been immunized with the partially purified material. Hybridomas have been prepared from their spleens and culture supernatants have been screened for binding to CA125 positive mucin using ^{125}I labeled rabbit anti-mouse immunoglobulin. Antibodies are further screened for a lack of inhibition of CA125 binding in the sandwich radioimmunoassay, as well as a lack of reactivity with pericardium and adult derivatives of the Müllerian duct. Three antibodies have been isolated which meet these criteria (Table 3). All three react with colon and bind to both mucinous and non-mucinous epithelial ovarian cancers. Whether these will provide more specific reagents in combination with OC125 remains to be seen.

RADIONUCLIDE IMAGING OF
EPITHELIAL OVARIAN CARCINOMA

Binding of ^{125}I labeled OC125 has been studied
with four different epithelial ovarian carcinoma cell
lines (36). Apparent affinities range from 6.0×10^{7}
to 3.1×10^{9}. The apparent number of antigenic
determinants ranges from 2.8×10^{5} to 1.0×10^{7}.
Importantly, binding of OC125 does not induce antigenic
modulation or internalization of the CA125 determinant.
Antibody remains associated with the cell surface for
at least 24 hours in cell culture. Dr. J. F. Chatal in
Nantes has used intact ^{131}I labeled OC125 to image more
than 20 patients with epithelial ovarian carcinoma.
Sites of tumor have been localized in the majority of
these individuals. In collaboration with Drs. Michael
Zalutsky and William Kaplan, radionuclide imaging with
smaller amounts of ^{131}I labeled OC125 F(AB')$_{2}$ injected
intravenously or intralymphatically has been attempted
in 8 patients with ovarian carcinoma at the Dana-Farber
Cancer Institute in Boston. In one of these
individuals, an axillary metastasis was successfully
imaged, but intra-abdominal disease has not been
visualized. Successful visualization of primary and
recurrent epithelial ovarian carcinoma has been
reported by Granowska et al (37) using the anti-milk
fat globule protein antibodies and by Symonds et al
(38) with an antibody raised against osteogenic
sarcoma. In both series, most patients could be
successfully imaged. The utility of this approach for
detecting diaphragmatic metastases and retroperitoneal
lymph node metastases remains to be determined.

TABLE 1

CA125 LEVELS IN OVARIAN CANCER PATIENTS

Investigators	Antigen Levels (U/ml)	# Positive	# Studied
Bast, et al, (1)	35	84/101	(83 %)
Chatal, et al, (11)	30	35/ 38	(92 %)
Sarmini, et al, (12)	35	14/ 27	(52 %)
Canney, et al, (13)	35	34/ 44	(77 %)
Crombach, et al, (14)	35	71/ 91	(78 %)
Auvray, et al, (15)	35	43/ 49	(83 %)
Kreienberg and Melchart, (16)	65	36/ 57	(63 %)
Lien, et al (17)	65	29/ 30	(97 %)
TOTAL		346/437	(79.2%)

TABLE 2

MONOCLONAL ANTIBODIES REACTIVE WITH EPITHELIAL OVARIAN CARCINOMAS

Source of immunogen	Antibody	Investigators
Ovarian Carcinoma	OC125	Bast, et al, (6)
	ID3	Bhattacharya, et al, (21)
	MOV-2	Colnaghi, et al, (22)
	OC133	Berkowitz, et al, (23)
	MD144	Mattes, et al, (24)
	MF61	Mattes, et al, (24)
	MF116	Mattes, et al, (24)
	632	Fleuren, et al, (25)
	OV-TL-3	Poels, et al, submitted (26)
Endometrial Carcinoma	MH55	Mattes, et al, (24)
	MH94	Mattes, et al, (24)
Colorectal Carcinoma	19-9	Koprowski, et al, (27)
Pancreatic Carcinoma	DU-PAN-2	Metzgar, et al, (28)
Breast Carcinoma	F36/22	Croghan, et al, (29)
Milk Fat Globule Protein	HMFG2	Epenetos, et al, (30)
	AUA1	
Laryngeal Carcinoma	CA-1	Woods, et al, (31)
Osteogenic Sarcoma	791-T/36	Embleton, et al, (32)

TABLE 3
MONOCLONAL ANTIBODIES TO COMPLEMENTARY
LINEAGE ASSOCIATED DETERMINANTS

Binding to CA125+ Mucin	Competition with OC125	Pericardium	Binding to Mullerian Duct Derivatives	Colon	Epithelial Ovarian Cancers
OC125 +	+++	+	+	-	26/35
OC3632 +	-	-	-	+++	8/10
OC3634 +	-	-	-	+++	7/ 7
OC3697 +	-	-	-	++	7/ 9

REFERENCES

1. Bast RC Jr, Klug TL, St. John E, Jenison E, Niloff J, Lazarus H, Berkowitz RS, Leavitt T, Griffiths CT, Parker L, Zurawski VR, Knapp RC (1983). A radioimmunoassay using a monoclonal antibody to monitor the course of epithelial ovarian cancer. N Engl J Med 309:883.
2. Niloff JM, Bast RC Jr, Schaetzl FM, Knapp RC (1985b). Predictive value of CA125 antigen levels at second look procedures in ovarian cancer. Am J Obstet Gynecol in press.
3. Bast RC Jr, Siegal FP, Runowicz C, Klug TL, Zurawski VR, Schonholz D, Cohen CJ, Knapp RC (1985). Elevation of serum CA125 prior to diagnosis of an epithelial ovarian carcinoma. Gyn Oncol in press.
4. Niloff M, Knapp RC, Schaetzl E, Reynolds C, Bast RC Jr (1985a). CA125 antigen levels in obstetric and gynecologic patients. Obstet Gynecol in press.
5. Einhorn N, Knapp RC, Zurawski VA, Bast RC Jr (1985). Preoperative evaluation of serum CA125 levels in patients with primary epithelial ovarian cancer. Obstet Gynecol in press.

6. Kohler G, Milstein C (1975). Continuous cultures of fused cells secreting antibody of predefined specificity. Nature 257:495.

7. Bast RC Jr, Feeney M, Lazarus H, Nadler LM, Colvin RB, Knapp RC (1981). Reactivity of a monoclonal antibody with human ovarian carcinoma. J Clin Invest 68:1331.

8. Kabawat SE, Bast RC Jr, Bhan AK, Welch WR, Knapp RC, Colvin RB (1983a). Tissue distribution of a coelomic epithelium related antigen recognized by the monoclonal antibody OC125. Int J Gyn Path 2:275.

9. Kabawat SE, Bast RC Jr, Welch WR, Knapp RC, Colvin RB (1983b). Immunopathologic characterization of a monoclonal antibody that recognizes common surface antigens of human ovarian tumors of serous, endometrioid and clear cell types. Am J Clin Path 79:98.

10. Klug TL, Bast RC Jr, Niloff JM, Knapp RC, Zurawski VR (1984). Monoclonal antibody immunoradiometric assay for an antigenic determinant (CA125) associated with human epithelial ovarian carcinomas. Cancer Res 44:1048.

11. Chatal JF, Ricolleau G, Fumoleau P, Kramer M, Curtet C, Douillard JY (1983). Radioimmunoassay of the CA12-5 antigen in epithelial ovarian carcinomas. Cancer Detection Prevention 6:624.

12. Sammini H, Scalet M, Pouillart P, Robinet D, Mazabraud A, Bon J, Funes A (1984). Study of CA125, CA19-9 and CEA levels in ovarian and breast cancer. International meeting on monoclonal antibodies in Oncology: Clinical applications. Nantes.

13. Canney P, Moore M, Wilkinson P, James R (1984). Ovarian cancer antigen CA12-5 sensitivity and variations with chemotherapy. International meeting on monoclonal antibodies in oncology: Clinical applications. Nantes.

14. Crombach G, Zippel HH, Wurz H (1983). Clinical significance of cancer antigen 125 (CA125) in ovarian cancer. Cancer Detection Prevention 6:623.

15. Auvray E, Kerbrat P, de Certaines J, Benoist C (1984). Seric CA12.5 radioimmunoassay in human ovarian carcinoma: Preliminary results from 49 patients. International meeting on antibodies in oncology: Clinical applications. Nantes.

16. Kreienberg R, Melchart F (1983). CA125-A new radioimmunoassay for monitoring patients with epithelial ovarian carcinoma. Cancer Detection Prevention 6:619.

17. Lien LC, Hu XF, Liu WS. A monoclonal antibody RIA for an antigeneic determinant (CA125) in ovarian cancer patients. Submitted for publication.

18. Niloff JM, Klug TL, Schaetzl E, Zurawski VR, Knapp RC and Bast RC Jr (1985c). Elevation of serum CA125 in carcinomas of the fallopian tube, endometrium and endocervix. Am J Obstet Gynecol in press.

19. Knapp RC, Lavin PT, Schaetzl E, Niloff JM, Bast RC Jr (1985). Elevation of CA125 prior to recurrence of ovarian cancer. Proc Soc of Gynecologic Oncology 16:30.

20. Knauf S, Urbach GI (1980). A study of ovarian cancer patients using a radioimmunoassay for human ovarian tumor associated antigen OCA. Am J Obstet Gynecol 138:1222.

21. Bhattacharya M, Chatterjee SK, Barlow JJ, and Fuji H (1982). Monoclonal antibodies recognizing tumor-associated antigen of human ovarian mucinous cyst-adenocarcinomas. Cancer Res 42:1650.

22. Colnaghi MI, Canaveri S, Dellatorre G et al (1982). Monoclonal antibodies directed against human tumors. Proc 13th Int Cancer Congress, p 55.

23. Berkowitz RS, Kabawat S, Lazarus H, Colvin RC, Knapp RC, Bast RC Jr (1983). Comparison of a rabbit heteroantiserum and a murine monoclonal antibody raised against a human epithelial ovarian carcinoma cell line. Am J Obstet Gynecol 146:607.

24. Mattes MJ, Cordon-Cardo C, Lewis JL Jr, Old LJ, Lloyd KO (1984). Cell surface antigens of human ovarian and endometrial carcinoma defined by mouse monoclonal antibodies. Proc Natl Acad Sci USA 81:568.

25. Fleuren G, Coerkamp E, Nap M, Warnaar S (1984). Immunohistological characterization of monoclonal antibody directed against non-mucinous ovarian carcinomas. International meeting on monoclonal antibodies in oncology: Clinical applications. Nantes.

26. Poels L. Personal communication.

27. Koprowski H, Steplewski Z, Mitchell K, Herlyn M, Herlyn D, Fuhrer JP (1979). Colorectal carcinoma antigens detected by hybridoma antibodies. Somatic Cell Genet 5:957.

28. Metzgar RS, Gaillard MT, Levine SJ, Tuck FL, Bossen EH, Borowitz MJ (1982). Antigens of human pancreatic adenocarcinoma cells defined by murine monoclonal antibodies. Cancer Res 42:601.

29. Croghan GA, Wingate MB, Gamarra M, Johnson E, Chu TM, Allen H, Valenzuela L, Tsukada Y, Papsidero LD (1984). Reactivity of monoclonal antibody F36/22 with human ovarian adenocarcinomas. Cancer Res 44:1954.

30. Epenetos AA, Mather S, Granowska M, Nimmon CC, Hawkins LR, Britton KE, Shepherd J, Taylor-Papadimitriou J, Durbin H, Malpas JS, Bodmer WF (1982). Targeting of iodine-123-labelled tumor-associated monoclonal antibodies to ovarian, breast and gastrointestinal tumours. Lancet 2:999.

31. Woods JC, Sprigas AI, Harris H, McGee JO'D (1982). A new marker for human cancer cells. 3. Immuno-cytochemical detection of malignant cells in serous fluids with the Ca-1 antibody. Lancet 2:512.

32. Embleton MJ, Gunn B, Byers YS, Baldwin RW (1981). Antitumor reactions of monoclonal antibodies against a human osteogenic sarcoma cell line. Br J Cancer 43:582.

33. Charpin C, Bhan AK, Zurawski V (1982). Carcino-embryonic antigen (CEA) and carbohydrate determinant 19-9 (CA19-9) localization in 121 primary and metastatic ovarian tumors: An immuno-histochemical study with the use of monoclonal antibodies. Int J Gynecol Path 1:231.

34. Bast RC Jr, Klug TL, Schaetzl E, Lavin P, Niloff J, Greber TF, Zurawski VR Jr, Knapp RC (1984). Monitoring human ovarian carcinoma with a combination of CA125, CA19-9 and carcinoembryonic antigen. Am J Obstet Gynecol 149:553.

35. Bast RC Jr, Klug T, Knapp RC, Zurawski VR Jr. CA19-9 can be expressed on the same mucin-like glycoprotein. Submitted for publication.

36. Masuho Y, Zalutsky M, Knapp RC, Bast RC Jr (1984). Interaction of monoclonal antibodies with cell surface antigens of human ovarian carcinomas. Cancer Res 44:2813.

37. Granowska M, Shepherd S, Mather S, Carroll MJ, Flatman WD, Nimmon CC, Taylor-Papadimitriou J, Ward B, Horne T, Britton KE (1984). A prospective study of radioimmunoscintigraphy with ^{123}I monoclonal antibody in 26 patients with suspected ovarian cancer. Proceedings of the European Nuclear Medicine Congress: "Nuclear Medicine in Research and Practice." Helsinki, Finland, August 14-17, 1984.

38. Symonds EM, Perkins AC, Pimm MV, Baldwin RW, Hardy JG, Williams DA (1984). Clinical implication for immunoscintigraphy in patients with ovarian malignancy. Brit J Obstet & Gynecol in press.

Monoclonal Antibodies and Cancer Therapy, pages 53–61
© **1985 Alan R. Liss, Inc.**

MONOCLONAL ANTIBODIES DIRECTED AGAINST
LYMPHOMAS OF THE MONOCYTE/RETICULUM CELL SYSTEM

Su-Ming Hsu, Mark D. Pescovitz,
Pei-Ling Hsu

Department of Pathology and
Laboratory Medicine,
University of Texas,
Houston, Texas 77030
and
the Immunology Branch,
National Cancer Institute,
Bethesda, Maryland 20205

ABSTRACT   Recently the use of monoclonal antibodies
(MoAb) has contributed significantly to the understanding of T and B cell lymphomas. However, a third group
of human lymphoma derived from monocytes/histiocytes/
interdigitating reticulum cells (IRCs) has not been yet
studied due to the lack of specific MoAbs.   We have
produced three MoAbs, 2H9, 1E9, and 1A2, that may facilitate the diagnosis of true histiocytic lymphoma (THL)
malignant hstiocytosis (MH) and Hodgkin's disease (HD).
These antibodies were made by immunizing mice with
SU-DHL-1 cells; cells that lack immunoglobulin gene
rearrangements, express neither B nor T cell markers,
but have features of, or share features with monocytes/
histiocytes.   All three MoAbs do not react with normal
B or T lymphocytes, or with B- or T-cell lymphomas.
However, two MoAbs, 2H9 and 1E9 react with the nuclear
membrane of histiocytes and IRCS in normal lymphoid
tissues. Both 2H9 and 1A2 also react with the cell
membrane of the neoplastic cells of HD and THL, whereas
1E9 stains the nuclear membrane of neoplastic cells of
THL and MH. The possible origins of THL, MH and HD are
studied using the current MoAbs and other monocyte
MoAbs. We conclude that THL, MH, and HD are likely the
neoplasms of fixed histiocytes, free histiocytes
(monocytes/ macrophages) and IRCs, respectively. Two

MoAbs, 1A2 and 2H9 may be useful for immuno-imaging or
-therapy because they react only with very rare cells
(1A2), or with only the nuclear membrane of cells
(2H9) in normal tissues.

INTRODUCTION

Lymphomas are proliferative disorders of the immune
system. Recently, studies of surface markers of lympoid
cells using monoclonal antibodies (MoAbs) have provided
abundant information on the nature of the proliferating
cells and new insights into the pathogenesis of lymphoproliferative disorders. To date, there are more than 25
different MoAbs that react with B or T cells. These MoAbs
have greatly facilitated the diagnosis of B cell- and
T cell lymphomas. Some of these antibodies have been con-
templated, and others have already been used for passive
immunotherapy. Examples include J5, BA-2 and T101 (1-3).
However, it is generally recognized that none of these
antibodies is completely suitable for in vivo therapy
because they also react with the cell membranes of numerous
normal tissues or cells (4-6).
    In addition to the lymphomas of B or T cell origins, a
third group of lymphoma related to IRCs, monocytes or histiocytes exists. The confirmation of this type of lymphoma
is generally very difficult due to the lack of sufficient
diagnostic criteria. Although, quite a few MoAbs reactive
with monocytes (7,8), only rare of these antibodies stain
the neoplastic cells of the histioccytes/monocytes-related
neoplasms.
    In normal lymphoid tissues, there are at least three
types of cells, namely, fixed histiocytes, free histiocytes
(macrophages) and interdigitating reticulum cells (IRCs),
thought to be related with monocytes (9). Therefore, there
may be more than one type of monocytes/histiocytes or
reticulum cells-related neoplasms. In our laboratory, we
have developed MoAbs that can be used to distinguish three
types of such neoplasms. The origins of these monocyte-
related lymphomas are traced by their comparable marker
expression with their presumable normal counterparts. A
fourth type of lymphoma derived from Langerhans cells (10),
called histiocytosis X (HX) is also studied because of the
possible link between IRCs and Langerhans cells (9). In
this paper, we summarize our preliminary results using
these and other MoAbs for lymphoma classification and

diagnosis. The possibility of using these antibodies for therapy is also discussed.

METHODS

PRODUCTION OF MONOCLONAL ANTIBODIES. Male BALB/c mice, 8 to 10 wk old, were immunized i.p. with 1×10^7 SU-DHL-1 cells on days 0, 8 and 15. On day 18, mouse spleens were harvested sterilely and fused with the myeloma line, SP2/0.Ag14 of BALB/c origin. Hybrids were selected in hypo-xanthine-aminopterin-thymidine medium. Ten to 14 days after fusion, supernatants from growth positive wells were screened for the binding to SU-DHL-1 cells by the immuno-peroxidase technique described below. Hybrids of interest were subsequently cloned. Three clones, 2H9, 1A2, and 1E9, were selected for detailed studies. All three MoAbs did not react with neoplastic cells in any of the T or B cell lymphomas (more than 40 cases) tested.

IMMUNOHISTOCHEMICAL STAINING.   The avidin-biotin-per-oxidase complex (ABC) method was used to study the pheno-typic expression of lymphomas. The MoAbs used include the 3 new MoAbs, 2H9, 1A2 and 1E9, and others, including OK M1 (Ortho Diagnsotic, NJ), Mo2 (Coulter Immunology, FL), Leu M1 and Leu M3 (Becton-Dickinson Monoclonal Inc., CA), Tac (anti-interleukin 2 receptor), HeFi-1 (anti-Hodgkin's neoplastic cells) and OK T6 (Ortho).

The staining technique in frozen sections has been described in detail previously (5,6). A total of 6 cases each of THL, MH and HD, and 2 cases of HX were studied for the marker expression. The staining using anti-Leu M1 was carried out in B5-fixed paraffin-embedded sections with or without neuramidase treatment (11).

RESULTS

DISTRIBUTION OF ANTIGENS IN LYMPHOMAS.   The distribu-and subcellular localization of various antigens on a variety of non-B and non-T lymphomas, including true histio-cytic lymphoma (THL), malignant histiocytosis (MH) and Hodgkin's disease (HD) is summarized in Table 1. Note that B and T cell lymphomas were not included in this table because they are consistently negative for these antigens.

Table.1. Antigenic Distribution on
Moncoytes/Histiocytes/IRCs/Langerhans cells-
Related Neoplasms.

	HD	THL	MH	HX
2H9	m+	m+	–	–
1E9	–	nm+	nm+	–
1A2	m+	m+	–	–
HeFi-1	m+	m+	–	–
Leu M1	m+	g+	g+	m+
OK M1	–	–	m+/–	–
Mo2	–	–	m+	–
Leu M3	–	–	m+/–	–
OK T6	–	–	–	m+

1. HD, Hodgkin's disease,
   THL, true histiocytic lymphoma,
   MH, malignant histiocytosis,
   HX, histiocytosis X.
2. m+, membranous staining;
   nm, nuclear membranous staining;
   g+, golgi staining.
3. anti-Leu M1 staining may require an
   enhancement with neuramidase treatment.

DISTRIBUTION OF ANTIGENS IN NORMAL LYMPHOID TISSUES.
In order to correlate the phenotypic expression of the
above neoplastic cells with their possible normal counterparts, the phenotypic expression of normal histiocytes,
Langerhans cells and IRCs were studied with the same MoAbs,
and the results are summarized in Table 2. Noteworthy
was that fixed histiocytes were distinct from free histiocytes by the abscence of monocyte markers, such as OK M1,
Mo2 and Leu M3.
    Free histiocytes show a marker expression very
similar to that of monocytes except for 1E9. The MoAb 1E9
stains the nuclear membrane of free histiocytes, whereas
it stains the cytoplasm of monocytes .

TABLE 2. Antigen Distribution in Normal
       Lymphoid tissues.

	IRCs	Histiocytes fixed	free	Langerhans cells
2H9	nm	nm	nm	-
1E9	nm	nm	nm	-
1A2	-	-	-	-
HeFi-1	-	-	-	-
Leu M1	m+	g+	g+	m+
OK M1	-	-	+	-
Mo2	-	-	+	-
Leu M3	-	-	+	-
OK T6	-	-	-	-

1. nm: nuclear membranous staining.
   g: golgi staining.
   m: cell membranous staining.
2. A positive Leu M1 staining may require a pretreatment of tissue sections with neuramidase.
3. The antigen distribution in monocytes is similar to
   Anti-Leu M1 may stain the membrane of monocytes.
   MoAb 1E9 reacts the cytoplasm in monocytes.

DISCUSSION

The great majority of lymphomas can be classified
according to their phenotypes. True " null" cell lymphomas
are extreme rare. There are four types of lymphoma that
are consistently negative for markers specific for T or B
cells, and they are considered to be related with histiocytes, IRCs and Langerhans cells. These include:
   1). Hodgkin's disease (HD),
   2). True histiocytic lymphoma (THL),
   3). Malignant histiocytosis (MH), and
   4). Histiocytosis X (HX).
In order to examine the nature, and to determine the
possible origins of these lymphomas, we studied the phenotypic expression with a panel of MoAbs (see table 1.2),
including three that were produced in this laboratory.
None of the MoAbs reacts with B or T lymphocytes. Although
OK M1 may stain some pre-B cell or hairy cell leukemias,

these antibodies, when used together, can specifically identify the monocyte-related neoplasms.

MoAbs, 1E9 and 2H9 react with the nuclear membrane of fixed histiocytes and IRCs. The similarity in the phenotypic expression of IRCs and fixed histiocytes shown in paper and others (9) suggests that both types of cells may share a common origin or differentiation pathway. It is reasonable to speculate that tumor cells derived from these two types of cells may also share common markers (see below).

Despite a similar distribution of 1E9 and 2H9 in normal histiocytes and IRCs, the expressions of these two antigens in HD, THL and MH are different. MoAB 1E9 reacts with the nuclear membrane of THL and MH tumor cells, whereas 2H9 stains the cell membrane of HD and THL tumor cells. The reason for this striking difference is not known. However, the exclusive association of these antigens with histiocytes and IRCs indicates a possible relationship between these cells and HD, THL and HD.

By the comparsion of markers among these cells, we may suggest that HD is probably a neoplasm related to IRCs, rather than fixed histiocytes. Note that both IRCs and Hodgkin's-Reed-Sternberg (H-RS) cells are characterized by surface Leu M1 expression, whereas histiocytes are charactterized by a golgi pattern with anti-Leu M1. Other evidences suggestive of relationship between H-RS cells and IRCs are summarized below (for review see also ref. 12).

(1). Both IRCs and H-RS cells express similar markers such as T200, HLA-Dr, OK T9, A1G3 and Leu M1.

(2). Both IRCs and H-RS cells possess similar lectin receptors; i.e., receptors for peanut agglutinin (PNA) and pisum sativum agglutinin (PSA), etc.

(3). Both express small amounts of acid phosphatase and nonspecific esterase with a punctate distribtuion.

(4). IRCs are localized in the thymus-dependent (T cell) zone. Similarly, H-RS cells tend to involve the T cell zone.

H-RS cells and IRCs however, differ in the expression of 1A2, HeFi-1 and 1E9. Although 1E9 is generally absent from H-RS cells in tissue sections, it can be detected in H-RS cells in short-term cultures (data not shown). The two antigens, 1A2 and HeFi-1 (13), appear to be relatively specific for H-RS cells, because they are absent from the great majority of normal histiocytes or IRCs.

THL cells are consistently negative for monocyte markers, such as OK M1, Mo2 and Leu M3. The absence of

these markers was also observed in a specific group of
normal histiocytes, namely fixed histiocytes, in lymphoid
tissues (9). Fixed histiocytes are present in germinal
centers and sinuses of lymph nodes, and red pulps of spleen
(9). They are probably derived from monocytes or their precursors. Both THL cells and fixed histiocytes express 2H9,
1E9, and a golgi typed-Leu M1. They are both negative for
OK M1, Mo2 and Leu M3. Therefore, THL is likely the neoplasm of fixed histiocytes. The neoplastic cells of THL
also express two markers, 1A2 and HeFi-1, known associated
with H-RS cells. The findings are compatible with an idea
that THL and HD are derived from cells closely realted,
i.e., fixed histiocytes vs IRCs.

   In contrast to IRCs and fixed histiocytes, the free
histiocytes in lymphoid tissues are characterized by the
expression of several monocyte markers, such as OK M1, Mo2,
and Leu M3 which are also present on monocytes. Thus, free
histiocytes are likely directly related to monocytes.
MH is characterized by the expression of monocyte/ free
histiocyte markers, especially Mo2 and golgi pattern of
Leu M1. Prelimiary study in our laboratory also shows
that the neoplastic cells of MH can be induced by phorbol
ester to express more monocyte/free histiocyte markers,
such as OK M1 and Leu M5. Therefore, MH is likely the
the neoplasm of free histiocytes.

   This study also included histiocytosis X - the neoplasm of Langerhans cells because a proposed relationship
between Langerhans cells and IRCs. HX sometimes shows a
a histopathology difficult to distinguish from HD and THL.
Both Langerhans cells and IRCs express surface Leu M1.
However, Langerhans cells are different from IRCs by the
expression of OK T6, and the absence of 1E9 and 2H9. A
diagnosis of HX can be easily confirmed by the expression of OK T6 and surface Leu M1 in tumor cells.

   In conclusion, this study identified four types of
monocytes/histiocytes/IRCs/Langerhans cells-related neoplasms. They can be easily distinguished by unique phenotypic expression despite a frequent similarity in morphology. This study does provide direct demonstration for
the origins of each tumor cells. However, the results
summarized in this paper can be used to indicate a possible relationship of these lymphomas with normal IRCs,
histiocytes, or Langerhans cells. Finally, the MoABs,
2H9 and 1A2 may be useful for immunotherapy and immuno-
imaging of THL and HD. MoAb 1A2 reacts with very rare
histiocytes and some granulocytes in normal lymphoid

tissues, whereas 2H9 stains only the nuclear membrane of IRCs, histiocytes and some normal nonlymphoid cells. Among these four types of lymphomas, MH is a high grade lymphoma, and patients usually die within 1 year after the onset of disease. MoAb Mo2 may be worth trying for immunotherapy despite its reactivity with monocytes.

REFERENCES

1. Ritz J, Pesando JM, Notis-McConarty J, Lazarus H, Schlossman SF (1980). A monoclonal antibody to human acute lymphoblastic leukemia antigen. Nature 283:583.
2. LiBien T, Kersey J, Nakazawa S, Minato K, Minowada J (1982). Analysis of human leukemia/lymphoma cell lines with monoclonal antibodies BA-1, BA-2 and BA-3. Leukemia Res 6:299.
3. Foon KA, Schroff RW, Mayer D, Sherwin SA, Oldham RK, Bunn PA, Hsu SM (1983). Monoclonal antibody therapy of chronic lymphocyic leukemia and cutaneous T-cell lymphoma: preliminary observations. In Boss BD, Langman R, Trowbridge I, Dulbecco R (eds): "Monoclonal Antibodies and Cancer," New York: Academic Press, Inc., p 39.
4. Metzgar RS, Borowitz MJ, Jones NH, Dowell BL(1981). Distribution of common acute lymphoblastic leukemia antigen in non-hematopoietic tissues. J Exp Med 154:1249.
5. Hsu SM, Zhang HA, Jaffe ES (1983). Monoclonal antibodies against human lymphoid, monocytic, and granulocytic cells: Reactivities with other tissues. Hybridoma 2:403.
6. Hsu SM, Cossman J, Jaffe ES (1983). Lymphocyte subsets in normal lymphoid tissues. Am J Clin Pathol 80:21.
7. Breard J, Rhinherz EL, Kung PC, Goldstein G, Schlossman SF (1980). A monoclonal antibody reactive with peripheral blood monocyte. J Immunol 124:1493.
8. Todd RF, Nadler LM, Schlossman SF (1981). Antigen on human monocytes by monoclonal antibodies. J Immunol 126:1435.
9. Hsu SM (1985). Phenotypic expression of histiocyte/reticulum/dendritic cells defined by monoclonal antibodies directed against monocyte and C3 complement receptors. Am J Clin Pathol, in press.
10. Murphy GF, Bhan AK, Sato S, Harrist TJ, Mihm MC Jr (1981). Characterization of Langerhans cells by the use

of monoclonal antibodies. Lab Invest 45:465.

11. Hsu SM, Jaffe ES (1982). Leu M1 and peanut agglutinin
    stain the neoplasic cells of Hodgkin's disease.
    Am J Clin Pathol 82:29.
12. Hsu SM, Yang K, Jaffe ES (1985). Phenotypic exprssion
    of Hodgkin's and Reed-Sternberg cells. Am J Pathol,
    in press.
13. Hecht TT, Longo DL, Cossman J, Bolen JB, Hsu SM,
    Israel M, Fisher RI (1985). Production and charac-
    terization of a monoclonal antibody that selectively
    binds Reed-Sternberg cells. submitted.

Monoclonal Antibodies and Cancer Therapy, pages 63–74
© **1985 Alan R. Liss, Inc.**

DU-PAN-2: A PANCREATIC ADENOCARCINOMA ASSOCIATED ANTIGEN[1]

Richard S. Metzgar, David M. Mahvi,
Michael J. Borowitz, Michael S. Lan,
William C. Meyers, H. F. Seigler, and
Olivera J. Finn

Departments of Microbiology and Immunology,
Surgery and Pathology, Duke University Medical
Center, Durham, North Carolina 27710

ABSTRACT DU-PAN-2 is a large mucin-like antigen
defined by a murine monoclonal antibody as well as
a polyclonal monospecific rabbit antiserum. The
antigen is expressed on a variety of normal and
neoplastic cells. The tissue distribution of the
antigen in the fetus is different from that seen
in the adult animal. Cord blood levels of DU-PAN-2
antigen as determined by a competition RIA are 10-
15 fold higher than that seen in adult serum. The
antigen is expressed in high levels in sera of patients with adenocarcinomas especially those of the
pancreas, stomach and gall bladder. Pancreatic
cancer patients with elevated serum DU-PAN-2 levels
and surgically resectable disease usually have
normal serum values 1-2 weeks after curative resection.
Patients receiving radiation and chemotherapy often
have normal DU-PAN-2 antigen levels during the early
phase of their treatment and then show increasing
levels with progressive or recurrent disease.

[1]This work was supported by grant IM-326 from the
American Cancer Society and CA 32672 from the National
Cancer Institute.

DU-PAN-2 is an antigen on human pancreatic adenocarcinoma cells defined by a murine monoclonal antibody
elicited to a human pancreatic ductal adenocarcinoma cell
line HPAF (1). The cell line was derived from the ascites
of a patient with pancreatic adenocarcinoma and also grows
as an adenocarcinoma in nude mice. The nude mouse xenograft is remarkably similar to human pancreatic ductal
adenocarcinoma at the light (1) and electronmicroscopic
level. Electron microscopic examination of the HPAF tumor
in nude mice revealed groups of epithelial cells with
basally-oriented nuclei and abundant cytoplasmic secretory product. The apical portions of the cells contained
abundant microvilli which sometimes appeared to arise from
a cytoplasmic stalk. The cells were arranged around well-
formed lumens which contained a large amount of secreted
material (Figure 1).

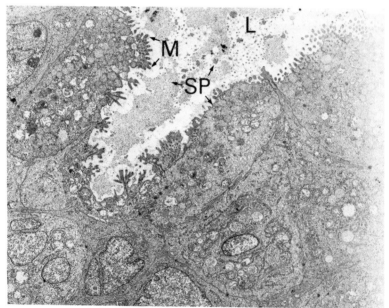

FIGURE 1. Transmission electron microscopy of HPAF
nude mouse tumor. L=lumen, SP=secretory product in lumen
and as granules in cells, M=microvilli.

Immunohistologic studies have indicated that the DU-
PAN-2 antigen is present on 16/16 pancreatic adenocarcinomas,

5/5 gall bladder or bile duct carcinomas, and on 18/21 gastric carcinomas. The antigen was infrequently expressed on adeno-carcinomas of the colon, lung, and breast. In the normal adult pancreas, the antigen was present on ductal cells, but not detected on acinar or islet cells (2). When fetal pancreas was tested with DU-PAN-2 antibodies by immunoperoxidase, a different cellular distribution was noted. A frozen section of pancreatic tissue from a 20 week fetus showed that DU-PAN-2 antigen was present in pancreatic acini as well as in the ductal epithelial cells (Figure 2A). This is in contrast to the pattern seen in the normal adult pancreas (Figure 2B) where staining was confined to the ductal epithelia, and was not detected in the acinar cells. However, we had earlier noted and commented on the immunoperoxidase staining with DU-PAN-2 antibody of acinar cells in areas of chronic pancreatitis and acini adjoining some pancreatic tumors (2). The DU-PAN-2 antigen is found as early as 8 weeks in fetal development. An oblique frozen section from an 8 week fetus, taken at the level of the developing small intestine, shows distinct immunoperoxidase staining of the epithelial layer of this portion of small bowel (Figure 3). There is also intense staining of the cartilage in the developing limb bud. In adults, cartilage does not express DU-PAN-2 antigen. The differential distribution of the DU-PAN-2 antigen between normal adult and fetal cells and its increased expression in tumors indicated that the antigen could be considered as oncofetal and might possibly be related to differentiation of one or more cell types.

Studies on the molecular properties of DU-PAN-2 antigen have indicated that the antigen is a large, mucin-like molecule that is sensitive to treatment with neuraminidase. The antigen has been detected by immunoblotting after electrophoresis in 1% agarose and by immunoprecipitation of metabolically labeled antigen with DU-PAN-2 antibody, followed by electrophoresis in 1% agarose. The antibody precipitates 2 distinct broad bands after labeling with radioactive monosaccharides and sulfate. The heavily glycosylated and polydispersed nature of this antigen and the results of various enzymatic digestions also suggest that the DU-PAN-2 antigen is expressed on a mucin-like molecule (3).

The DU-PAN-2 monoclonal antibody does not bind antigen well after purification and immobilization on an insoluble matrix. This is largely due to its IgM isotype. To overcome this problem, we immunized a rabbit with DU-PAN-2 antigen that was purified by ammonium sulfate fractionation (50-75%), chromatography on Affi-Gel Blue and then cesium bromide density gradient centrifugation (3). The rabbit antiserum immunoprecipitated an antigen with the same electrophoretic mobility in 1% agarose as that noted with the DU-PAN-2 murine monoclonal antibody (Figure 4). The rabbit antiserum does not specifically precipitate any

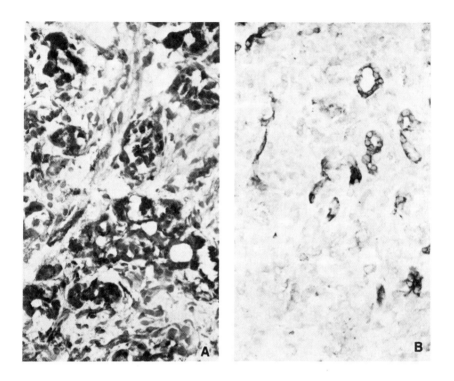

FIGURE 2.   Frozen sections of pancreas from a 20 week old fetus (A) and from an adult (B) stained by immunoperoxidase with monoclonal antibody DU-PAN-2. There is diffuse staining of both ducts and acini in the fetal pancreas, but only ductular epithelium stains in the adult.   Immunoperoxidase, hematoxylin counterstain X250.

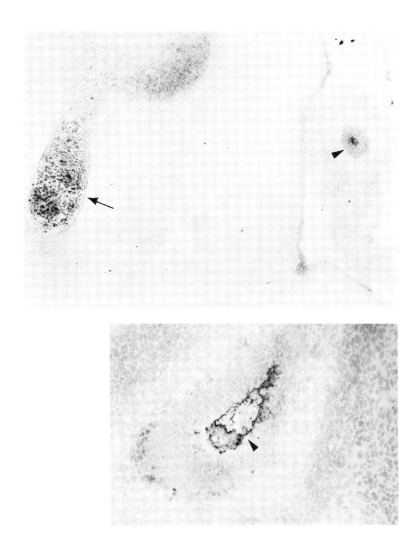

FIGURE 3. Frozen oblique sections from an 8 week fetus
stained by immunoperoxidase with monoclonal antibody DU-
PAN-2. There is strong staining of cartilage in the developing limb bud (arrow) and in the loop of developing small
bowel (arrowhead). The undifferentiated mesenchyme does
not stain. At high magnification (bottom) the bowel staining can be seen to be along the lumen. Immunoperoxidase,
hematoxylin counterstain X68 (top); X170 (bottom).

other radiolabeled antigens from HPAF cells. We are currently using immunodepletion of labeled HPAF cell lysate with DU-PAN-2 monoclonal antibody and sequential immunoprecipitation of the depleted lysate with the rabbit antiserum in order to establish the relationship between the populations of DU-PAN-2 molecules recognized by the two reagents.

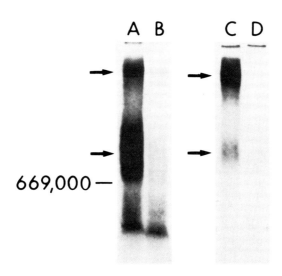

FIGURE 4. Radioimmunoprecipitation of DU-PAN-2 antigen from cell lysates of HPAF cells labeled with $[^3H]$ glucosamine. Radiolabeled antigens were immunoprecipitated with rabbit antiserum to DU-PAN-2 antigen (lane A), normal rabbit serum (lane B), murine monoclonal antibody DU-PAN-2 (lane C), and murine IgM monoclonal antibody to a myeloid cell antigen (lane D).

DU-PAN-2 antigen was noted to be readily released or shed by HPAF cells into the tissue culture medium and could be detected in a soluble form in the ascitic fluid of the patient from which the HPAF cell line was derived. Using crude soluble DU-PAN-2 antigen from these sources, we were able to develop a competition radioimmune assay for the detection of the DU-PAN-2 molecule (4). Preliminary studies using this assay for the detection of antigen in serum and ascites of patients with adenocarcinoma were recently published (4). The competition RIA utilized partially purified antigen attached to polyvinyl chloride 96 well plates by poly-L-lysine. Binding of the DU-PAN-2 to the antigen coated wells was determined by binding of ^{125}I labeled F (ab')$_2$ fragments of a goat antiserum to mouse IgM. Antigen in body fluids was determined by its ability to complex or bind DU-PAN-2 monoclonal antibody before it was added to the antigen coated plates. The amount of antigen in serum or ascites was compared to a standard antigen preparation and expressed as arbitrary units/ml (U/ml) (4). Serum from 126 normal adult donors had a mean DU-PAN-2 level of 81 U/ml, whereas serum from 89 pancreatic carcinoma patients had a mean of 4,888 U/ml. Approximately 68% of the pancreatic cancer patients tested in this initial study had elevated levels of DU-PAN-2 antigen (>300 U/ml), whereas none of the normal donors or patients with stage III melanoma, pediatric lymphoma, and solid tumors, and patients with nasopharyngeal or ovarian tumors had values >300 U/ml. Some patients with acute pancreatitis, gastric, and colorectal carcinomas also had elevated DU-PAN-2 levels (4).

To investigate further the oncofetal or developmental nature of DU-PAN-2 antigen cord blood serum samples were tested for DU-PAN-2 antigen (Table 1). The mean DU-PAN-2 level (1,142 U/ml) was significantly elevated compared to serum values from adult volunteers (81 U/ml). When serum samples from small numbers of infants from 1 month to 1 year of age were tested, a gradual decrease in DU-PAN-2 U/ml were noted during this time period (Table 1). The DU-PAN-2 values after 11 months were just below one of the arbitrary cutoff values (300 U/ml) selected for discrimination between serum from normal and malignant donors (4). The elevated serum DU-PAN-2 values from cord blood, neonates, and infants less than 6 months of age are supportive of the oncofetal nature of the DU-PAN-2 antigen which was suggested by the immunohistology.

Serial studies of DU-PAN-2 serum antigen levels in patients with pancreatic cancer are currently being conducted in order to see if the DU-PAN-2 competition RIA could be used as a clinical management aid in this disease similar to that reported for the CEA antigen (5). Some of these studies were retrospective, thus there were often difficulties in having serum samples available for serological testing at the various clinical stages of the

patient's disease. In addition, it was often difficult to
establish the exact clinical status and tumor burden of a
patient on the date a serum sample was available for study.
More recently, some patients' samples have been collected
in a prospective manner. Several interesting findings
have been obtained from these preliminary studies.

TABLE 1
DU-PAN-2 ANTIGENS IN CORD BLOOD AND NEWBORN
SERUM COMPARED TO SERUM VALUES FROM ADULT
VOLUNTEERS

Serum source	Number of samples tested	Mean DU-PAN-2 U/ml[1]	Standard deviation U/ml
Adult	126	81	22
Cord blood	25	1,142	435
Infants (age)			
1 month	4	1,108	82
2 months	10	806	556
3 months	5	765	1045
6 months	7	518	159
8 months	4	260	79
11 months	6	229	15

[1]U/ml = arbitrary units/ml as defined in reference (4).

When patients with surgically resectable pancreatic
adenocarcinomas were studied, those patients with elevated
DU-PAN-2 serum levels at the time of surgery usually had
serum values within the normal range within 6 weeks post
resection (Table 2). Patients (1-4) that had one or more
samples available for testing within 4 postoperative weeks
showed a return to normal within that period. The earliest
samples available for testing from patients #5 and #6 were
6 and 7 weeks respectively and at that time they were well
within the normal range. DU-PAN-2 levels in serial serum
samples from patient 4 of Table 2 are shown in Figure 5.

TABLE 2

CHANGES IN DU-PAN-2 ANTIGEN LEVELS IN SERA OF
PANCREATIC ADENOCARCINOMA PATIENTS WITH SURGICALLY
RESECTABLE DISEASE

Patient	DU-PAN-2 level[1] Before surgery	After surgery	Weeks to return to normal range[2]
1	400	43	2
2	1424	128	4
3	356	190	1
4	1312	196	1
5	600	150	6
6	750	120	7

[1]Arbitrary units/ml as described in reference (4).
[2]Normal range defined as less than 300 units/ml.

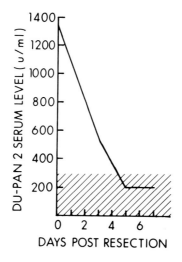

FIGURE 5.   DU-PAN-2 levels in pre and post-operative
serum samples from a patient with surgically resectable
pancreatic adenocarcinoma.   Day 0 represents pre-operative
sample. Diagonal lines depict normal serum range (0-300 U/ml).

Several patients have been followed prospectively past resection. At times the DU-PAN-2 levels increased before the patient was judged to have progressive disease, while at other times, it was concomitant with documented progressive disease. In many instances, the interval between sample collection and clinical visits was too long to ascertain whether the test was capable of early prediction or detection of progressive disease.

Serial serum samples from patients with non-resectable exocrine pancreatic cancer were also studied retrospectively. These patients all received irradiation and/or chemotherapy. In many instances, a pre-treatment sample was not available for study or comparison. However, it was clear that irradiation and chemotherapy were able to either decrease the DU-PAN-2 antigen levels to a normal range within a short time after therapy was initiated, or that this treatment maintained DU-PAN-2 levels in the normal range. Approximately 80% of these nonoperable patients whose values were in the normal range during early treatment had elevated levels when their disease progressed. The DU-PAN-2 antigen levels in serial serum samples from a representative patient with pancreatic adenocarcinoma treated with irradiation and 5 fluorouracil is given in Figure 6. Levels of DU-PAN-2 in the earliest samples available for testing from this patient were in the normal range, but increased to abnormal levels concomitant with progressive disease. The serial serum studies of DU-PAN-2 antigen emphasize a shortcoming in the interpretation of single sample studies in estimating the percentage of patients in a cancer or disease category which have elevated antigen levels. This percentage is markedly affected by the stage of the disease and treatment studies of the patient at the time the sample is collected.

Although these clinical management studies are preliminary, DU-PAN-2 serum antigen determinations may help to predict and monitor progressive disease in patients with pancreatic adenocarcinoma. The findings also indicate that effective surgical therapy or irradiation-chemotherapy can reduce levels of this antigen to the normal range. DU-PAN-2 levels inevitably rise with progressive disease. Even if DU-PAN-2 or other tumor markers are early indicators of recurrent or progressive disease, at the present time there is very little the oncologist can offer the patient as a therapeutic modality which can alter the course of their disease. Thus, we are strongly motivated to focus

our research on a better understanding of the basic molecular
biology of pancreatic exocrine cell differentiation and
transformation, as well as on therapeutic approaches which
can utilize antibodies or immune cells in this regard.

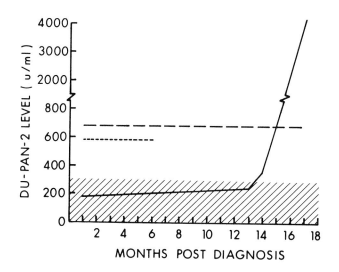

FIGURE 6. DU-PAN-2 levels in serial serum samples
from a patient with non-resectable disease irradiated
with a total of 4,400 rads (short horizontal dashed lines)
and intermittent 5 fluorouracil (long horizontal dashed
lines). Normal adult serum range of 0 to 300 U/ml is
indicated by diagonal lines.

ACKNOWLEDGEMENTS

The authors wish to gratefully acknowledge 1)
Dr. Robert C. Bast of the Department of Medicine, Duke
University Medical Center for providing some of the
serum samples from patients with pancreatic cancer treated
at the Dana Farber Cancer Institute 2) Professor H. F.
Kern of the Department of Anatomy and Cell Biology at
Phillips University in Marburg, Federal Republic of
Germany for the electron photomicrograph of the HPAF
nude mouse tumor, 3) Mr. Francis Tuck and Mr. David
Phillips for performing the competition RIA and immuno-
peroxidase studies and 4) Mrs. Teresa Hylton and Mrs.
Kathy Greenwell for their secretarial assistance and
patience in preparing this report.

REFERENCES

1.   Metzgar RS, Gaillard MT, Levine SJ, Tuck FL,
     Bossen EH, Borowitz MJ (1982). Antigens of human
     pancreatic adenocarcinoma cells defined by murine
     monoclonal antibodies. Cancer Res. 42:601.
2.   Borowitz MJ, Tuck FL, Sindelar WF, Fernsten PD,
     Metzgar RS (1984). Monoclonal antibodies against
     human pancreatic adenocarcinoma: Distribution of
     DU-PAN-2 antigen on glandular epithelia and adeno-
     carcinomas.JNCI 72:999.
3.   Lan MS, Finn OJ, Fernsten PD, Metzgar RS (1985).
     Isolation and properties of a human pancreatic
     adenocarcinoma-associated antigen, DU-PAN-2.
     Cancer Res. 35:305.
4.   Metzgar RS, Rodriguez N, Finn OJ, Lan MS, Daasch
     VN, Fernsten PD, Meyers WC, Sindelar WF, Sandler
     RS, Seigler HF (1984). Detection of a pancreatic
     cancer-associated antigen (DU-PAN-2 antigen) in
     serum and ascites of patients with adenocarcinoma.
     Proc. Natl. Acad. Sci. 81:5242.
5.   Zamcheck N, Kupchik HZ (1980). Summary of clinical
     use and limitations of the carcinoembryonic antigen
     assay and some methodological considerations. In
     Rose NR, Friedman H (eds): "Manual of Clinical
     Immunology", Washington, D. C.: American Society
     of Microbiology, p. 919.

II. HUMAN-HUMAN HYBRIDOMAS

Monoclonal Antibodies and Cancer Therapy, pages 77-96
© **1985 Alan R. Liss, Inc.**

THE EBV-HYBRIDOMA TECHNIQUE AND ITS
APPLICATION TO HUMAN LUNG CANCER[1]

S.P.C. Cole[2], D. Kozbor[3] and J.C. Roder[4]

Department of Microbiology & Immunology
Queen's University, Kingston, Ontario, Canada K7L 3N6

ABSTRACT   A detailed   comparison of hybridization frequencies, yield of antigen-specific hybridomas, immunoglobulin   secretion   levels, cloning   efficiencies, division times, and stability(1) leads to the conclusion
that the EBV-hybridoma system described here is near
optimal and approaches the murine system in efficiency
with mean fusion frequencies of 1.54 x 10^{-5} in four
independent studies and secretion levels of > 5 µg/ml
specific antibody in vitro and > 1000 µg/ml in vivo.
Lymphocytes from lymph nodes, tonsils, bone marrow and
peripheral blood of hyperimmune, healthy donors or
cancer patients, or in vitro immunized cultures, have
been fused effectively and human monoclonal antibodies
against M. leprae, tetanus toxoid and lung tumor cells
have been generated in our lab.   A plasmacytoma-like
fusion partner has been constructed and we have successfully adapted our human hybridomas for growth in

[1]This work was supported by a grant to Dr. Roder from
the Terry Fox Program of the National Cancer Institute of
Canada and from the National Sciences and Engineering Research Council.   Dr. Kozbor is a fellow of the National
Cancer Institute of Canada.
[2]Present address: The Ontario Cancer Treatment &
Research Foundation, Kingston Regional Centre, King Street
West, Kingston, Ontario, Canada K7L 2V7
[3]Present address: The Wistar Institute of Anatomy &
Biology, Thirty-Seventh Street at Spruce, Philadelphia, Pen-
nsylvania 90026
[4]Present address: Mount Sinai Research Institute,
Mount Sinai Hospital, 600 University Avenue, Toronto,
Ontario, Canada M5G 1X5

serum-free medium in vitro or as ascites tumors in nude mice. We are currently developing a non-Ig-secreting fusion partner. The EBV-hybridoma technique offers a high degree of flexibility since the use of EBV (i) immortalizes the donor B cells for future use and repeated fusions, (ii) aids the expansion of rare antigen-specific B cells in the peripheral blood prior to fusion, and (iii) increases hybridization frequencies over 10-100-fold. One limitation of the system is that the majority of hybridomas obtained in this way secrete antigen-specific IgM, rather than IgG. Recent developments may allow induction of an IgM to IgG switch in these hybrids with UV light or using gene transfer. We hope that human monoclonal antibodies produced by the EBV-hybridoma technique will become useful tools for the diagnosis and treatment of human diseases including cancer.

INTRODUCTION

Human monoclonal antibodies (MABs) will become essential for the prophylaxis and treatment of human disease. There are three conceptual approaches to producing human MABs including (i) transformation of antigen specific B lymphocytes by Epstein-Barr virus (EBV), as first carried out by Steinitz et al.(2), (ii) hybridization of 6-TG^r human plasmacytomas or lymphoblastoid fusion partners to immune human lymphocytes, as first demonstrated in the mouse by Kohler and Milstein(3) and adapted to the human by Olsson and Kaplan(4) and Croce et al.(5), and (iii) a combination of the EBV and hybridoma techniques which combines the strengths of each system alone and avoids the weaknesses, as first shown by Kozbor et al(6). We have reviewed the human hybridoma system in other papers(1) and in this report we will summarize our own experience with the EBV and EBV-hybridoma systems for producing human MABs against lung carcinoma cells.

RESULTS AND DISCUSSION

I. EBV Immortalization

Epstein-Barr virus (EBV) is a Herpes virus originally isolated in 1964 from a cultured cell line derived from an

African Burkitt's lymphoma biopsy(7) and has been shown to be the etiological agent of infectious mononucleosis(8). Rosen et al.(9) demonstrated that direct in vitro infection of purified human blood lymphocytes with EBV stimulated polyclonal secretion of immunoglobulin.

Within the lymphoid system, EBV is specific for small resting B cells(10) bearing EBV receptors which are closely associated with, but distinct from, C3 receptors(11,12). The infection in vitro of B lymphocytes leads to permanent stimulation of cell growth, a phenomenon termed 'transformation', or 'immortalization'. This 'immortalization' preserves the characteristics of the original B cells, including EBV receptors, complement receptors, surface immunoglobulin and secretory immunoglobulin. Those cells which grow out in vitro and carry EBV-DNA are termed lymphoblastoid cell lines (LCLs).

All such LCLs express the EBV specific nuclear antigen (EBNA) and the amount of EBNA is directly proportional to the average number of EBV-genomes per cell(13). Normally, some EBV infected B cells should also express both early (EA) and late antigens (VCA) of the viral cycle and release virus particles. However, the EBV recommended in hybridoma work is derived from the B95-8 marmoset cell line and is defective(14) in that it induces transformation in human B lymphocytes but does not induce early viral protein synthesis. Consequently viral replication is blocked, presumably as a result of a 12 Kb deletion in an EcoR1 fragment in the 3' end of the molecule(15).

Thus, in vitro transformation with EBV may be employed to obtain LCLs secreting antibodies to selected antigens. In fact, this method has been exploited successfully in numerous laboratories since the first report of Steinitz et al.(2) who established anti-hapten antibody-producing human cell lines after preselection for hapten binding followed by EBV transformation. LCLs secreting specific human MABs against streptococcal carbohydrate A(16), Rhesus antigen D, (17-19) and tetanus toxoid(20) - to mention but a few - have been established this way. As summarized previously(1), EBV does not appear to bias the immune repertoire since (i) specific antibodies against a wide range of antigens have been obtained, representing chemically defined haptens, proteins, carbohydrates and nucleic acids, and (ii) antibodies of both IgM, IgG, and kappa and lambda types are represented. However, little information is available on the affinity of antibodies produced by EBV lines.

An alternative strategy involves the EBV transformation

of the total B cell population (i.e. no preselection) followed by cloning and testing for specific antibody-producing cultures. This method has been used to isolate LCLs producing MABs against diptheria toxoid(21), acetylcholine receptor(22), tetanus toxoid(20,23,24), phosphorylcholine(25), melanoma antigens(26,27), bacterial(28) and viral(29,30) antigens, as well as many other antigens.

A major disadvantage of the EBV-imortalization technique is that bulk cultures of EBV-transformed lines frequently lose their ability to produce specific antibody after long-term culture(20,29). The reason for this instability is not clear but may be due, at least in part, to the overgrowth of non-producing cells within the culture. Thus, in some cases, early cloning by limiting dilution has been reported to result in a stable antibody-producing cell line(18,20,28,29). Several investigators have reported varying successes in cloning EBV-transformed cell lines. This variation is largely unexplained but may be influenced by the immune status of the donor and the tissue from which the lymphocytes were derived, as well as the source of feeder layer cells used in cloning(18,31,32). However, more complex intracellular events likely also play a role in the stabilization of specific antibody production since cloning does not always stabilize the lymphoblastoid cell lines(20,32). We have found that one anti-tetanus toxoid clone produced specific monoclonal antibody for 8 months of culture and then suddenly shut off light chain synthesis, thereby precluding recovery of antigen binding activity in culture supernatants(20). In addition to the instability of specific antibody production, a second limitation of the EBV immortalization technique is that low quantities of antibody (< 1 µg/ml) are generally produced. In combination with EBV immortalization, cell fusion (hybridoma) techniques may be employed to rescue high levels of stable MAB production from EBV lines.

II. Selection of Antigen-Specific Cells

In the EBV technique, as in the hybridoma procedure, it is important to use lymphocytes of individuals who have previously been immunized with the antigens and have increased numbers of specific antibody-producing cells in their circulation. The EBV procedure involves two steps: (1) the enrichment of cells with receptors for the given antigens, and (2) immortalization of these cells by EBV

infection.   Preselection of antigen-specific cells may
facilitate the establishment of specific cell lines since
even after immunization in vivo, only a small fraction
(10^{-4}) of the B lymphocytes produce the desired anti-
body(33).   Several methods of pre-selection have been tried,
including: (i) antigen-specific lymphocytes were enriched
by rosetting with antigen-coupled erythrocytes, followed by
separation on a density gradient(1,16,17,34-36), (ii) biotinylated antigen was bound to the surface of the antigen-
specific cells and those cells binding fluorescein coupled
avidin   were   subsequently   separated   electronically   on   a
fluorescence-activated cell sorter (FACS)(20), (iii) antigen
was bound to solid surfaces in a panning technique(32), and
(iv) cells which did not bind antigen were removed(20).
This   negative preselection technique was first performed in
the mouse by Walker et al.(37), and is based on the observation that B cells, upon binding to antigen, usually shed
their surface Ig receptors and become nude or stripped.   In
the human, the B cell-enriched fractions were obtained by
the removal of monocytes and cells rosetting with SRBC.
Those B cells not binding antigen, and therefore maintaining
their surface Ig, are removed by rosetting with sheep erythrocytes coated with the $F(ab')_2$ fragment of anti-human Ig.
The non-rosetting B cells remaining are then EBV infected
and the resulting antigen-specific cell line is cloned
within 3 weeks by limiting dilution on a feeder layer or
fused directly with a TG^r, Oua^r fusion partner such as KR-4.

III.   In Vitro Immunization

    One limitation of EBV and human hybridoma technology is
the requirement, thus far, to use lymphocytes from hyper-
immunized donors.   Sources of parental cells have included
peripheral blood lymphocytes (PBL) from measles virus-
infected, subacute sclerotizing panencephalitis patients(5),
spleen cells from dinitrochlorobenzene-sensitized Hodgkin's
patients(4), tumor-infiltrating lymphocytes(38) and tonsils
from tetanus-vaccinated donors(39).   It is apparent that PBL
from humans offer the only readily available source of
normal lymphocytes for fusion.   However, only 1 in 10 PBL
are B cells.   As reported by Stevens et al.(33), the
frequency of B cells in the circulation capable of respond-
ing to pokeweed mitogen (PWM) by producing anti-tetanus
toxoid (TT) antibody of the IgG class was only 1×10^{-4}, 2-4
weeks after booster injection.   This low number, together

with typical fusion frequencies of 10-6 and a B cell frequency of 10^{-1}, makes the chance of obtaining a specific hybridoma in the order of 10^{-11}, or 10^{-9} if we allow for an estimated 100-fold greater fusion frequency with antigen-stimulated B cells than resting B cells.   It is clear that further improvements are necessary to increase the yields and proportions of immune B cells.

We have compared the usefulness of specific antigens (TT) and two polyclonal mitogens (PWM, EBV) in stimulating cultures of PBL prior to fusion.(40) Stimulation with EBV yielded cells with much higher frequencies of hybrid for-mation (36×10^{-7}) compared to unstimulated PBL (10^{-7}) or cells cultured with PWM (6×10^{-7}) or TT antigen (3×10^{-7}). The proportion of hybridomas (approximately 1%) producing anti-TT antibody was similar in EBV and TT-stimulated cult-ures, although one would expect that antigen driven cultures would yield higher affinity antibodies. Preselection of EBV subcultures for high anti-TT production prior to fusion resulted in a five-fold increase in TT-specific hybridomas (p < 0.001).   Most (20/21) specific hybrids produced IgM anti-TT, whereas one (1/21) produced IgG anti-TT, possibly due to the immature stage of differentiation in EBV-stimulated parental cells.   Immunized cultures can be tran-sformed with EBV and used for hybridoma construction (un-published observations).   The ability to choose an antigen, immunize and expand the rare antigen-specific B cells from PBL in vitro prior to EBV immortalization and fusion, should yield an increasing spectrum of human monoclonal antibodies for diagnostic, therapeutic or basic studies.

IV.   Selection of a Fusion Partner

Many human fusion partners are available for study(1). Lines should be chosen which yield high fusion frequencies, high levels of specific immunoglobulin production, high proportions of antigen specific hybridomas, and long term stability.   If high yields of monoclonal antibody are need-ed, then a line is preferred which has a proven ability to form hybridomas that grow as ascites tumors in nude mice. The fusion partner must be HAT sensitive and it is suggested that cells be rendered resistant to 6-thioguanine (6-TG^r) rather than 8-azaguanine (8-AG^r). The fusion partner should also have a dominant selectable marker such as ouabain or neomycin resistance to allow fusion with EBV transformed donor lymphocytes, a procedure which improves hybridization

frequencies 10-100 fold.   KR-4 is one line which meets   all
of these requirements.   It is a cell line originally derived
from a 6-TG^r variant of GM1500, by a procedure which may be
of general use for deriving Oua^r mutants of other fusion
partners as well(6).   The concentration of ouabain required
to kill 50%$_7$ of the Oua^r KR-4 cells was 5 x 10^{-3} M, compared
to 5 x 10^{-7} M for non-mutagenized parental cells, normal
human lymphocytes, and EBV-transformed lymphoblastoid cell
lines.   This   represents a remarkable level of drug resistance (10,000 fold) and ouabain can now be used at high
concentrations as a very effective selective agent for
hybridomas.   The Oua^r marker was stable in these lines in
the absence of ouabain.

V. Human Hybridomas Constructed with EBV Lines

        The first human hybridomas were constructed in 1980 by
Olsson and Kaplan(4) and by Croce et al(5).   However, the
efficiency of these systems was low and they were not adapted for general use.   As described in other reviews(1),
most of the human fusion partners developed since also have
serious deficiencies. EBV transformed cell lines and clones
have also provided a source of human monoclonal antibodies
since the pioneering work of Steinitz et al. in 1977(2),
but poor stability and low rates of Ig secretion have posed
limitations to the approach.   In our laboratory, we have
combined both the EBV immortalization method and conventional hybridoma technology to develop a system which we
feel combines the strengths and overcomes the weaknesses
inherent in each system alone(6).   We simply hybridize our
plasmacytoma, or LCL fusion partner, with donor lymphocytes
that have been transformed by EBV and established as a cell
line.   In this system, both parental cells are immortal and
therefore it was necessary to have a fusion partner with
appropriate drug markers to counterselect against the parental cells.   Thus, thioguanine-resistant GM-1500 lymphoblastoid cells were rendered ouabain-resistant, as discussed
in section IV, and the resulting line was designated KR-4.
In our first study(6), KR-4 was fused with an EBV-
transformed, anti-tetanus toxoid producing clone, B6, and
hybrids selected in HAT:ouabain containing medium.   The
hybridomas produced 8-fold more anti-tetanus toxoid antibody
at a much higher rate, and cloned more efficiently than the
parental B6 line. Furthermore, specific antibody production
has remained stable for more than two years.   Our total

experience with the system is summarized in Table 1.

In a second study(41) we have established EBV-immortalized cells lines from lymphocytes derived from peripheral blood, tumor-draining lymph nodes, bone marrow aspirates, tumors and pericardial effusions from lung cancer patients. Clones from a number of these lines were screened for tumor-specific antibody production but none were positive, suggesting that B lymphocytes specific for tumor antigens are rare in lung cancer patients. These results are in agreement with those of other investigators (42). The EBV lines were then fused with KR-4 in an attempt to rescue low frequency B cell precursors specific for tumor cells. More than 8% of hybridomas screened showed significant levels of activity although most were not tumor cell specific since they also reacted with EBV-infected cells from the lymphocyte donor. Two hybridomas showed apparent specific binding early after fusion but this activity was lost upon continued growth although, in general, hybrids continued to secrete high levels (up to 50 µg/ml) of IgM, in some cases, beyond 18 months in culture. Recently, we have produced several hybridomas, all derived from the same patient, which react with a number of tumor cell lines but not with normal PBLs. These hybridomas have been cloned and are now being fully characterized. Thus the EBV-hybridoma system should be useful for rescuing low frequency tumor-reactive B cell precursors.

We have also constructed human hybridomas which produce antibodies against a number of antigen preparations of Mycobacterium leprae(43). EBV-transformed cell lines from lepromatous leprosy patients were fused with KR-4 and hybrids screened for antibodies against three antigen preparations of armadillo-derived M. leprae, including (i) a soluble sonicate antigen, (ii) a detergent extract of insoluble sonicated M. leprae, and (iii) a phenolic glycolipid antigen. A number of reactive MABs were obtained which were further screened for specificity on a panel of antigens from four other mycobacteria. A total of nine cloned stable hybrids have been obtained with specificity for M. leprae. In comparison, 10,000 EBV-transformed lymphocyte clones from lepromatous leprosy patients were screened for anti-M. leprae antibody production and all the 42 clones that were initially positive lost their ability to produce antibodies within 6 weeks in culture. These results suggest that the EBV-hybridoma system is superior to the EBV system for production of human MABs from leprosy patients.

TABLE 1

A COMPARISON OF THE EBV AND EBV-HYBRIDOMA SYSTEMS FOR PRODUCING HUMAN

MONOCLONAL ANTIBODIES

Lympho-cyte Source	Selec-tion	Donor	EBV trans	Fusion Partner	# of hy-brids or clones screened	Anti-gen	Fusion Freq. (x 10-7)	% antigen specific hybrids or clones	Specific Ig-secre-tion (µg/ml)	Ig Class	Clon-ing Eff. (%)	Stab-bil-ity (mo)	Ref.
PBL	+	vacc.	+	none	96	TT	NA[n]	3.1	0.7	IgM	30	6	20
PBL	+	vacc.	+	P3x63Ag8	200	TT	100	70.0[o]	1.8	IgM	ND[p]	6	44
PBL	+	vacc.	+	KR-4	395	TT	112	94.0	4.2	IgM	64	>24	6
PBL	-	vacc.	+	KR-4	936	TT	36	0.7	2.6	M/G	ND	>6	40
PBL	-	vacc.	-	KR-4	20	TT	2	0.0	0.0	-	ND	ND	6,40
tonsil	-	vacc.	-	KR-4	32	TT	8	0.0	0.0	-	ND	ND	40
PBL	-	lepr.	+	KR-4	4,400	lep.	126	8.2	10.0	IgM	90	>12	43
PBL	-	lepr.	-	KR-4	5	lep.	2	0.0	0.0	-	ND	ND	43
PBL	-	lepr.	+	none	10,000	lep.	NA	0.42	0.0	ND	ND	ND	43
PBL,LN,BM,TIL,PE	-	Ca	+	KR-4	4,500	tum.	166	8.0	44	IgM	20	2	41
PBL,LN,BM,TIL,PE	-	Ca	+	none	140	tum.	NA	0.7	ND	ND	1	>12	41
PBL	-	neuro	+	none	300	MAG	NA	0.6	ND	ND	ND	ND	41

(Continued)

Table 1 (Continued)

aSource of lymphocytes: PBL, fresh peripheral blood lymphocytes; Pokeweed mitogen stimulated tonsilar lymphocytes; LN, draining lymph node cells; BM, bone marrow cells, TIL, tumor infiltrating lymphocytes; PE, pericardial effusion cells.

bEBV lines were selected for anti-tetanus toxoid reactivity and one clone, B6, from such a line was used on the donor cell in hybridization experiments.

cNormal donors were vaccinated with Tetanus Toxoid 2-3 weeks prior to fusions. Lepromatous leprosy patients were selected with high levels of circulating antibody against M. leprae. Lung cancer patients with small cell, large cell, adeno, squamous and bronchoalveolar carcinoma were also used as lymphocyte donors. Peripheral neuropathy patients with IgM paraproteinemia and high titers of anti-myelin-associated glycoprotein antibody were also used as PBL donors.

dLymphocytes were transformed with Epstein-Barr virus (B95-8).

eDonor lymphocytes were fused with a Thg^r murine plasmacytoma P3 x 63Ag8.653 or a Thg^r, Oua^r human lymphoblastoid cell line, KR-4, for hybridoma studies or were not fused for studies of EBV clones.

[f]Number of hybrids or clones screened for reactivity with antigen in an enzyme-linked immunosorbent assay (ELISA). Hybridization was confirmed by analysis of chromosomes and co-dominant expression of phenotypic markers in selected hybridomas. Clonality was confirmed by isoelectric focussing of secreted immunoglobulins in selected cases.

[g]TT, purified tetanus toxoid; lep., glycolipid or protein extracts from Mycobacterium leprae; tum., glutaraldehyde-fixed human lung tumor cells; MAG, purified human myelin-associated glycoprotein (M.W. 110,000).

[h]Fusion frequency (f.f.) was calculated from the following formula using 96-well plates with less than the Poisson number (66%) of wells positive for growth:

$$f.f. = \frac{\ln\frac{\Delta}{96}}{\chi}$$

where Δ is the number of wells negative for growth

and χ is the number of cells plated per well 2 since equal numbers of lymphocytes and fusion partner cells were hybridized.

[i]The proportion of all wells positive for growth which secreted antibody reacting with the antigen in question.

(Continued)

Table 1 (Continued)

[j]The quantity of antigen reactive antibody secreted from 10^5 hybridoma cells grown in a logarithmic fashion over a 7-day growth period. Values are mean from several high producing hybridomas selected for further study.

[k]Most hybridomas secreted antigen specific antibody of the IgM class, although occasionally (1/20) IgG hybridomas were also found.

[l]Cloning was performed by limiting dilution on feeder layers and cloning efficiency was calculated using the formula in h above.

[m]The length of time in continuous culture that hybridomas or EBV clones continued to produce specific antibody before becoming unstable and ceasing specific Ig secretion. > signifies that an endpoint was not reached and cultures secreted antibody beyond the time indicated.

[n]NA, not applicable.

[o]Only 1/5 of these were stable for the 6-month period of study.

[p]ND, not done.

VI.   Interspecies Hybrids

Mouse x human hybrids have been described that secrete human antibody against tetanus toxoid(44,45), human tumor-associated antigens(46-48), multiple endocrine organs (49), and other antigens.   A limitation of interspecies hybrids lies in their preferential segregation of human chromosomes and thus stable hybrids secreting specific human antibodies are generally difficult to obtain.   However, stable produc-tion of human anti-tetanus antibody from an interspecies hybrid for more than 8 months after fusion has been reported at least in one case(50).   Loss of human chromosomes from mouse x hybrids does not appear random;   human chromosomes 14 (heavy chain) and 22 (light chain-λ) are preferentially retained whereas chromosome 2 (light chain-ϰ) is pre-ferentially lost(51,52).   The stability of the chromosomal constitution is much greater in hybrids derived from par-ental cells of the same species;   thus, to produce stable human x human hybridomas, establishment of fusion partners of human origin became necessary.

VII.   Large Scale Production of Human MABs

Ascites Production.   One of the problems remaining in human MAB technology is that of bulk production.   Mouse hybridomas may be grown as ascites tumors in mice, increas-ing the yield of antibody up to 1000-fold.   With human hybridomas, the use of immunodeficient mice is required to avoid xenograft rejection.   Instead, we and others(53) have found it necessary to passage the hybridoma in nude mice as a subcutaneous solid tumor, followed by in vitro culture, before intraperitoneal inoculation of the cells to grow as ascites (Fig.   1) (54).   In our studies, the appearance of ascites was not significantly affected by pristane-pretreatment of mice alone nor by depletion of natural killer cells with anti-asialo GM$_1$.   On the other hand, irradiation of the mice together with pristane enhanced tumor takes and ascites growth of human hybridomas.   With some hybridomas, ascites growth was observed in 50% of the mice injected and re-passage of cells recovered from the ascites resulted in a two-fold increase in human Ig produc-tion by EBV hybridomas(55).   Aproximately half of the total human Ig detected in the ascites fluid was specific for tetanus toxoid.   The other half probably represents produc-

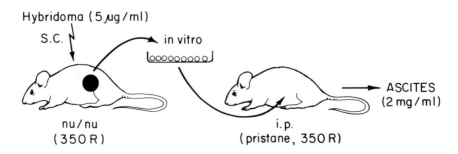

FIGURE 1.   Ascites growth of human hybridomas.
Human hybridoma cells (10⁷) are injected s.c.   into 350R-
irradiated Balb/c nu/nu mice and after 3-4 wks the tumor is
removed and established in tissue culture.   When sufficient
cells have grown up, they are harvested and injected i.p.
into irradiated (350R) Balb/c nude mice, pre-injected with
0.5 ml pristane 2 wks prior.   Approximately half the mice
will develop ascites fluid which can be recovered as a
highly concentrated source of human monoclonal antibodies.

tion of human parental chains by the KR-4 and KR-12 fusion
partners.   It should be noted that we have been unable to
adapt some hybridomas to ascites growth.   The reason for
this variability is presently unknown but may have to do
with chromosome segregation patterns of each particular
clone.   It may be necessary to lose suppressor chromosomes
for full expression of the malignant phenotype in these
hybrids (Kozbor, unpublished results).

   Serum-Free Culture.   As an alternative to ascites
production, hybridomas may be grown in large scale tissue
culture systems.   However to be practical and economically
feasible, a serum-free culture system is essential.   Furthermore, elimination of serum would facilitate rapid purification of human immunoglobulins.   Several systems have
been described for growing human lymphocytes under serum-
free conditions(56,57).   We have adapted several human
hybridomas to grow in serum-free RPMI 1640 medium in a
step-wise fashion(58).   The hybrids did not grow well when
the percentage of fetal bovine serum was decreased to less
than 5%, and failed to thrive at 1% FCS.   However, the cells
readily adapted to growth in RPMI 1640 medium supplemented

with 0.5% bovine serum albumin, transferrin (10 μg/ml) and 2-mercaptoethanol (5 x 10^{-5} M). Attempts to grow human hybrids in completely protein-free culture medium are in progress. Thus it appears entirely feasible to grow human hybridomas in serum-free culture and it is possible that this will become the method of choice for large scale production of human MABs.

IX.   Limitations and Future Developments

An issue that has frequently been raised relates to the presence of either EBV or retroviruses in monoclonal antibody preparation intended for human use. Xenotropic retroviruses which are known to be infectious for human cells (59) are present in mouse plasmacytomas and are found in hybrids descending from the mouse myeloma cells(60,61). We have not observed retrovirus particles either in human fusion partners KR-4 and KR-12 or hybridomas, but discovery of a human C-type virus, HTLV, in certain T-cell leukemias/lymphomas(62,63) warrants a closer look at human fusion partners. Indeed, recent results suggest that HTLV may be associated with a broader range of host cells than previously recognized. For example, human T cell leukemia virus type II (HTLV-II) was found to be capable of infecting both B and T cells(64). HTLV-I has been isolated from a HTLV-transformed B-lymphocyte clone from a patient with HTLV-associated adult T-cell leukemia(65). A strain of lymphadenopathy-associated retrovirus (LAV) passaged in vitro was used to infect a lymphoblastoid cell line, and the virus produced from this line (B-LAV) was also able to grow in some other LCLs as well as a Burkitt lymphoma line. There is no information on presence of C- and A-type virus particles in human plasmacytomas or LCLs used as fusion partners, or human x human hybridomas. Thus far, the only human plasmacytoma studied, RPMI-8226, was found to be positive for retrovirus designated RPMI-8226V, which is identical to squirrel monkey virus and should be classified in the group of type D oncornaviruses(66). The most permissive cells for its propagation were bat (CCL88) and mink (CCL64) (67).

The EBV used for human hybridoma work is derived from the B95-8 marmoset cell line(14). The virus transforms human B lymphocytes in vitro and the EBV nuclear antigen, EBNA, is expressed but the viral cycle is not completed. Consequently, infectious virus is not released, although the possibility of contaminating hybridoma supernatants with transforming viral DNA does exist at least in theory. However, virus and viral DNA can easily be inactivated or removed form antibody preparations(68) which can be monitored by sensitive B-cell transformation tests or DNA hybridization techniques. Of considerable interest is the recent report (69) that a number of hybrids generated from an EBV-transformed cell line and a heteromyeloma did not retain the EBV genome. Thus it would seem possible that once specific hybrids are obtained, clones could be selected which do not carry viral DNA.

It should be remembered that hyperimmune serum from hepatitis patients is currently used for γ-globulin prophylaxis after removal of contaminating virus. As an additional safeguard, potential recipients of human monoclonal antibodies could be screened for serum antibodies to EBV. Most adults in Western countries are positive, having been exposed to infectious mononucleosis. Only in the very rare x-linked lymphoproliferative syndrome(70) would EBV infection be life-threatening. Some patients have already been exposed to EBV-carrying human hybridomas growing in patients within implanted, cell-impermeable chambers (44). As in all novel therapies, the potential benefits to the patient will have to be weighed against any potential risks.

The application of recombinant DNA techniques to the production of human monoclonal antibodies is just beginning. Jonak et al.(71) have immortalized splenocytes derived from mice immunized with human cells by transfection with human leukemia DNA. Several transfectants obtained secreted mouse antibodies reacting with the human cells used for immunization and with other human cell types. Whether this type of approach may be adapted to the production of human monoclonal antibodies remains to be determined. Other systems, such as electrofusion, may in theory produce higher affinity monoclonal antibodies and should be investigated(72).

Using a different application of recombinant DNA technology, several laboratories have reported immunoglobulin light chain(73-77) and heavy chain(78,79) expression after transfection of various cell types with cloned light and heavy chain genes, respectively. In addition, Ochi et al.(80) have demonstrated functional mouse IgM production after transfection of cloned immunoglobulin heavy and light chain genes into selected murine lymphoid cells; these cells possessed all the biochemical machinery for IgM production except the structural genes for the μ and κ chains. Most recently, Boulianne et al.(81) have obtained functional chimeric antibodies consisting of mouse V regions and human C regions. Thus is now appears possible to produce whole mouse immunoglobulin molecules by recombinant DNA methods and the technology is being adapted to human monoclonal antibody production.

ACKNOWLEDGEMENTS

We thank Dr. B. Campling, of the Department of Radiation Oncology, and Dr. J. Pym, of the Department of Surgery at Queen's University, for supply of patient materials, and Peggy Pritchard for typing the manuscript. The expert technical assistance of Els Vreeken and Ingrid Louwman is gratefully acknowledged.

REFERENCES

1. Roder JC, Cole SPC and Kozbor D (1985). In Di Sabato G, Langone JJ and van Vunakis H (eds): "Immunochemical Techniques" a volume in "Methods In Enzymology," FLA, Academic Press (in press).
2. Steinitz M, Klein G, Koskimies S and Makela O (1977). Nature 269:420.
3. Kohler G and Milstein C (1975). Nature 256:495.
4. Olsson L and Kaplan HS (1980). Proc Natl Acad Sci 77: 5429.
5. Croce CM, Linnenbach A, Hall W, Steplewski Z and Koprowski H (1980). Nature 288:488.
6. Kozbor D, Lagarde A and Roder JC (1982). Proc Natl Acad Sci 79:6651.
7. Epstein MA, Achong BG and Barr YM (1964). Lancet i: 702.
8. Henle G, Henle W and Diehl V (1968). Proc Natl Acad Sci 59:94.
9. Rosen A, Britton S, Gergely P, Jondal M and Klein G (1977). Nature 267:52.
10. Aman P, Ehlin-Henriksson B and Klein G (1984). J Exp Med 159:208.
11. Jondal M, Klein G, Oldstone MBA, Bokish V and Yefenof E (1976). Scan J Immunol 5:401.
12. Yefenof E and Klein G (1977). Int J Cancer 20:347.
13. Shapiro IM, Luka J, Andersson-Anvert M and Klein G (1979). Intervirol 12:19.

14. Miller G and Lipman M (1973). Proc Natl Acad Sci 70: 190.
15. Bornkamm GW, Delius H, Zimber U, Hudewentz J and Epstein MA (1980). J Virol 35:603.
16. Steinitz M, Seppala F, Eichman K and Klein G (1979). Immunobiology 156:41.
17. Boylston AW, Gardner B, Anderson RL and Hughes-Jones NC (1980). Scand J Immunol 12:355.
18. Crawford DH, Barlow MJ, Harrison JF, Winger L and Huehns ER (1983). Lancet i:386.
19. Koskimies S (1980). Scand J Immunol 11:73.
20. Kozbor D and Roder JC (1981). J Immunol 127:1275.
21. Tsuchiya S, Yokoyama S, Yoshie O and Ono Y (1980). J Immunol 124:1970.
22. Kamo I, Furukawa S, Tada A, Mano Y, Iwasaki Y and Furuse T (1982). Science 215:995.
23. Zurawski VR, Haber Jr. E and Black PM (1978). Science 199:1439.
24. Zurawski VR, Spedden Jr. SE, Black P and Haber E (1978). Curr Top Microbiol Immunol 81:152.
25. Yoshie O and Ono Y (1980). Cell Immunol 56:305.
26. Irie RF, Sze LL and Saxton RE (1982). Proc Natl Acad Sci 79:5666.
27. Watson DB, Burns GF and MacKay IR (1983). J Immunol 130:2442.
28. Rosen A, Persson K and Klein G (1983). J Immunol 130: 2899.
29. Crawford DH, Callard RE, Muggeridge MI, Mitchell DM, Zanders ED and Beverley PCL (1983). J Gen Virol 64:697.
30. Seigneurin JM, Desgranges C, Seigneurin D, Paire J, Renversez JC, Jacquemont B and Micouin C (1983). Science 221:173.
31. Stein LD, Ledgley CJ and Sigal NH (1983). J Immunol 130:1640.
32. Winger L, Winger C, Shastry P, Russell A and Longe-necker M (1983). Proc Natl Acad Sci 80:4484.
33. Stevens RH, Macy E, Morrow C and Saxon A (1979). J Immunol 122:2498.
34. Kozbor D, Steinitz M, Klein G, Koskimies S and Makela O (1979). Scand J Immunol 10:187.
35. Steinitz M, Izak G, Cohen S, Ehrenfeld M and Flechner I (1980). Nature 287:443.
36. Steinitz M and Tamir S (1982). Eur J Immunol 12:126.
37. Walker SM, Meinke GC and Weigle WO, J Exp Med 146:445.
38. Sikora K, Alderson T, Phillips J and Watson JV (1982).

Lancet i:11.

39. Chiorrazzi N, Wasserman RL and Kunkel HG (1982). J Exp Med 156:930.

40. Kozbor D and Roder JC (1984). Eur J Immunol 14:23.

41. Cole SPC, Campling BG, Louwman IH, Kozbor D and Roder JC (1984). Cancer Res 44:2750.

42. Hirohashi S, Shimosata Y and Ino Y (1982). Br J Cancer 46:802.

43. Atlaw T, Kozbor D and Roder JC (1984) Inf Immun (submitted).

44. Kozbor D, Roder JC, Chang TH, Steplewski Z and Koprowski H (1982). Hybridoma 1:323.

45. Gigliotti F and Insel RA (1982). J Clin Invest 70:1306.

46. Sikora K and Wright R (1981). Br J Cancer 43:696.

47. Sikora K and Phillips J (1981). Br J Cancer 43:105.

48. Schlom J, Wunderlich D and Teramoto YA (1980). Proc Natl Acad Sci 77:6841.

49. Satoh J, Prabhakar BS, Haspel MV, Ginsberg-Feblner F and Notkins AL (1983). N Engl J Med 309:217.

50. Levy R, Dilley J, Brown S and Bergman Y (1980). In Herberman RB (ed.): "Monoclonal Antibodies. Hybridomas: A New Dimension in Biological Analysis" New York: Plenum, p 137.

51. Croce CM, Shander M, Martinis J, Circurel L, d'Ancoma GG and Koprowski H (1980). Eur J Immunol 10:486.

52. Erikson J, Martinis J and Croce CM (1981). Nature 294:173 (1981).

53. Truitt KE, Larrick JW, Raubitschek AA, Buck DW and Jacobson SW (1984). Hybridoma 3:195.

54. Cole SPC, Campling BG, Atlaw T, Kozbor D and Roder JC (1984). Mol Cell Biochem 62:109.

55. Kozbor D, Abramow-Newerly W, Tripputi P, Cole SPC, Weibel J, Roder JC and Croce C (1985) J Immunol (submitted).

56. Sharath MD, Rincerknecht SB and Weiter JM (1984). J Lab Clin Med 103:739.

57. Rarrant J, Newton CA, North ME, Weyman C and Brenner MK (1984). J Immunol 68:25.

58. Cole SPC, Vreeken EH and Roder JC (1985). J Immunol Meth (in press).

59. Weiss RA (1982). Immunol Today 3:292.

60. Shen-Ong GLC and Cole MD (1982). J Virol 42(2):411.

61. Stavrou D, Bilzer T, Jsangaris J, Durr E, Steinecke M and Anzil AP (1983). J Cancer Res Clin Oncol 106(1):77.

62. Poiesz BJ, Rusceth FW, Gazdar AF, Bunn PA, Minna JD and Gallo RC (1980). Proc Natl Acad Sci 77:7415.

63. Miyoshi I, Kubonishi E, Yoshimoto S, Akagi T, Ohtsrki Y, Shiraishr Y, Nagata K and Hinuma Y (1981). Nature 294:770.

64. Chen IS, Quann SG and Golge DW (1983). Proc Natl Acad Sci 80:7006.

65. Longo DL, Gelmann EP, Cossman J, Young RA, Gallo RC, O'Brien SJ and Matis LA (1984). Nature 310:505.

66. Shikova EE (1983). Vopr Virusol 6:714.

67. Grofova M, Matoska J, Lizonova A and Altstein AD (1983). Arch-Geschwulstforsh 53(6):551.

68. Crawford DH, Huehns ER and Epstein MA (1983). Lancet i:1040.

69. Bron D, Feinberg MB, Teng NNH and Kaplan HS (1984). Proc Natl Acad Sci 81:3214.

70. Sullivan JL, Byron KS, Brewster FF and Purtilo D (1980). Science 210:543.

71. Jonak ZL, Braman V and Kennett RH (1984). Hybridoma 3:107.

72. Lo M, Tsong T, Conrad M, Strittmatter S, Hester L and Snyder S (1984). Nature 310:792.

73. Ochi A, Hawley RG, Shulman M and Hozumi N (1983). Nature 302:340.

74. Oi VT, Morrison SL, Herzenberg LA and Berg P (1983). Proc Natl Acad Sci 80:825.

75. Rice D and Baltimore D (1982). Proc Natl Acad Sci 79:7862.

76. Falkner FG and Zachau HG (1983). Nature 298:286.

77. Picard D and Schaftner W (1983). Proc Natl Acad Sci 80:417.

78. Gillies SD, Morrison SL Oi VT and Tonegawa S (1983). Cell 33:717.

79. Neuberger MS (1983). Embo J 2:1373.

80. Ochi A, Hawley RG, Hawley T, Shulman M, Traunecher A, Kohler G, Hozumi N (1983). Proc Natl Acad Sci 80:6351.

81. Boulianne G, Hozumi N and Shulman M (1984). Nature 312:643.

Monoclonal Antibodies and Cancer Therapy, pages 97–109
© **1985 Alan R. Liss, Inc.**

HUMAN MONOCLONAL ANTIBODIES TO HUMAN CANCER CELLS

Mark C Glassy, S.A. Gaffar. Robert E. Peters and Ivor Royston

U.C. San Diego Cancer Center, T-011
Department of Medicine
University of California, San Diego
San Diego, CA 92103

ABSTRACT UC 729-6, A 6-thioguanine resistant human lymphoblastoid B cell line, developed in our laboratory, fuses with human B cells to produce stable hybridomas secreting human MoAbs. Since cancer patients make antibodies reactive with their own tumors we have used UC 729-6 to fuse with lymphocytes from lymph nodes draining tumors and thereby immortalize B cells making putative anti-tumor antibodies. Using lymph nodes from patients with cancer of the cervix, prostate, vulva, and kidney we have made a series of human-human hybridomas producing both IgM and IgG antibodies which have broad reactivity profiles with human carcinoma cells but do not react with hematopoietic or fibroblast cell lines and normal peripheral blood leukocytes. These human hybridomas grow in serum free media with enhanced production of Ig synthesis (1-9 ug/ml). One IgG MoAb, termed VLN3G2, precipitated a 2 subunit glycoprotein of 60K and 18K M.W. from an NP-40 extract of A431 human epidermoid carcinoma cells. Our studies to date have shown that (1) UC 729-6 is a suitable cell line for producing human-human hybridomas and immortalizing human B cells and (2) regional draining lymph nodes of cancer patients contain B cells whose Ig is reactive with tumor-associated antigens.

INTRODUCTION

A major problem with the repeated in vivo use of murine monoclonal antibodies (MoAb; Ref. 1) in man is the host immune response to these foreign proteins. One potential means of obviating this problem is by producing clinically useful human MoAbs which are allotypically matched to the patient. Recently, human MoAbs have been produced (2,3), some of which react to human tumor-associated antigens (4-12). This is based on the premise that tumor patients mount both cell mediated and humoral immune responses to their tumors (13). Earlier studies from Lloyd Old's group (14) have provided some basis for this type of reasoning by demonstrating that the sera of cancer patient's do contain antibodies to their own tumors. Therefore, by immortalizing human B cells producing such anti-tumor antibodies, a steady supply of the MoAb will be available.

Unlike murine MoAbs, which are produced from xenogeneic immunizations, human MoAbs to human tumors are produced from lymphocytes of cancer patients without prior intentional immunizations. As such, humans may recognize novel tumor specific antigens that are, if at all, weakly immunogenic in the mouse. Schlom et al. (4) demonstrated, and others confirmed (5,8,12) that B lymphocytes in the regional draining lymph nodes of cancer patients are primed to synthesize antibodies against tumor antigens. Therefore, the immortalization of these lymphocytes through the now classical hybridoma technique will yield human MoAbs reactive with tumor antigens. In addition, from a more basic aspect, we are also interested in learning more about the spectrum of the human B cell repertoire and as more human MoAbs are produced this goal will be achieved.

Our laboratory has focused on a human hybridoma system consisting of (i) the development of the genetically stable UC 729-6 cell line (8), shown to be useful in producing human hybridomas (15,16); (ii) enzyme immunoassays (EIA) that are rapid, sensitive, and simple in detecting human immunoglobulin (9); (iii) and the generation of immunoreactive human MoAbs (8-12).

MATERIALS AND METHODS

Cells and Tissues. Cell lines used in this study were
UC 729-6 (see Table 1 for some general chracteristics),
myelomas SKO-007 and 8226, lymphomas Nalm-6 and 8402,
leukemias Molt-4 and CEM, melanomas M21 and Sk-MEL-28,
colon HT-29 and T-84, lung T293, NCI-69, Calu-1, and
Sk-MES-1, stomach AGS, Kato-III, MKN-74, and MNK-28, prostate DU 145, PC-3, and Ln-Cap, cervix HeLa and CaSki,
bladder T24 and Scaber, kidney Caki-2, vulva A431, normal
fibroblasts 350Q and WI-38, and murine P3-NS-1-Ag4-1 (NS-1).
Peripheral blood lymphocytes were obtained from ficoll-hypaque preparations of normal healthy volunteers.

Fresh frozen and paraffin embedded human tissue sections were obtained and processed as described (12).

All lymph nodes used for this study were obtained
from cancer patients and received within 3 hr of surgery.

Fusion, Selection, and Cloning of Hybridomas.

Regional lymph nodes draining cancers of the cervix,
kidney, prostate, and vulva were processed for polyethylene
glycol fusion as described (8). Isolated lymphocytes from
the cervix, kidney, and vulva lymph nodes were fused with
UC 729-6 as described (8). Lymphocytes isolated from a
prostate lymph node were fused with murine NS-1 cells as
described (12).

All hybridomas were cloned by limiting dilution (1
cell/3 wells) without the use of feeder layers.

TABLE 1

GENERAL CHARACTERISTICS OF UC 729-6

1.) Human lymphoblastoid B cell line derived from
     parental WIL-2 cells.
2.) 6-thioguanine resistant and dies in HAT media
     within 10 days.
3.) Fc receptor negative.
4.) HLA profile: HLA-A1, A2, B5, B17, DR4, DR7.
5.) Diploid with a $21p^+$ chromosome marker.
6.) Secretes $\leq$ 20-50ng $IgM/10^6$ cells/ml/day.
7.) Doubles every 17 hours.

In this study we describe 3 IgM secreting human-human hybridomas termed 8A1, CLNH5, and VLN1H12, 2 IgG secreting human-human hybridomas termed VLN3G2 and VLN3F10, and one IgM secreting mouse-human hybridoma termed MHG7. Some of their general characteristics are outlined in Table 2.

Enzyme Immunoassay. An enzyme immunoassay (EIA), previously described (9,10) was used to determine human IgM and IgG concentrations and to determine the reactivity of the human MoAbs with their target cell associated antigens.

Cytofluorographic Analysis of DNA Content. Cells and hybridomas were stained by the propidium iodide method for the determination of relative cell DNA content and analyzed by cytoflourometry as described (17).

Immunofluorescence Analysis. Formalin fixed, paraffin embedded, and fresh frozen tissue sections were prepared for immunofluorescence analysis using reagents and procedures as described (12).

Antigen Characterization. Approximately 5×10^6 mid-log phase A431 cells were intrinsically labelled with 100uCi of ^{35}S-methionine (New England Nuclear) for 18 hrs in methionine-free RPMI-1640 media supplemented with 10% FCS. Cells were scraped off with a rubber policeman,

TABLE 2

GENERAL CHARACTERISTICS OF HUMAN HYBRIDOMAS

Hybridoma	Source of B Lymphocytes	Human Ig secreted*
8A1	Chronic lymphocytic leukemia	3-5ug IgM
CLNH5	Cervical lymph node	3-5ug IgM
MHG7	Prostate lymph node	2-3ug IgM
VLN1H12	Vulva lymph node	1-3ug IgM
VLN3G2	Vulva lymph node	1ug IgG
VLN3F10	Vulva lymph node	0.5ug IgG

*values are expressed as $ug/10^6$ cells/ml/day.

washed twice (500 x g for 10 min/wash in serum-free RPMI-1640 media), and lysed with NP-40 detergent (0.5% NP-40, 1mM PMSF, 5mM EDTA, 50mM TRIS, pH 7.4) for 1 hr at 4°C. Extracted macromolecules were ultracentrifuged (100,000 x g for 1 hr), precleared with affinity purified irrelevant human IgG overnight at 4°C, and washed twice in a microfuge. To the cleared supernatant, 30ug of affinity purified VLN3G2 were added, incubated for 2 hr at 4°C, and precipitated with Pansorbin (2 hr at 4°C). After three washes, the samples were prepared for SDS-gel electrophoresis as described (18).

RESULTS

In over 100 fusions performed in our laboratory with UC 729-6, greater than 80% of the hybrids generated have secreted human Ig. Approximately 90% of these hybrids have mitotic cycles of between 25-35 hours and are routinely passaged twice a week with dilutions of 10^5 cells/ml for optimal growth. Fusion frequencies of UC 729-6 varies, depending upon the source of human B lymphocytes, ranging from 5 to 50 hybrids per 10^7 cells fused. Lymphocytes obtained from peripheral blood or spleen gave the poorest fusion yield, whereas those from lymph nodes or tonsils gave the highest number of hybrids. Since the routine maintenance of UC 729-6 in 100 uM 6-thioguanine eleminates HGPRT[+] revertant subclones, none have been observed. Cryopreservation and thawing of UC 729-6, normal B cells, or

TABLE 3

CYTOFLUOROGRAPHIC ANALYSIS OF HUMAN HYBRIDOMA DNA

Cell Type	Relative DNA Content[1]				
	2months	4mo	8mo	12mo	24mo
UC 729-6	45± 2	44± 2	45± 2	45± 2	45± 2
CLNH5	83± 3	82± 2	83± 3	83± 3	82± 3
VLN3G2	80± 3	81± 3	80± 4	80± 3	ND
MHG7	74± 2	68± 3	55± 3	54± 3	51± 2
VLN1H12	82± 3	81± 3	81± 3	ND	ND

[1]Relative DNA contents of UC 729-6, human human hybrids, and the mouse-human hybrid MHG7 were obtained by the propidium iodide method (17). At the indicated times after fusions the DNA contents of the cells were recorded.
ND - not determined.

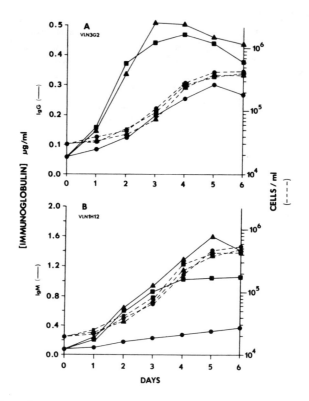

FIGURE 1.   Growth of human-human hybridomas in serum -
free media.   Cells were washed three times in serum-free
RPMI-1640 media and resuspended in HB101 (■), HB102 (▲),
and RPMI-1640 supplemented with 10% FCS and glutamine (●).
At 24 hr intervals, both viable cell number (-- -) and Ig
concentration (——) were determined.   A, VLN3G2 and IgG. B,
VLN1H12 and IgM.

hybridomas has not resulted in any deleterious effects in
stability, secretion, or fusion frequencies.
    Relative DNA contents of UC 729-6 and human Ig-secret-
ing hybridomas are shown in Table 3.   Over the time periods
indicated, the tetraploid hybridomas CLNH5 and VLN3G2 and
the heteroploid mouse-human hybrid, MHG7, were compared
with the diploid UC 729-6.   The DNA contents of UC 729-6,
CLNH5 and VLN3G2 have been relatively stable in culture
while MHG7 has lost a significant number of chromosomes
over the same time frame.

TABLE 4
EIA REACTIVITY WITH HUMAN MoAbs*

Cell Types		IgM			IgG	
		8A1	CLNH5	MHG7	VLN3G2	VLN3F10
Myeloma:	SKO-007	-	-	-	-	-
	8226	-	-	-	-	-
Lymphoma:	Nalm-6	-	-	-	-	-
	8402	-	-	-	-	-
Leukemia:	Molt-4	-	-	-	-	-
	CEM	-	-	-	-	-
Melanoma:	M21	-	N.T.	-	2	-
	SK-MEL-28	-	2	N.T.	1-2	-
Colon:	HT-29	-	-	-	1-2	-
	T-84	N.T.	2	2	3	-
Lung:	T293	-	3-4	2-3	5-6	4
	NCI-69	-	-	-	-	-
	Calu-1	-	2-3	-	3	-
	SK-MES-1	-	3	-	-	-
Stomach:	AGS	N.T.	-	-	5	-
	Kato-III	-	1-2	3	3	3
	MKN-74	-	-	-	4	4
	MKN-28	-	-	-	6	-
Prostate:	DU 145	-	-	-	3	-
	PC-3	-	-	2-3	4-5	2-3
	LN-Cap	-	2-3	3	3	3
Cervix:	Hela	-	4	-	3	-
	CaSki	-	4	-	6	2
Bladder:	T24	-	N.T.	-	4-5	-
	Scaber	-	-	-	2-3	2-3
Kidney:	Caki-2	N.T.	-	-	2	-
Vulva:	A431	-	4	3	6-7	4-5
Fibroblasts:	350 Q	-	-	-	1-2	-
	WI-38	-	-	-	1-2	-
Normal Lymphocytes:	PBL	-	-	-	-	-

*Cells were used in the EIA (see Materials and Methods) at 2.0×10^5/well. The Reactivity Index values were calculated from the following formula:

$$\text{Reactivity Index} = \frac{\text{O.D.}_{490} \text{ test MoAb} - \text{O.D.}_{490} \text{ background}}{\text{O.D.}_{490} \text{ control MoAb} - \text{O.D.}_{490} \text{ background}}$$

The control MoAbs were either an irrelevant affinity purified human IgG or an IgM. Negatives were unreactive. N.T., not tested.

Serum Free Culture Conditions. The growth of human Ig secreting hybridomas in commercially available serum free media (Hana Biologics) was assessed and shown in Figure 1. Over a 6 day period there was no significant change in the growth curves of the human hybridomas when cultured in RPMI-1640 media (supplemented with 10% FCS and glutamine) or in serum-free HB101 or HB102 (used according to manufacturer's instructions). However, there was an enhanced secretion of both IgG (Fig 1A) and IgM (Fig 1B) in serum free conditions, as compared to serum supplemented growth. Maximum IgG levels of VLN3G2 were observed during days 3-4 in HB102, whereas maximum IgM levels of VLN1H12 were observed on day 5 in HB102.

Enzyme Immunoassay Reactivity. Human MoAbs which bind greater than two-fold the optical density of an irrelevant chromatographically purified control Ig myeloma protein to a cell line are assumed positive in preliminary tests. These human MoAbs are then tested against an expanded panel of human carcinoma cell lines. The reactivities of the MoAbs from 5 isolated hybridomas are shown in Table 4. The results shown in this table are compiled from several EIA's and reflect the consistency of the reactivity index (see footnote, Table 4) over several experiments. 8A1 was unreactive with all cell types tested, CLNH5 was reactive with 10 cell types, MHG7 was reactive with 6 cell types, VLN3G2 was reactive with 21 cell types, and VLN3F10 was reactive with 8 cell types. None of these human MoAbs were reactive by EIA with any of the hematopoietic cells tested, including peripheral blood lymphocytes.

High reactivity indices were obtained with the MoAbs with cell lines of the same type as the patient's cancer. MHG7 was very reactive with the prostate cell lines Ln-Cap and PC-3; CLNH5 and high reactivity with cervical cell lines HeLa and CaSki; and VLN3G2 and VLN3F10 were very reactive with the vulva carcinoma cell line, A431.

Antigen Characterization. A summary of the data describing some of the general biochemical chacteristics of the antigen(s) recognized by VLN3G2 is given in Table 5. Under non-reducing conditions, a single band was identified with an apparent MW of 78,000 (78K) daltons was identified from the A431 cell line that under reducing conditions became two subunits with molecular weights of 60,000 (60K) and 18,000 (18K) daltons. T293 cells however, yielded a single band with an apparent MW of 66,000 daltons (66K), which was composed of two subunits with molecular weights of 48K and 18K.

The pI of the intact antigen from the A431 cell line was 5.85 whereas the antigen from the T293 cell line was 5.0.

TABLE 5
MOLECULAR PARAMETERS OF ANTIGENS
RECOGNIZED BY VLN3G2

Experimental Condition	A431 Cell Line	T293 Cell Line
Reducing[1]	60K & 18K	48K & 18K
Non-Reducing[2]	78K	66K
Isoelectric point	5.85	5.0

[1] 10% SDS-PAGE with B-mercaptoethanol

[2] 10% PAGE

DISCUSSION

Our aim is the further understanding of the human immune response to autologous tumor antigens. To achieve this goal we have developed a human-human hybridoma system. Our fusion partner, UC 729-6 (8), serves as the genetically stable vector by which we immortalize human lymphocytes. We also exploit the use of regional draining lymph nodes of cancer patients, which contain B lymphocytes sensitized to their own tumor antigens (4,5,8,11). These lymphocytes were immortalized by polyethylene glycol mediated somatic cell hybridization with UC 729-6 resulting in a continuous supply of the anti-cancer MoAb.

Of the human IgM and IgG MoAbs generated in our laboratory thus far, none have reacted with normal and malignant hematopoietic cells. These human MoAbs have, however, reacted with a broad range of non-hematopoietic malignant cell types. For example, the CLNH5 and MHG7 IgM MoAbs react with a diverse cell population of adherent cell lines of malignant origin in addition to the cervix and prostate cell lines, respectively, and therefore, are not cervix and prostate specific. However, since they were unreactive with normal fibroblasts they may recognize putative tumor-associated antigens. Likewise, the VLN3G2 and VLN3F10 IgG MoAbs may also recognize tumor-associated antigens, since they reacted strongly with the allogeneic A431 carcinoma of the vulva cell line and weakly, if at all, with normal fibroblasts.

The human IgG MoAbs we have produced in our laboratory are inherently more interesting since they have a higher affinity for their respective antigens and are easier to work with than the generally lower affinity IgM's. Because of the higher affinity of the IgG's we have been able to precipitate their antigens from NP-40 cell lysates. The antigen recognized by VLN3G2 IgG is a two subunit structure composed of 60K and 18K species from A431 and 48K and 18K species from T293 cells. The 12K difference in the apparent molecular weight of the larger subunit is most likely due to post-translational modifications, such as glycosylation heterogeneity. This is based on the knowledge that when these cells are incubated in the presence of tunicamycin, an inhibitor of glycosylation, there is a decrease in the cell expression of the antigen, indicative of it being a glycoprotein (unpublished observations). Furthermore, since the pI of the antigen is decreased in the T293 cells then a significant number of charged residues are contributing to this difference, possibly occuring during the above mentioned metabolic modifications. Questions still unresolved are whether the VLN3G2 IgG MoAb recognizes the larger or the smaller subunit and what affect each subunit has on the biological and chemical properties of the intact antigen.

Genetic stability of the human hybridomas is a crucial element to assure long term production of the identified MoAbs. The human-human hybridomas derived from UC 729-6 have remained tetraploid for at least one year in culture whereas the MHG7 mouse-human hybridoma has lost a significant number of chromosomes. This is typical of mouse-human hybrids which characteristically eliminate human chromosomes (19,20). Long term growth of these mouse-human hybrids will eventually lead to the cessation of immunoglobulin secretion. However, with diligent frequent subcloning a continuous supply of the MoAb may be achieved.

Under serum-free growth conditions our human hybridomas secreted significantly increased amounts of Ig. VLN3G2 secreted about 2 to 3 fold more IgG in serum-free media compared to RPMI-1640 media, while VLN1H12 secreted about 4 to 5 fold more IgM under similar conditions. It is tempting to speculate that serum-free conditions provide the appropriate milieu for the increased level of Ig secretion in that there are no suppressor or inhibitory type factors which may be in fetal calf serum that retard the rate of Ig secretion. The absence of these "factors" in serum-free media would allow Ig secretion to occur unimpeded.

Human MoAbs reactive with human cancers may have advantages over MoAbs from other species, particularly those of murine origin. First, murine MoAbs are xenogeneic foreign proteins and, when used clinically patients have encountered some difficulties ranging from minor allergic reactions to anaphylaxis (21). MoAb inhibition has also occurred due to an endogenous anti-mouse immune response. Also, mice, when immunized with a human antigen, usually recognize highly immunogenic determinants. However, human tumor antigens may be weakly immunogenic and do not elicit a significant enough immune response in mice. Humans, on the other hand, may easily recognize these novel antigens and mount an immune response against them. Furthermore, human MoAbs will tell us more about human polymorphic antigens, such as HLA, than MoAbs from other species. This technology provides investigators an opportunity to study the spectrum of the human B lymphocyte repertoire, particularly those to tumor antigens, and may open up new areas of investigation facilitating the diagnosis and treatment of human cancers. As long as these human MoAbs do not have different allotypic determinants, we predict that such antibodies will be used repeatedly without a host immune response.

The final practical problem we face in the clinical applications of human MoAbs to human cancers, both therapeutics and imaging, is the availability of sufficient amounts (usually in the gram range) of the MoAb. Others, including ourselves, have had sporadic success in generating ascites in nude mice and is currently not an optimal method. Fortunately, mass tissue culture techniques employed by a variety of commercial companies are currently available to produce sufficient quantities for in vivo administration. As such, hybridomas which are high producers of human MoAbs, though esthetically pleasing, are not critical due to this mass culture technology.

ACKNOWLEDGEMENTS

We would like to thank Dorothy Kwiat for her expert preparation of this manuscript.

REFERENCES

1. Kohler G and Milestein C (1975). Nature 256:495.
2. Olssen L and Kaplan HS (1980). Proc Natl Acad Sci USA 77:5429.
3. Croce C, Linnenbach A, Hall W, Steplewski Z, and Koprowski H (1980). Nature 288:488.
4. Schlom J, Wunderlich D, and Teramoto YA (1980). Proc Natl Acad Sci USA 77:6841.
5. Sikora K and Wright R (1981). Brit J Cancer 43:696.
6. Cote RJ, Morrissey DM, Houghton AN, Beattie EJ Jr, Oettgen HF, and Old LJ (1983). Proc Natl Acad Sci USA 80:2026.
7. Houghton AN, Brooks H, Cote RJ, Taormina MC, Oettgen HF, and Old LJ (1983). J Exp Med 158:53.
8. Glassy MC, Handley HH, Hagiwara H, and Royston I (1983). Proc Natl Acad Sci USA 80:6327.
9. Glassy MC, Handley HH, Cleveland PH and Royston I (1983). J Immunol Meth 58:119.
10. Glassy MC and Surh C (1985). J Immunol Meth (in press).
11. Glassy MC, Handley HH, and Royston I (1985). In: Human Hybridoma and Monoclonal Antibodies. Ed. by EG Engleman, SJ Foung, JW Larrick, and A Raubitschek. New York: Plenum Pub Corp (in press).
12. Lowe DH, Handley HH, Schmidt J, Royston I, and Glassy MC (1984). J Urol 132:780.
13. Hellstrom KE and Brown JP (1979). In: The Antigens, Vol 5. Ed. by M Sela. New York: Academic Press, p 1-82.
14. Old LJ (1981). Cancer Res 41:361.
15. Abrams PG, Knost JA, Clarke G, Wilburn S, Oldham RK, and Foon KA (1983). J Immunol 131:1201.
16. Thielemans K, Maloney DG, Meeker T, Fujimoto J, Doss C, Warnke RA, Bindl J, Gralow J, Miller RA, and Levy R (1984). J Immunol 133:495.
17. Taylor IW (1980). J Histochem Cytochem 28:1021.
18. Davis BJ (1964). Ann NY Acad Sci 121:404.

19. Ruddle FH (1973). Nature 242:165.
20. Glassy MC and Ferrone S (1982). Cancer Res 42:3971.
21. Dillman RO (1984). CRC Crit Rev Oncology/Hematology 1:357.

III. MONOCLONAL ANTIBODY THERAPY IN PATIENTS WITH LEUKEMIA AND LYMPHOMA

Monoclonal Antibodies and Cancer Therapy, pages 113–120
© 1985 Alan R. Liss, Inc.

TREATMENT OF RELAPSED NON-HODGKIN'S LYMPHOMA UTILIZING
PURGED AUTOLOGOUS BONE MARROW

Tak Takvorian, Kenneth C. Anderson,
Jerome Ritz, and Lee M. Nadler

Departments of Medical Oncology and Tumor Immunology
Dana-Farber Cancer Institute
Boston, MA 02115

ABSTRACT Eleven patients with relapsed non-Hodgkin's
lymphoma of B-cell origin were treated with intensive
cyclophosphamide and whole body irradiation, and
received autologous bone marrow which had been treated
in vitro with the B-cell specific monoclonal antibody
anti-B1 and rabbit complement. All patients had failed
multiple primary therapies and were treated to a minimal disease state (including less than 5% bone marrow
involvement with lymphoma) prior to transplantation.
No excessive acute or chronic toxicity has been seen
and there were no treatment deaths. All 11 patients
achieved a complete response but five patients relapsed
within 6 months of transplantation. Six patients (55%)
are alive and well in a disease-free, unmaintained
remission from 7+ to 27+ months (median 14+ months).
This study demonstrates that anti-B1 treated bone
marrow will engraft and provides preliminary evidence
that this approach may be useful in B-cell lymphoma.

INTRODUCTION

Certain conclusions can be drawn from a review of
the published experience on bone marrow transplantation
(syngeneic, allogeneic and autologous) for relapsed non-
Hodgkin's lymphoma (1-7).
Despite relapse from multiple combination chemotherapy
regimens and radiation therapy, many of the non-Hodgkin's
lymphomas are still sensitive to a variety of intensive
combination chemotherapy and combined modality preparative
regimens which utilize bone marrow transplantation either
for reconstitution or support of the attendant myelo-

suppression. Response rates are in the range of fifty to one hundred percent. However, there is a toxic death rate ranging from 20-33% due primarily to opportunistic infection, pneumonitis which may be radiation induced when whole body radiation is part of the preparative regimen, and graft-versus-host disease in the setting of allogeneic bone marrow transplantation. Long term survival hovers around 25% of all patients coming to transplantation (1,2). Late relapses (>1 year post-transplantation) are rare, and disease recurs primarily in sites of former bulk disease. Most series to date have not made an attempt at debulking patients prior to entry onto these programs. A variety of bone marrow purge techniques have been tried (8,9,10) but the necessity for this has not been addressed by any of the published series.

Bone marrow involvement with non-Hodgkin's lymphoma at initial diagnosis is approximately 40%. One might well surmise that the incidence of tumor involved marrow at a time of relapse is considerably higher. Furthermore, new tissue culture techniques enable lymphoma cell lines to be grown from bone marrow apparently histologically uninvolved with tumor in the order of 15% (11).

Therefore, we designed a treatment program for relapsed non-Hodgkin's lymphoma of B cell origin utilizing intensive combined modality therapy with autologous marrow support. All patients were debulked and treated into a minimal disease state prior to entry onto this program. Since a number of studies in both animals and man (8) indicate that small numbers of tumor cells can be selectively eliminated with monoclonal antibody and complement without inhibiting subsequent hematopoietic engraftment, autologous bone marrow in our patients was purged free of tumor with anti-B1 monoclonal antibody and rabbit complement in vitro and used to support the attendant myelosuppression of the systemic ablative regimen.

METHODS

The method for generation, and the phenotypic and biochemical characterization of the B1 monoclonal antibody (murine IgG2a), which recognizes a B cell differentiation antigen within the hematopoietic system, have been previously described in detail (12). Bone marrow at the time of histologic remission was harvested from the iliac crests of patients under general anesthesia and collected

in RPMI 1640 media with preservative free heparin, filtered
through stainless steel mesh, and washed with an IBM cell
washer. The mononuclear cells were then isolated by Ficoll-
Hypaque gradients and treated three times with anti-B1
antibody and rabbit complement. Cells were suspended at a
concentration of 2×10^7 cells per milliliter and were
incubated for thirty minutes with antibody (1:10 dilution)
at 20°C followed by incubation at 37°C for thirty minutes
with complement (1:10 dilution). After three successive
treatments, these cells were cryopreserved in medium
containing 10% dimethyl sulfoxide and 90% autologous serum
at -196°C in the vapor phase of liquid nitrogen. Before
infusion, the cryopreserved marrow was rapidly thawed and
cells were diluted in medium containing twenty five IU/ml
DNAase to minimize clumping.

Eleven patients, median age 50 years (range 30 to 58
years), with recurrent non-Hodgkin's lymphoma of B-cell
origin were entered onto protocol. There were seven
patients with diffuse histiocytic lymphoma in the Rappaport
classification, three with diffuse poorly-differentiated
lymphocytic lymphoma, and one with diffuse-mixed non-
Hodgkin's lymphoma. No patient had evidence of central
nervous system lymphoma. All patients were advanced
(stages 3 and 4), had failed multiple prior combination
chemotherapy and radiation therapy programs, and all were
treated into a minimal disease state (nodal disease less
than 2 centimeters in diameter) with varying chemotherapeutic and local radiation therapy regimens at the time of
entry onto protocol. Although bone marrow had been
involved at some time during the history of each of these
patients, marrow was only harvested at a time of histologically inapparent involvement with tumor after systemic
cytoreduction. Following bone marrow harvest, the patients
were treated with cyclophosphamide at 60 milligrams per
kilogram intravenously on each of two successive days.
This was followed by whole body radiation, 1200 rads mid-
plane dosage delivered as fractionated radiation therapy
twice daily for the next three consecutive days. The
previously harvested, treated and cryopreserved autologous
bone marrow was thawed and infused through a central venous
catheter within 24 hours of the completion of whole body
irradiation.

RESULTS

The preparative regimen was well tolerated by all 11

patients and minimal toxicity was seen. All patients had
some degree of nausea and vomiting which was controlled with
intravenous Trilafon and Nembutol. All but two patients
had some degree of mucositis, but severe sloughing of the
oral mucosa was seen in only three patients. Despite
alimentation support, patients lost approximately 10% of
their pre-treatment basal body weight and stabilized at
this level. The length of myelosuppression was comparable
to other series of autologous marrow transplantation without a purge technique (13). Marrow engrafted in all of the
patients with the first evidence of white cell recovery
generally by day 7, with a stable poly count greater than
$500/mm^3$ by day 21 post infusion of marrow, and a stable
untransfused platelet count greater than $20,000/mm^3$ by day
28 post marrow infusion. Low-grade fever without a
cultured source developed in ten of eleven patients and
responded to broad spectrum antibiotics. There were no
treatment related deaths.

Reconstitution of B lymphocytes was reflected by the
number of B1+ cells in peripheral blood as well as by
serum immunoglobulin levels. The first B1+ cells in peripheral blood were detected between 35 and 57 days post
transplant. However, normal numbers of B1+ mononuclear
cells (approximately 5%) could be consistently detected
only after 2-3 months. Normal circulating immunoglobulin
levels occurred considerably later than the appearance of
B1+ cells. Circulating IgM and IgG levels, which dropped
to less than 25% of normal after transplantation, slowly
returned to normal within 3-6 months without passive
immunization.

T lymphocytes which co-expressed the T3, T11, T12,
and Ia antigens were the first to appear. Although T
cells from peripheral blood also normally co-express T3,
T11, and T12, the Ia antigens are normally seen on cells
after activation. In all patients, the ratio of the
number of T cells which express the T8 antigen (cytotoxic/
suppressor) and the T4 antigen (helper/inducer) was
reversed. This abnormality has persisted for over 6
months in all patients and has gradually only returned to
normal by the end of the first year. Of interest is the
number of cells which express the 901 antigen which is
restricted in its expression to natural killer cells. The
901 antigen was found on approximately 10-15% of peripheral blood mononuclear cells in the first 3 weeks post
autologous bone marrow transplantation.

A complete response with the absence of all measure-

able disease was attained in all eleven patients. However,
five patients subsequently relapsed. Four of the five
patients relapsed at 3 months or less post entry onto this
protocol and one patient relapsed at 6 months. Four of
these five patients relapsed in sites of former bulk
disease (as defined under Methods above). Six patients
are alive and well in a disease-free unmaintained remission,
ranging from 7+ to 27+ months (median 14+ months).

Chronic toxicity has included five cases of dermatomal
Herpes zoster and one case of Herpes simplex, occurring
approximately 3 months post-transplantation. Two patients
have had pneumonitis (one diffuse and one localized) with
no identifiable infectious source on biopsy which was
self-limited. One patient developed a diffuse dermatitis
without clear etiology, which resolved within 2 months.
Another patient is suffering with a chronic sinusitis of
3 months duration which may be related to altered immunity.

DISCUSSION

We draw the following preliminary conclusions from
the study. This study was designed as a phase 1 trial
to determine the toxicity of the preparative regimen
and the ability of bone marrow treated with anti-B1
monoclonal antibody and rabbit complement in vitro to
engraft in vivo. The transplanted bone marrow engrafted
in each case and was not tardy in its hematologic reconstitution as compared with non-manipulated bone marrow.
The toxicity of the ablative regimen has been acceptable
and minimal despite an older population as compared with
other series in the literature and there were no toxic
deaths. In a limited series of selected patients who are
capable of being reduced into a minimal state of disease
after relapse from multiple intense chemotherapy and
radiation therapy treatments, we have had a 100% complete
response rate with cyclophosphamide and whole body
irradiation. Furthermore, there is a hint of benefit
in terms of survival in 6 of the 11 patients treated (55%)
with a median disease free survival of 14+ month (range
7+ to 27+ months).

Future directions need to focus on better systematic
therapy and better marrow tratment as well. More effective
systemic treatment might be gained from combination chemotherapy rather than a single alkylating agent and the
improved use of fractionated radiation therapy, which
allows for an increased dosage. Also, one would expect

a greater sensitivity to this therapy at a treatment time earlier in the course of disease before resistance and bulk disease have developed. Most importantly, bulk disease must be eliminated prior to transplantation in order to eradicate sites of potential recurrence.

In addition, more effective and selective elimination of tumor cells from the bone marrow need to be developed. This would involve a new generation of monoclonal antibodies, perhaps used in combination as guided by the phenotypic markers identified on the individual patient's tumor cells. Monoclonal antibodies can also be used as a delivery agent by conjugation with cell poisons or radiopharmaceuticals as an alternative to tumor cell lysis with heterologous complement.

The issue of the necessity for bone marrow purging was not addressed by our study. Since we are impressed that many patients with non-Hodgkin's lymphoma have bone marrow involvement and since our study demonstrates no lack or tardiness of engraftment, or toxicity imparted by the in vitro treatment of the bone marrow with a monoclonal antibody capable of lysis with complement, we intend to continue to purge bone marrow. Although a number of studies report patients transplanted with autologous bone marrow which has not been manipulated to purge tumor cells, the number of long-term survivors is small and the issue not addressed (2): it will require a prospective, randomized study to answer the question definitively as to whether there is a necessity for bone marrow purging prior to autologous transplantation. Since patients were not debulked in other series and relapse first occurred in sites of bulk disease, it is possible that the effects of tumor-involved bone marrow did not have time to be expressed. However, until better systemic therapy is available, the issue of marrow purging is a secondary issue.

REFERENCES

1. Appelbaum FR, Thomas ED (1983). Review of the use of marrow transplantation in the treatment of non-Hodgkin's lymphoma. J Clin Onc 1:440-447.

2. Phillips GL, Herzig RH, Lazarus HM, et al. (1984). Treatment of resistant malignant lymphoma with cyclophosphamide, total body irradiation, and transplantation of cryopreserved autologous marrow. N Eng J Med 310:1557-61.

3. Nadler LM, Takvorian T, Botnick L, et al. (1984). Anti-B1 monoclonal antibody and complement treatment in autologous bone-marrow transplantation for relapsed B-cell non-Hodgkin's lymphoma. Lancet 2:427-431.

4. Gorin NC, David R, Stachowiak J, et al. (1981). High dose chemotherapy and autologous bone marrow transplantation in acute leukemias, malignant lymphomas and solid tumors. Europ J Cancer 17:557-568.

5. O'Leary M, Ramsay NKC, Nesbit ME Jr, et al. (1983). Bone marrow transplantation for non-Hodgkin's lymphoma in children and young adults. Am J Med 74:497-501.

6. Philip T, Biron P, Hervé P, et al. (1983). Massive BACT chemotherapy with autologous bone marrow transplantation in 17 cases of non-Hodgkin's malignant lymphoma with a very bad prognosis. Eur J Cancer Clin Oncol 19: 1371-79.

7. Spitzer G, Dicke K, Zander AR, et al. (1984). High-dose chemotherapy with autologous bone marrow transplantation. Cancer 54:1216-1225.

8. Bast RC Jr, Ritz J, Lipton JM, et al. (1983). Elimination of leukemic cells from human bone marrow using monoclonal antibody and complement. Cancer Res 43: 1389-94.

9. Muirhead M, Martin PJ, Torok-Storb B, Uhr JW, Vitetta ES (1983). Use of an antibody-ricin A-chain conjugate to delete neoplastic B cells from human bone marrow. Blood 62:327-32.

10. Sharkis SJ, Santos GW, Colvin M (1980). Elimination of acute myelogenous leukemia cells from marrow and tumor suspensions in the rat with 4-hydroperoxycyclophosphamide. Blood 55:521-523.

11. Benjamin D, Magrath IT, Douglass EC, Corash LM (1983). Derivation of lymphoma cell lines from microscopically normal bone marrow in patients with undifferentiated lymphomas: evidence of occult bone marrow involvement. Blood 61:1017-19.

12. Stashenko P, Nadler LM, Hardy R, Schlossman SF (1980). Characterization of a human B lymphocyte specific antigen. J Immunol 125:1678-1685.
13. Appelbaum FR, Herzig GP, Ziegler JL, et al. (1978). Successful engraftment of cryopreserved autologous bone marrow in patients with malignant lymphoma. Blood 52:85-95.

Monoclonal Antibodies and Cancer Therapy, pages 121–131
© 1985 Alan R. Liss, Inc.

OBSERVATIONS ON THE IN VIVO FATE OF CELLS COATED
WITH MURINE MONOCLONAL ANTIBODIES[1]

Paul J. Martin,[2,3] Cliff Astley,[4] Albert Giorgio,[5]
Barbara Weiblen,[5], C. Robert Valeri,[5] and
John A. Hansen[2,3,6]

Fred Hutchinson Cancer Research Center,[2] Seattle,
Washington 98104; Department of Medicine[3] and Regional
Primate Research Center,[4] University of Washington,
Seattle, Washington 98195; Puget Sound Blood Center,[6]
Seattle, Washington 98104; Naval Blood Research
Laboratory[5], Boston University School of Medicine,
Boston, Massachusetts 02118

ABSTRACT The question regarding the in vivo fate of
cells coated with unmodified monoclonal antibodies
has major importance in considering the application
of such reagents in the treatment of malignancies.
Our data suggest that the ability to facilitate
cytolysis through cell-dependent mechanisms represents an unusual property of murine monoclonal
antibodies which may depend critically on the
precise epitope of the specific antigen recognized.
Moreover, recent observations in bone marrow transplant patients and experiments in nonhuman primates

[1] This work was supported by the office of Naval
Medical Research under contracts N00014-82-K-0660
and N-00014-79-C0168 with funds provided by the
Naval Medical Research Command and by grants
CA18029, CA30924, CA29548 and RR00166 from the
National Institutes of Health, Department of
Health and Human Services. The opinions or
assertions contained herein are those of the
authors and are not to be construed as official
or reflecting the view of the Navy Department or
the Naval Service at large.

have suggested that the reticuloendothelial system may have a limited capacity to eliminate antibody sensitized cells. From our data, there appears to be little basis for expecting significant clinical benefit from treating cancer patients with unmodified murine monoclonal antibodies. Our findings give impetus to efforts to produce and evaluate drug-antibody conjugates and toxin-antibody conjugates.

INTRODUCTION

When techniques were introduced for the generation of monoclonal antibodies, it was immediately recognized that these new reagents might prove valuable in therapeutic applications. For the treatment of malignancies, investigators were originally encouraged by observations that under certain experimental conditions, in vivo administered monoclonal antibodies could have antitumor effects in mice. Monoclonal antibody therapeutic trials in patients with malignancies, however, have met with limited success, with antigenic modulation, circulating free antigen and immunization to mouse immunoglobulin representing some of the difficulties encountered (2-4). Incomplete antibody penetration and inaccessibility of effector cells or complement components in tissues may represent additional limitations.

On the other hand, tumor regression has occurred in certain patients (5, 6) and it has been observed repeatedly that infusions of monoclonal antibodies can cause clearance of antigen-positive cells from the circulation (7). In some situations, the number of antigen-positive cells in circulation remains decreased only for a period of hours, after which cells reappear in the circulation despite the continued presence of saturating amounts of antibody. In other situations, however, more durable effects have been observed. For example, in patients treated with monoclonal antibody OKT3 for renal allograft rejection, lymphopenia occurs within minutes after administration of the antibody and persists for days if antibody infusions are continued (8). Cells gradually reappear in circulation when therapy is discontinued or when the patient becomes immunized to the murine immunoglobulin. These observations have raised the issue of whether the disappearance of cells from circulation represents cell death or merely cell redistribution.

IN VITRO STUDIES OF ANTIBODY EFFECTS

The question regarding the in vivo fate of cells coated with unmodified monoclonal antibodies has major importance in considering the application of such reagents in the treatment of malignancies. Binding of antibodies in and of itself does not ordinarily cause cell death, although certain antibodies can inhibit cell proliferation (9). Lysis of antibody-sensitized nucleated cells can be mediated by complement fixation. However, the process of complement-mediated lysis of nucleated cells follows multi-hit kinetics and occurs inefficiently compared to lysis of erythrocytes because nucleated cells have a membrane repair capacity (10, 11). Most of the anti-human T cell murine monoclonal antibodies we have tested did not appear to be capable of mediating efficient cytolysis with human serum as a source of complement, although some antibodies could fix human C3. Certain murine and rat monoclonal antibodies, however, have been described to cause cell killing together with human complement (12, 13).

Lysis of antibody-sensitized cells might also occur through cell-mediated effector mechanisms, either by opsonizing cells for clearance and elimination in the reticuloendothelial system (RES) or by triggering antibody-dependent cytotoxic cells (K cells) (14). We have screened 159 monoclonal anti-human T cell antibodies from the Second International Workshop on Leucocyte Differentiation Antigens for activity in antibody-dependent cell-mediated cytotoxicity (ADCC) against HPB-MLT, a leukemic T cell line known to express most human T cell associated antigens. Most of these antibodies caused a slight but significant degree of target cell lysis. Only two antibodies proved capable of mediating ADCC as effectively as the rabbit anti-thymocyte globulin (ATG) positive control (Figure 1). One of the active antibodies was an IgG2b immunoglobulin specific for CD2, the E-rosette receptor of human T lymphocytes. The other active antibody was an IgG3 specific for an epitope of CD2 that is preferentially expressed on activated T cells. None of the other 22 anti-CD2 antibodies present in the Workshop panel, including seven IgG1, four IgG2a, one IgG2b, three IgM and seven antibodies of undetermined isotype, had any effect in ADCC assays against HPB–MLT cells.

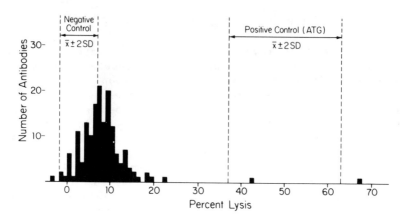

FIGURE 1. Frequency distribution of antibody-dependent cell-mediated cytotoxicity (ADCC). Workshop antibodies were dispensed in microwells along with 10^5 51-Cr labeled HPB–MLT cells. Peripheral blood mononuclear cells (PBL) were added at an effector:target ratio of 100:1. After four hours incubation at 37°C, cell-free supernates were harvested, and released 51-Cr was quantitated by gamma counting. Percent lysis was determined according to the formula: (A – C/B – C) x 100%, where A = cpm released in test wells, B = cpm released by detergent lysis, and C = cpm released spontaneously. "Negative control" represents results from 12 replicates tested in the absence of antibody. "Positive control" represents results from 12 replicates tested in the presence of rabbit anti-thymocyte globulin.

We have also tested whether cultured human macrophages are capable of mediating lysis of targets sensitized with murine monoclonal antibodies (15). The proliferation of murine SL-2 cells was inhibited by cultured human macrophages in the presence of a murine IgG2b monoclonal anti-Thy 1.1 antibody, but the proliferation of human HPB–MLT cells was unaffected by effector cells in the presence of any of five IgG2a antibodies tested. Taken together, these data suggest that the ability to facilitate cytolysis through cell-dependent mechanisms represents an unusual property of murine monoclonal antibodies which may depend critically on the precise epitope of the specific antigen recognized. A relationship between antibody isotype and activity in cell-mediated cytolysis assays was not evident.

IN VIVO STUDIES OF ANTIBODY EFFECTS

Prevention of Graft-versus-Host Disease

Observations that murine monoclonal antibodies can clear from circulation antigen-positive target cells in the absence of complement activation or ADCC activity in vitro have suggested that the RES in man may be capable of recognizing and eliminating some antibody-sensitized cells independent of these other effector mechanisms. The ability of the RES to clear antibody-sensitized cells has been tested clinically as a result of recent attempts to prevent acute graft-versus-host disease (GVHD) after allogeneic bone marrow transplantation by removing mature T cells from the graft with the use of murine monoclonal antibodies. In human bone marrow transplantation, the donor marrow is obtained through multiple aspirations from the iliac crests and contains on the order of 10^{10} nucleated cells, of which 10-20% or approximately 10^9 are mature T cells. After intravenous administration of the marrow, stem cells migrate to the marrow spaces where the microenvironment allows proliferation and differentiation to bring about hematopoietic reconstitution. Thus, the attempt to prevent GVHD by treatment of donor marrow with antibody alone can be viewed as a test of the ability of the RES to eliminate approximately 10^9 antibody-sensitized T cells from the vascular compartment. This represents a "best case" situation in which delivery of antibody to the target and accessibility of effector cells in tissues are not limiting and the mass of cells to be eliminated is small (approximately 1 gm). Although initial results were encouraging, it appears that treatment of donor marrow with a single monoclonal antibody, OKT3, in the absence of exogenous complement had no effect on GVHD (16, 17).

One additional study carried out in Seattle tested the hypothesis that an insufficient amount of surface-bound antibody was responsible for the lack of success when a single antibody was used (18). Thus, donor marrow cells were incubated with a combination of eight monoclonal antibodies that bind noncompetitively to seven

different human T cell antigens. Three of six evaluable
patients had severe GVHD and one of the patients died of
hepatic failure caused by GVHD. A subsequent study has
demonstrated that two-three log depletion of T cells by
treatment of donor marrow with the same combination of
antibodies together with rabbit serum as an exogenous
source of complement can decrease the incidence and
severity of GVHD (Martin et al, submitted). Thus it
appears that in vivo mechanisms at least in these patients were not sufficient to eliminate antibody-coated T
cells with an efficiency required for prevention of GVHD.

It remains possible that the human RES is capable of
eliminating antibody-sensitized cells but that other
factors were responsible for the observed failure to
prevent GVHD. First, antibody may not have remained
bound to the T cell surface for a time period sufficient
to allow interaction with the RES. The kinetics of
antibody clearance from the cell surface has been tested,
and the results indicate that for most antibodies, less
than 25% of the antibody remains on the cell surface
after 24 hr at 37°C (19). The loss of surface-bound
antibody probably represents the combined effects of
antigenic modulation and antibody dissociation. Second,
the cytotoxic chemotherapy and total body irradiation
included in the marrow transplant preparative regimen may
have impaired the function of effector cells required for
the clearance of antibody-sensitized T cells (20).
Finally, antibodies other than the ones that we have
tested may be capable of more efficient opsonization of
nucleated cells.

Studies in Nonhuman Primates

Experimental systems for addressing these issues
have been developed in non-human primates. In one
approach, baboon peripheral blood mononuclear cells were
labeled with ^{111}In-oxine, sensitized in vitro with an
IgG2a murine monoclonal antibody specific for CD2 (the
E-rosette receptor) and infused intravenously. Lymphocyte migration was then monitored by external scanning
and compared to results with radiolabeled cells that were
not treated with antibody. The antibody had little
effect on the distribution of radioactivity between five
minutes and 48 hours after infusion of cells, although
the antibody did cause slight enhancement of up-take in
the liver during the first two hours. In addition,

radiolabel appeared in axillary and inguinal lymph nodes at 24 and 48 hours after infusion of either antibody-sensitized or unsensitized cells. The disappearance of radiolabel from the blood was unaffected by the antibody. Similar results were found when 20 mg doses of antibody were administered intravenously just before and 24 and 48 hours after the radiolabeled cells were infused in order to assure that antibody binding sites on circulating cells remained saturated. Despite the lack of effect on the distribution of radiolabel, the antibody infusions did cause transient decrements in the absolute number of circulating lymphocytes. These data suggest that the clearance of antibody-reactive cells from circulation often observed after intravenous infusion of monoclonal antibodies cannot be reliably interpreted to indicate cell destruction.

A second approach for determining the capability of the RES to eliminate antibody-sensitized cells has been developed with the use of baboons in which an extra-corporeal shunt was placed between the thoracic duct in the chest and the inferior vena cava. Thoracic duct lymphocytes were collected for 24 hours and labeled with fluorescein isothyocyanate (FITC) or tetramethyl rhoda-mine isothyocyanate (TRITC) (21-22). When equivalent numbers of FITC and TRITC-labeled cells were co-infused intravenously, approximately equal numbers of FITC and TRITC-labeled cells were detected in the thoracic duct lymph between one and seven days later (Figure 2A), indicating that short term cell viability was not affect-ed by the labeling procedure. In contrast, when the TRITC-labeled cells were pre-sensitized with horse anti-human thymocyte globulin which crossreacts with 100% of baboon lymphocytes, the number of TRITC-labeled cells that appeared in the thoracic duct lymph was reduced (Figure 2B). From the ratio of TRITC and FITC-labeled cells, it was calculated that only 5-10% of the expected number of antibody-sensitized cells succeeded in cir-culating from peripheral blood to thoracic duct lymph. It could not be determined whether the antibody-sensi-tized cells were permanently removed or merely seques-tered out of circulation for a prolonged period since antibody could be detected on in vitro cultured cells for more than seven days. In either case, the results suggest that the RES may have a limited capacity to eliminate antibody-sensitized cells because appreciable numbers of TRITC-labeled cells did continue to circulate.

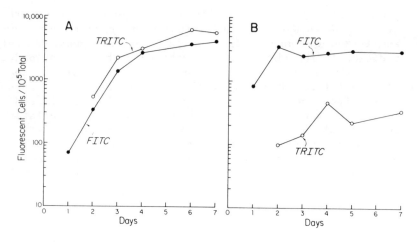

FIGURE 2. Effect of antithymocyte globulin on circulation of baboon lymphocytes. Panel A: Equal numbers (1×10^8/kg) of FITC and TRITC-labeled thoracic duct lymphocytes were infused intravenously and the number of fluorescent cells in thoracic duct lymph was monitored. Panel B: Results when TRITC-labeled cells were pretreated with horse anti-human thymocyte globulin (ATGAM, Upjohn, Kalamazoo, MI).

CONCLUSION

From our data, there appears to be little basis for expecting significant clinical benefit from treating cancer patients with unmodified murine monoclonal anti-bodies. It remains possible that certain monoclonal antibodies might be capable of activating human cytolytic effector mechanisms to a degree sufficient for producing tumor regression. Screening strategies and in vitro assay systems that could increase the likelihood of generating and identifying such antibodies prospectively are especially needed. Alternatively, it might be possible to identify antibodies capable of modifying the biologic behavior of malignant cells in vivo either by interfering with proliferation or by inducing differ-entiation. More importantly, our findings give impetus for efforts to produce and evaluate drug-antibody conju-gates and toxin-antibody conjugates (23).

Even if clinical benefit might not be expected, there does remain a rationale for trials with unmodified monoclonal antibodies in cancer patients. Much remains to be learned about the pharmacology and bio-distribution of monoclonal antibodies. In particular, there is little quantitative information about the ability of monoclonal antibodies to penetrate noninflamed tissues or regions with poor blood supply. Finally, the problem of immunization by foreign proteins remains to be surmounted, except perhaps in patients whose underlying disease produces severe immunosuppression. Otherwise, therapy with drug-antibody conjugates or toxin-antibody conjugates will have to be delivered as a single course of treatment given in a relatively short period of time.

ACKNOWLEDGMENTS

We thank Gary Longton, Gloria McDowell and Karen Ramberg-Laskaris for excellent technical assistance, and Pauline Marsden for assistance in preparation of the manuscript.

REFERENCES

1. Bernstein ID, Tam MR, Nowinski RC (1980). Therapy with monoclonal antibodies against a thymus differentiation antigen. Science 207:68.
2. Nadler LM, Stashenko P, Hardy R, Kaplan WD, Button LN, Kufe DW, Antman KH, Schlossman S. (1980). Serotherapy of a patient with a monoclonal antibody directed against a human lymphoma-associated antigen. Cancer Res 40:3147.
3. Pesando JM, Ritz, J, Lazarus H, Tomaselli KJ, Schlossman SF (1981). Fate of a common acute lymphoblastic leukemia antigen during modulation by monoclonal antibody. J Immunol 126:540.
4. Ritz J, Pesando JM, Sallen SE, Clavell LA, Notis-McConorty J, Rosenthal P, Schlossman S (1981). Serotherapy of acute lymphoblastic leukemia with monoclonal antibody. Blood 58:141.
5. Miller RA, Levy R (1981). Response of cutaneous T-cell lymphoma to therapy with hybridoma monoclonal antibody. Lancet 2:226.
6. Miller RA, Maloney DG, Warnke R, Levy R (1982). Treatment of B-cell lymphoma with monoclonal anti-idiotype antibody. N Engl J Med 306:517.

7. Miller RA, Maloney DG, McKillop J, Levy R (1981). In vivo effects of murine hybridoma monoclonal antibody in a patient with T-cell leukemia. Blood 58:78.

8. Cosimi AB, Colvin RB, Burton RC, Rubin RH, Goldstein G, Kung PC, Hansen WP, Delmonico FL, Russell PS (1981). Monoclonal antibodies for immunologic monitoring and treatment in recipients of renal allografts. N Engl J Med 305:308.

9. Trowbridge IS, Domingo DL (1981). Anti-transferrin receptor monoclonal antibody and toxin-antibody conjugates affect growth of human tumour cells. Nature 294:171.

10. Ramm LE, Whitlow MB, Koski CL, Shin ML, Mayer MM (1983). Elimination of complement channels from the plasma membranes of U937, a nucleated mammalian cell line: Temperature dependence of the elimination rate. J Immunol 131:1411.

11. Mayer MM, Imagawa DK, Ramm LE, Whitlow MB (1983). Membrane attack by complement and its consequences. In Yamamura Y, Tada T (eds): "Progress In Immunology V," Tokyo: Academic Press Japan, Inc., p 427.

12. Hale G, Bright S, Chumbley G, Hoang T, Metcalf D, Munro AJ, Waldmann H (1983). Removal of T cells from bone marrow for transplantation: A monoclonal antilymphocyte antibody that fixes human complement. Blood 62:873.

13. Stepan DE, Bartholomew RM, LeBien TW (1984). In vitro cytodestruction of human leukemic cells using murine monoclonal antibodies and human complement. Blood 63:1120.

14. Herlyn D, Koprowski H (1982). IgG2a monoclonal antibodies inhibit human tumor growth through interaction with effector cells. Proc Natl Acad Sci USA 47:61.

15. Martin PJ, Hansen JA, Storb R, Thomas ED (1985). Applications of monoclonal antibodies for prevention of graft-versus-host disease. In Grignani F (ed): "Monoclonal Antibodies in Haematopathology," Rome: Serono Symposia, in press.

16. Prentice HG, Janossy G, Skeggs D, Blacklock HA, Bradstock KF, Goldstein G, Hoffbrand AV. (1982). Use of anti-T-cell monoclonal antibody OKT3 to prevent acute graft-versus-host disease in allogeneic bone marrow transplantation for acute leukaemia. Lancet 1:700.

17. Filipovich AH, McGlave P, Ramsay NKC, Goldstein G, Warkentin PI, Kersey JH (1982). Pretreatment of donor bone marrow with monoclonal antibody OKT3 for prevention of acute graft-versus-host disease in allogeneic histocompatible bone marrow transplantation. Lancet 1:1266.

18. Martin PJ, Hansen JA, Thomas ED (1984). Preincubation of donor bone marrow cells with a combination of murine monoclonal anti-T-cell antibodies without complement does not prevent graft-versus-host disease after allogeneic marrow transplantation. J Clin Immunol 4:18.

19. Martin PJ, Hansen JA, Remlinger K, Torok-Storb B, Storb R, Thomas ED (1983). Murine monoclonal anti-human T cell antibodies for the prevention and treatment of graft-versus-host disease. In Gale RP (ed): "Recent Advances in Bone Marrow Transplantation," New York: Alan R. Liss, p. 313.

20. Miller RA, Oseroff AR, Stratte PT, Levy R (1983). Monoclonal antibody therapeutic trials in seven patients with T-cell lymphoma. Blood 62:988.

21. Butcher EC, Weissman IL (1980). Direct fluorescent labeling of cells with fluorescein or rhodamine isothiocyanate. I. Technical aspects. J Immunol Method 37:97.

22. Butcher EC, Scollay RG, Weissman IL (1980). Direct fluorescent labeling of cells with fluorescein or rhodamine isothiocyanate. II. Potential application to studies of lymphocyte migration and maturation. J Immunol Method 37:109.

23. Uhr JW (1984). Immunotoxins: Harnessing nature's poisons. J Immunol 133:i.

Monoclonal Antibodies and Cancer Therapy, pages 133–146
© 1985 Alan R. Liss, Inc.

CLINICAL TRIAL OF 24 HOUR INFUSIONS
OF T101 MURINE MONOCLONAL ANTIBODY[1]

Robert O. Dillman,[2] Jacquelyn Beauregard, Daniel
L. Shawler, Maurie Markman, Samuel E. Halpern,
Maureen Clutter, Kevin P. Ryan

University of California San Diego School of
Medicine and Cancer Center and Veterans
Administration Medical Center, San Diego,
California 92161

ABSTRACT We conducted a study involving 56 24-hour
infusions of murine monoclonal antibody (MoAb) T101
in 6 patients with chronic lymphocytic leukemia (CLL)
and 10 with cutaneous T cell lymphoma (CTCL) at doses
of 10, 50, 100, or 500 mg. Direct side effects of
therapy included fever, sweats, and chilling, but
there was also a 15% frequency of allergic manifesta-
tions including pruritis and urticaria. In vivo binding of T101 to target cells in blood, skin, lymph
nodes, tumor masses, and bone marrow was demonstrated.
Antigenic modulation occurred rapidly. Serum T101
levels were related to tumor burden and dose as well
as to the presence of antimouse antibodies which were
demonstrated in 5/10 CTCL and 0/6 CLL patients. All
appeared to have an anti-idiotype component to their
antimouse response. Sustained, but limited, clinical
benefit was observed in 4/10 CTCL and 2/6 CLL patients. The antitumor effects of T101 alone appear
limited and useful antitumor effects may be achievable
only with cytotoxic immunoconjugates.

[1]This work was supported by the Biological Response
Modifiers Program of the National Cancer Institute, the
Veterans Administration, and the UCSD Cancer Center.
[2]Department of Medicine, Division of Hematology/On-
cology, San Diego VAMC-V111E, San Diego, California 92161.

INTRODUCTION

Because of their specificity, MoAbs may provide an important alternative approach to cancer therapy. Despite the fact that T101 produced only limited direct cytotoxic effects with human complement or human effector cells (1), pilot studies with murine antihuman T cell MoAbs showed some evidence of an antitumor effect in CLL and CTCL (2,3). However, it appeared that toxicity was a problem at higher doses using rapid infusion rates (2,4) and it was difficult to confirm in vivo binding outside of circulating cells at lower doses. Therefore, we initiated a clinical trial of 24-hour infusions of T101 over the dose range of 10-500 mg after initial studies suggested a possible clinical advantage for the longer infusion rate and higher doses (5).

METHODS

T101 Monoclonal Antibody.

T101 is an IgG2A murine MoAb which immunoprecipitates a 65 kd glycoprotein antigen (T65) present on T lymphocytes, thymocytes, and CLL cells (6). T101 does not react with myeloid or erythroid progenitor cells although it does suppress colony formation by T cells and CLL cells in clonogenic assays (7,8). T101 was produced and purified as previously described (5) and was provided by Hybritech, Inc. (La Jolla, CA).

Human subjects. Patients with advanced CLL or CTCL who had failed or declined standard effective therapeutic options were eligible. The presence of malignant cells bearing the T65 antigen was confirmed in each patient prior to therapy. Informed consent was obtained as per protocols on file with the institutional review boards of the University of California San Diego School of Medicine and the San Diego VA Medical Center.

Administration of T101. Patients received 1-8 24-hour infusions of T101 at doses of 10, 50, 100, or 500 mg in 1000 ml of normal saline, at intervals of 1-4 weeks depending on response. Patients were closely monitored for untoward reactions by a clinical research nurse specialist and/or the nursing staff of the Clinical Research Center at University Medical Center, and of the third floor medicine wards at the VA Medical Center.

Study Parameters.

   Toxicity. Vital signs were monitored every 15-30
minutes during the first 2 hours of all infusions. Complete blood cell (CBC) counts, electrolytes, and renal and
hepatic function and urinalyses were monitored weekly
while patients were on study. In addition, EDTA blood for
CBC and differential, heparinized blood for peripheral
blood lymphocyte typing, and serum for T101 levels and antimouse antibody levels were obtained at various time
points.

   Expression of T65 antigen and binding of T101. Direct and indirect immunofluorescence assays were used to
ascertain the expression of T65 antigen and the binding of
T101 to circulating target cells as previously described
(5,9). To measure in vivo binding of T101 following
treatment, peripheral blood mononuclear cells were incubated directly with antimouse antibody. Saturation of
circulating target cells was determined by comparing the
proportion of cells that bound T101 in vivo to the binding
of T101 after incubation with additional T101 in vitro.
Thus, complete in vivo saturation produced a value of 1.0
while incomplete saturation produced a value of less than
1.0. This saturation index correlated well with the
fluorescence intensity of the fluorescein-conjugated anti-
mouse antibody. To assess in vivo modulation of T65,
other peripheral blood mononuclear cell surface markers
(Ia antigen for CLL and Leu-4 for CTCL) were also measured. A modulation ratio was calculated as the ratio of
$T101^+$ cells to either Ia^+ or $Leu-4^+$ cells (5,9). In 5 patients, 111-Indium-conjugated T101 was given during the
first or last hour of infusion. Serial whole-body and regional radionuclide scans were obtained at various intervals and interpretations made by a nuclear medicine specialist (SEH).

   Clinical effect. Peripheral WBC and lymphocyte
counts were monitored serially following each infusion.
Specific measurements of circulating target cells were determined by multiplying WBC X % lymphocytes X % $T101^+$
cells. Serial measurements of lymph nodes and skin lesions were made, and standard criteria applied, for determining response (10,11).

   Serum levels of T101. Quantitative measurements of
serum T101 were determined by a solid-phase enzyme-linked
immunosorbent assay (ELISA) as previously described (5).

Antimouse antibodies. Serum was also analyzed for endogenous antimouse antibodies by a solid-phase ELISA. IgG
and IgM antimouse levels were determined using goat anti-
IgG or anti-IgM secondary antibodies. The specificity of
antimouse antibodies for T101 was determined by comparing
binding to, and absorption by other murine IgG2A antibodies.

RESULTS

Table 1 summarizes the results obtained in this trial.
There were 10 patients with CTCL who received 38 courses of
T101 and 6 patients with CLL who received 18 courses. Three
patients with CTCL and 3 with CLL were treated at more than
one dose. As can be seen, there was a tremendous variation
in circulating target cell levels which had a significant
impact on the various cell and serum levels measured. Some
degree of side effects or toxicity was seen in nearly every
patient. Although in vivo binding and decreases in circulating cells were demonstrated in all patients except the
two CLL patients at the 10 mg level. Endogenous antimouse
antibodies were detected in 5/10 CTCL, but 0/6 CLL patients.

As summarized in Table 1, in vivo saturation and modulation were observed in nearly all cases. The clear association between these is exemplified in Fig. 1. In that
patient with CLL and a very high lymphocyte count, saturation and modulation were not seen at 10 mg, but were evident at 100 mg. Rapid modulation was also demonstrated in
bone marrow, tumor nodules, and cutaneous lesions in various patients. In all 5 patients who received 111-Indium-
T101, uptake was seen in lymph nodes, liver, and spleen.
Fig. 2 exemplifies the scans obtained in patients with
CTCL. This sharp delineation of lymph nodes is probably
T101-T cell specific as we have not seen such uptake in
lymph nodes uninvolved with tumor in other radioimmunodetection studies (12,13).

Table 2 summarizes the toxicities seen. Fever,
chills, and diaphoresis appeared to be predictable side
effects associated with the elimination of circulating target cells. The only time these effects were not seen was
in the presence of antimouse antibodies which had a block-
int effect, and in 2 patients in whom pretreatment with
prednisone seemed to abrogate this effect even though circulating cells were removed. Allergic reactions including

TABLE 1
SUMMARY OF RESULTS BY DISEASE AND DOSE

Dose in mg	Diagnosis	Age	Sex	T101+ cells x 10³/ul	Courses	Toxicity	Clinical Response	Decrease Circulating T cells	In vivo Saturation	Antigenic Modulation	Antimouse Antibodies
10	CTCL	81	M	0.24	4	1	PD	+	+	+	−
10	CTCL	67	M	0.80	4	1	MR	+	+	+	+
10	CTCL	82	F	--	4	1	SD	+	UE	UE	+
50	CTCL	67	M	0.76	4	2	SD	+	+	+	+
50	CTCL	54	M	0.47	4	1	MR	+	+	+	−
50	CTCL	56	M	5.40	3	2	MR	+	+	+	−
50	CTCL	65	M	41.4	1	1	SD	+	+	+	−
100	CTCL	58	M	6.53	4	2	SD	+	+	+	+
100	CTCL	54	M	0.44	4	1	PD	+	+	+	−
100	CTCL	22	M	2.97	2	1	UE	+	+	+	−
100	CTCL	65	M	45.1	1	1	PD	+	+	+	−
500	CTCL	58	M	1.69	2	1	MR	+	+	+	+
500	CTCL	44	M	1.55	1	1	PD	+	+	+	+
10	CLL	67	M	218.0	4	1	SD	+	−	−	−
10	CLL	67	M	52.7	1	0	SD	+	−	−	−
50	CLL	67	M	68.6	3	2	SD	+	+	+	−
100	CLL	67	M	42.4	2	2	MR	+	+	+	−
100	CLL	67	M	66.7	1	2	SD	+	+	+	−
100	CLL	73	F	39.5	2	3	PD	+	+	+	−
100	CLL	43	F	13.7	2	1	MR	+	+	+	−
150	CLL	61	M	15.5	1	2	SD	+	+	+	−
150	CLL	43	F	7.69	1	1	SD	+	+	+	−
500	CLL	58	M	6.53	1	0	PD	+	+	+	−

TABLE LEGENDS:
Toxicity: 0 = none, 1 = minimal, 2 = mild, 3 = moderate,
           4 = severe or life threatening
Response: SD = stable disease, PD = progressive disease,
           MR = minimal response
Modulation & Anti-Mouse Level: UE = unevaluable

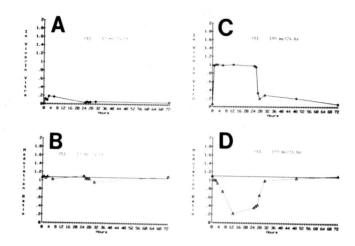

FIGURE 1. Saturation of circulating CLL cells with T101 and modulation of T65 antigen during and following 10 and 100 mg doses of T101 in the same patient. At 10 mg (A) shows absence of saturation while (B) shows absence of modulation (ratio of $T101^+/Ia^+$ is 1.0). At 100 mg (C) shows immediate saturation persisting for 24 hours of infusion followed by a rapid drop, while (D) shows reciprocal modulation which persists only for duration of infusion.

pruritis and urticaria occurred in about 1/3 of all courses. These were not harbingers of more severe toxicity and anaphylaxis was not seen. The most significant toxicities encountered were bronchospasm in one CLL patient and serum sickness in one CTCL patient following a second treatment with 500 mg T101. Three of 6 CLL patients had increases in liver transaminases during the time on treatment, but all had also received multiple blood transfusions previously.

Fig. 3 shows the effect of various T101 doses on circulating lymphocytes. In CTCL, the levels of circulating cells were so low that no clear dose/response was evident. However, in CLL, such a difference in response was apparent. The sharp increase seen in all curves between 1 and 4 hours after initiation of each infusion was associated with the entry into the circulation of T65-modulated cells. Cell counts generally returned to baseline levels within

2-3 days, but some patients had persistently decreased levels up to 4 weeks after treatment. Unfortunately, these changes in circulating cell count were rarely associated with significant clinical improvement. Using standard response criteria, including maintenance of the response for at least 1 month, there were only 6 responses, 4 in CTCL and 2 in CLL, and all were less than a partial response. In CTCL, some responses were very dramatic and bordered on complete responses, but could not be sustained for 1 month (5).

Serum concentrations of T101 depended on several variables, including T101 dose, circulating target cell number, total tumor burden, and the presence of antimouse antibodies. Fig. 4 illustrates the levels for various doses of T101. Much higher levels were reached in CTCL than in CLL, presumably because of lower circulating tumor burden, and the decline in levels was more rapid in CLL. A graph of 500 mg T101 for CTCL is not shown because mean concentrations of over 80 ug/ml were reached in the 2 patients. The curves suggest a rapid distribution and saturation followed by a steep rise in levels which peak at the end

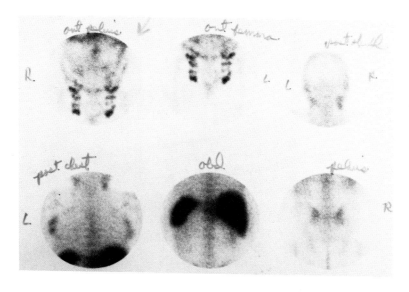

FIGURE 2. Uptake of 111-In-T101 in lymph nodes, liver and spleen of a patient with cutaneous T cell lymphoma.

TABLE 2
TOXICITIES ASSOCIATED WITH T101 INFUSIONS

	CLL		CTCL	
	% of Patients (6)	% of Courses (18)	% of Patients (10)	% of Courses (38)
Fever	67	44	80	32
Rigors/ Chills	67	39	80	32
Diaphoresis	83	44	60	24
Pruritis	50	33	80	34
Urticaria	67	39	30	8
Nausea	33	11	30	8
Vomiting	17	6	20	5
Diarrhea	17	6	20	5
Dyspnea	17	6	50	18
Broncho- spasm	17	6	0	0
Liver Enzymes	50	--	10	--
Hypotension	0	0	0	0
Anaphylaxis	0	0	0	0

of the 24 hour infusion, followed by a rapid decline and then a slower rate of decline toward baseline.

Antimouse levels were detected in 5/10 CTCL and 0/6 CLL patients. Fig. 5 shows the increasing levels seen in one patient who received 8 treatments over a 3 month period. He also had IgM antimouse antibodies as well. The appearance of antimouse antibodies was associated with a shortened interval of decreased circulating cells, a decreased duration of saturation and modulation, and much lower serum T101 levels. In this patient, the appearance of antimouse antibodies was unassociated with any toxicity. In fact, he actually had decreased side effects once the antimouse levels were formed because of the limited effect on circulating target cells. The proportion of anti-T101 specific antiglobulin increased with each treatment in this patient suggesting that this "immunization" schedule might optimize the production of anti-idiotype antibodies. Fig. 6 shows the IgG levels over time

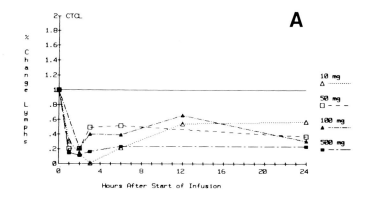

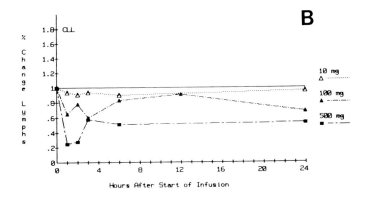

FIGURE 3.   Relationship of change in lymphocyte count (as proportion of original lymphocyte count) during infusions of various doses of T101 for CTCL (A) and CLL (B). Values are means from first treatment at each dose level so that results are unaffected by antimouse antibodies, modulation, persistent T101 levels, or sustained changes in lymphocytes after previous treatments.

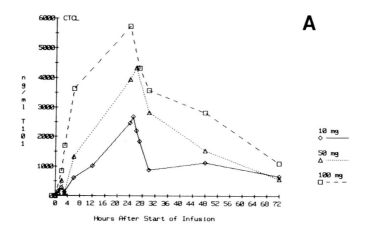

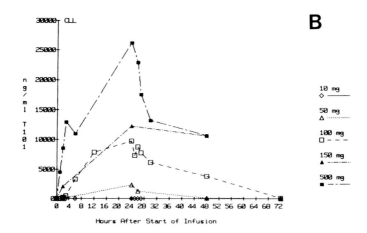

FIGURE 4. Serum T101 levels in ng/ml during and following 24 hour infusions of various doses of T101 for CTCL
(A) and CLL (B). Values are means for 2 or more patients
at each dose for first treatment at each dose level so that
results are unaffected by antimouse antibodies, modulation,
or persistent T101 levels.

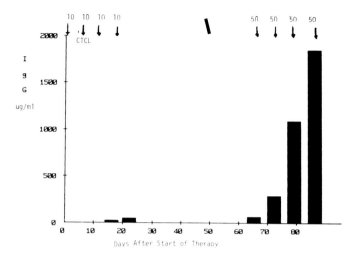

FIGURE 5.   The serum IgG antimouse levels in a patient with CTCL and relation to T101 treatments and time
after initiating treatment.

for all patients mounting an antimouse response on a log
scale which enables identification of a very low background "antiglobulin level".   It is interesting that in 3
of the 5 patients, this background level dropped at 1 week
prior to a rapid increase in anti-T101 levels.

DISCUSSION

This report describes the apparent limited therapeutic potential of T101 as passive immunotherapy in cancer
patients, but illustrates the large amount of information
which can be obtained in a clinical trial with a murine
monoclonal antibody.   The major specific observations are
discussed below.

T101 can be given with acceptable, but universal, direct side effects due to the biological activity of T101
and with a significant frequency of allergic reactions
which may be of considerable consequence in some patients.

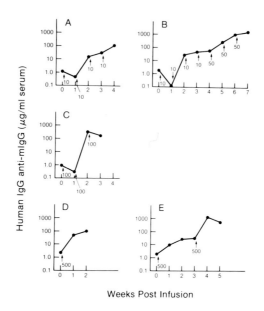

Human IgG anti-mIgG (µg/ml serum)

Weeks Post Infusion

FIGURE 6.   Plots of antimouse levels on log scale for all CTCL patients who developed antimouse antibodies. Note decrease in pre-existing background levels 1 week after treatment in 3 of 5 patients.

T101 clearly binds to circulating target cells and tissue depots of target cells in various parts of the body. However, other than in the circulation itself, there is no convincing evidence that T101 is toxic to targeted cells. This may be because T101 produces negligible cytotoxicity in the presence of human complement or human effector cells, or because of the rapid rate of antigenic modulation, or because of both. These may also explain the lack of a significant dose/response effect for T101. Once modulation has occurred, the remainder of the infusion may, in effect, be wasted. The function of the T65 antigen is unknown, but it is apparent that tumor cell burden is relatively unaffected despite long periods of T65 suppression during modulation.
    In those patients who had a tumor response, the explanation may reside in a leukophoresis-like effect to mo-

bilize skin and lymph node cells. In other words, peripheral cells appear to be eliminated and, presumably, homeostatic factors stimulated cells from tissues to enter the circulation to take their place. Inasmuch as they were already modulated in terms of T65, additional cell removal did not take place. Thus, in CLL, significant, sustained antitumor effects were not achieved and in CTCL, only brief responses were seen and these were often curtailed by the development of antimouse antibodies.

On a more positive note, specificity, affinity, and modulating capacity of T101 may be beneficial for immunoconjugate therapy. Because of the production of antimouse antibodies, future trials with T101 conjugates should concentrate on repeated therapy during a 2 week period, although repeated therapy of longer duration may be possible in CLL. Because of antigenic modulation, there may be no rationale for sustaining high serum levels of T101 for a prolonged period of time. With the knowledge gleaned from this study, we hope to embark on clinical trials with T101-immunoconjugates in the same disease groups in the near future.

ACKNOWLEDGMENTS

We would like to especially thank Paul Shragg of the University Hospital Clinical Research Center for his assistance in data management and analysis, and Kathleen Meyers for her invaluable technical assistance. We would also like to acknowledge the contributions of Steve Baird, Dennis Frisman, and Joe Volen of Pathology, Ivor Royston, and John Mendelsohn of UCSD Medical Oncology, Tammy MacCallister for laboratory assistance, and Dennis Carlo, Jim Frincke, and Richard Bartholomew of Hybritech.

REFERENCES

1. Dillman RO, Sobol RE, Collins H, Beauregard J, Royston I (1982). T101 monoclonal antibody therapy in chronic lymphocytic leukemia. In Mitchell MS, Oettgen HF (eds): "Hybridomas in the Diagnosis and Treatment of Cancer," New York: Raven Press, Prog Cancer Research Ther 21: p 151.
2. Dillman RO, Shawler DL, Sobol RE, Collins HA, Beauregard JC, Wormsley SB, Royston I (1982). Murine mo-

noclonal antibody therapy in two patients with chronic lymphocytic leukemia. Blood 59:1036.

3. Miller RA, Levy R (1981). Response of cutaneous T cell lymphoma to therapy with hybridoma monoclonal antibody. Lancet 2:226.

4. Dillman RO, Beauregard JC, Shawler DL, Sobol RE, Royston I (1983). Results of early trials using murine monoclonal antibodies as anticancer therapy. In Peeters H (ed): "Protides of the Biological Fluids", New York: Pergamon Press, 30: p 353.

5. Dillman RO, Shawler DL, Dillman JB, Royston I (1984). Therapy of chronic lymphocytic leukemia and cutaneous T cell lymphoma with T101 monoclonal antibody. J Clin Oncol 2:881.

6. Royston I, Majda JA, Baird SM, Meserve BL, Griffiths JC (1980). Human T cell antigens defined by monoclonal antibodies: The 65,000 dalton antigen of T cells (T65) is also found on chronic lymphocytic leukemia cells bearing surface immunoglobulin. J Immunol 125: 725.

7. Taetle R, Royston I (1980). Human T cell antigens defined by monoclonal antibodies: Absence of T65 on committed myeloid and erythroid progenitors. Blood 56: 943.

8. Perri RT, Royston I, LeBien TW, Kay NE (1983). Chronic lymphocytic leukemia progenitor cells carry the antigens T65, BA-1 and Ia. Blood 61:871.

9. Shawler DL, Miceli MC, Wormsley SB, Royston I, Dillman RO (1984). Induction of in vitro and in vivo antigenic modulation by the antihuman T cell monoclonal antibody T101. Cancer Res 44:5921.

10. Miller AB, Hoogstraten B, Staquet M, Winkler A (1981). Reporting results of cancer treatment. Cancer 47:207.

11. Silver RT, Sawitsky A, Rai K, Holland JF, Glidewell O (1978). Guidelines for protocol studies in chronic lymphocytic leukemia. Am J Hematol 4:343.

12. Dillman RO, Beauregard JC, Sobol RE, Royston I, Bartholomew RM, Hagan PS, Halpern SE (1984). Lack of radioimmunodetection and complications associated with monoclonal anti-CEA antibody crossreactivity with an antigen on circulating cells. Cancer Res 44:2213.

13. Halpern SE, Dillman RO, Witztum KF, Shega JF, Hagan PL, Burrows WM, Dillman JB, Clutter M, Sobol R (1985). Radioimmunodetection of melanoma utilizing 111-In-96.5 monoclonal antibody: a preliminary report. Radiology, in press.

IV. MODULATION OF EFFECTOR CELLS BY MONOCLONAL ANTIBODIES

Monoclonal Antibodies and Cancer Therapy, pages 149-164

ANTIBODY-DEPENDENT CELLULAR CYTOTOXICITY TO HUMAN MELANOMA ANTIGENS[1]

Karl Erik Hellström[2,3], Ingegerd Hellström[2,4], Gary E. Goodman[5], and Vera Brankovan[2]

ABSTRACT   Monoclonal mouse IgG3 antibodies 2B2, IF4, and MC-21, which recognize a GD3 ganglioside antigen expressed at the surface of human melanoma cells, mediate antibody-dependent cellular cytotoxicity (ADCC) when tested with lymphocytes from healthy human subjects as effector cells, using a 4-hr ^{51}Cr-release test, and antibody MG-21 also gives strong complement-dependent cytotoxicity with human serum. Antibody 2B2, which gives ADCC also with mouse effector cells, can inhibit the outgrowth of human melanoma in nude mice.   Lymphocytes from patients with disseminated melanoma, when combined with antibodies 2B2 or MG-21, were found to give much lower ADCC than lymphocytes from healthy subjects, while lymphocytes from two patients with no evidence of growing tumor were almost as reactive as lymphocytes from healthy controls.   In vitro treatment of lymphocytes with T cell growth factor can increase their effectiveness in ADCC assays. Antibody MG-21 is cytotoxic also when sera from patients with widespread melanoma are employed as the source of complement.

[1]This work was supported by National Cancer Institute grant CA 38011

[2]Present address: ONCOGEN, 3005 First Avenue, Seattle, WA 98121

[3]Department of Pathology, and

[4]Department of Microbiology and Immunology, University of Washington, Seattle, WA 98195

[5]Tumor Institute, Swedish Hospital Medical Center, Seattle, WA 98104

INTRODUCTION

Several human melanoma-associated antigens have been identified and characterized by using monoclonal antibodies. Their specificity for tumor is relative rather than absolute with the more specific antigens expressed in 20-fold or greater amounts in melanomas than in normal adult tissues (1).

Three melanoma-associated antigens are of particular interest, p97 (2,3,4), a proteoglycan (5), and a GD3 ganglioside (3,6). They are expressed, in large amounts, at the surface of cells from most melanomas and, in smaller amounts, in some carcinomas, while adult human tissues only contain trace amounts. All three antigens are of the onco-fetal of differentiation type, that is, they are relatively strongly expressed in certain embryonic cells.

Antibodies to these three antigens localize to tumor when injected intravenously into patients (7,8,9, and un-published findings) which implies that the antigens may be used as targets for therapy. Several possible such thera-peutic uses may be considered. A pilot study with [131]-labelled Fab fragments specific for either p97 or the proteoglycan antigen showed that large doses of radio-activity can be delivered to tumors with few side effects, and some clinical responses were observed (10,11). Anti-melanoma antibodies have been coupled with toxins (12,13), or drugs (14) to produce conjugates selectively toxic to antigen-positive cells, and anti-idiotypic antibodies (15), tumor antigens and synthetic peptides may be employed for active immunization. The simplest, but not necessarily the least attractive, therapeutic approach is, however, to use the antibodies as they are, without further modification. This requires antibodies which have strong anti-tumor effects either by themselves, or in the presence of com-plement or effector cells such as K cells or macrophages.

We have produced three monoclonal IgG3 antibodies to the melanoma-associated GD3 antigen, 2B2, IF4, and MG-21, which give strong antibody-dependent cellular cytotoxicity (ADCC) when tested against melanoma cells in the presence of human lymphocytes (16). Antibody MG-21, but not the others, is also cytotoxic to melanoma cells in the presence of human serum as a source of complement. We present data here which have a bearing on the potential therapeutic use of these and similar antibodies.

MATERIALS AND METHODS

Human subjects. Two types of donors of human blood
lymphocytes and sera were tested. First, we used healthy,
adult human subjects, 25-45 years of age. Second, we
tested patients with melanoma. After the blood samples
were drawn using 20 units heparin/ml of blood, lymphocytes
were separated on Ficoll-Hypaque (17).

Most tests were done on lymphocytes frozen in a mixture
of 10% dimethylsulfoxide (DMSO); 20% fetal calf serum and
RPMI culture medium (Grand Island Biological Company, Grand
Island, NY) as previously described (17) and were thawed at
37°C prior to testing.

Tumors. Five different human cell lines were used,
which had been established from metastatic melanoma, and
all of which, except one, M-2634, express high levels of
the GD3 antigen according to binding assays which were
carried out as previously described (6,18). Four of the
lines, SK-MEL 28 (2), M-2669 clone 13, M-2634, and M-2765,
were propagated in vitro. The fifth line, M-2586, which
failed to grow in vitro, was serially transplanted in nude
mice where it grew better than any of the other lines. All
the in vitro data presented in the Tables were derived from
studies on a cloned melanoma line, M-2669 cl 13.

Human lung (bronchial) carcinoma line CH27, which does
not express detectable GD3 antigen, was used as a control
for antibody specificity.

Antibodies. Hybridomas 2B2, MG-21, and IF4 were
derived from the spleens of BALB/c mice immunized with
SK-MEL 28 cells, using NS-1 cells as the fusion partner and
make antibodies which are IgG3 according to gel diffusion.
Antibody specificity for melanoma has been established by
binding assays with cultured cells and by immunohistological studies on frozen sections (19).

Two other antibodies, 96.5 and 48.7, were used for
comparison. The former is directed to p97 (4), and the
latter is specific for a proteoglycan antigen expressed by
most melanomas (20). Neither antibody has given
significant ADCC or inhibition of human melanomas in nude
mice.

Antibodies were affinity purified on a column of
Staphylococcal protein A covalently linked to Sepharose
CL-4B (Pharmacia Fine Chemicals, Uppsala, Sweden) and
eluted with 0.1 M citrate buffer, pH 3.5 or 4.5 (4).

Antibody-dependent cellular cytotoxicity (ADCC). A short-term ^{51}Cr-release test was used (16,21). Peripheral blood lymphocytes from healthy human subjects were separated on Ficoll-Hypaque (17) to provide effector cells and were prescreened for low NK cell reactivity against the target used for a given test. Unless otherwise stated, 100 lymphocytes were added per target cell; spleen lymphocytes from normal BALB/c mice were tested in two experiments. Target cells (10^6) were labelled by incubation with 100 µCi ^{51}Cr for 2 hr at 37°C, after which they were washed 3 times and resuspended in medium. The labelled cells were seeded, 2×10^4 cells/well in 20 µl volume, into Microtiter V-bottom plates (Cat. #1-220-25X, Dynatech Laboratories, Inc. Alexandria, VA). Purified antibody (at various dilutions, see Results), 100 µl/well, was added, followed by 2×10^5 lymphocytes/well in 100 µl. The mixtures were incubated for 4 hr, after which the plates were centrifuged at 400 g and the supernatants removed and counted in a gamma counter (100 µl/sample). There were 2 replicates per group; the variation between replicates was less than 10%. Spontaneous release was defined as the number of counts released into the medium from target cells exposed to neither antibodies nor lymphocytes, and total release as the number of counts released from target cells that were osmotically lysed at the end of the assay. Percent cytotoxicity was calculated as

$$100 \times \frac{\text{Experimental group release} - \text{spontaneous release}}{\text{Total release} - \text{spontaneous release}}$$

Complement-mediated cytotoxicity. The ^{51}Cr-release assay was also used to test the ability of antibodies to kill melanoma cells in the presence of human serum as a source of complement. It was carried out similarily to the assays for ADCC, except that 100 µl of undiluted, unheated, human serum was added per microtest well, instead of a suspension of effector cells.

Test of antibody activity in nude mice. Athymic "nude" (nu/nu) 2-3 month-old male mice were grafted subcutaneously, on both flanks, with a 1 x 1 mm diameter piece of melanoma M2586, which expresses both p97 (2) and the GD3 (6) antigens. Each experimental group comprised 5 mice. This represented 10 "sites", since the mice were grafted on both sides. The control group had 10 mice (20 "sites").

On the day following grafting, and on each third day thereafter, the mice were injected intravenously, via the tail vein, with 1 mg antibody in phosphate-buffered saline (PBS); this dose was chosen to provide excess of antibody in the treated mice. Separate groups received antibody 2B2, IF4, 96.5 or a combination of the three; the last group was injected with one third of the dose of each antibody. A total of 6 antibody injections was given. The control group was injected with culture medium, in the same amounts and at the same times.

The mice were inspected 3 times weekly over a period of 6 months. Two perpendicular diameters of each tumor were measured; we refer to a tumor as palpable when its mean diameter was 2 mm or larger.

Characterization of effector cells. Tests were performed in which lymphocyte preparations obtained by separation on Ficoll-Hypaque were incubated for 1 hr at 37°C in plastic culture flasks to remove adherent cells, after which they were passed through a nylon wool column (22); the cells in the column effluents were used as a source of effector cells. In other tests, the Ficoll-Hypaque-purified lymphocytes were incubated for 1 hr at 37°C with a mixture of anti-Leu-11b antibody (Becton-Dickinson, Mt. View, CA) at a concentration of $0.1 \, \mu g/10^6$ lymphocytes and rabbit serum diluted 1:5 (as a source of complement); this was done in order to abolish reactivity mediated by natural killer (NK) cells (23).

Treatment with T cell growth factor (TCGF). Peripheral blood lymphocytes (10^6/ml) were incubated in vitro for 5 days in the presence of 10% human TCGF (Cellular Products, Inc., Buffalo, NY), 20% human AB serum and 70% RPMI culture medium.

RESULTS

ADCC with lymphocytes from healthy human subjects. Table 1 presents an experiment which illustrates the data obtained. Mixtures of human lymphocytes, antibodies and ^{51}Cr-labelled M-2669 cl 13 melanoma cells were incubated for 4 hrs. A cytolytic effect was observed when a combination of antibody MG-21 and lymphocytes was tested, while antibody alone had no significant effect and lymphocytes alone gave only 7% cytotoxicity. Similar findings were obtained with antibody 2B2 (data not shown).

TABLE 1

ADCC WITH ANTIBODY MG-21 AND LYMPHOCYTES FROM A HEALTHY
HUMAN SUBJECT TESTED AGAINST M-1669 cl 13 MELANOMA CELLS.

Number of effector cells per target cell	Antibody concentration µg/ml	^{51}Cr-release* counts	% cytotoxicity**
100	50	137,890	60
100	10	123,972	56
100	None	25,043	7
10	50	63,346	26
10	10	67,105	28
10	None	14,215	2
None	50	10,289	0
Spont. release	None	None	10,310
Total release			212,729

* Means of results with 2 replicates/group; there was less than
  10% variation between the 2 replicates.
** % cytotoxicity was calculated by the formula:

$$100 \times \frac{\text{Experimental group release } - \text{ spontaneous release}}{\text{Total release } - \text{ spontaneous release}}$$

Table 2 summarizes experiments in which antibodies 2B2
and MG-21 were tested (at 10 µg/ml and 1 µg/ml) against
M-2669 clone 13 cells, using three different lymphocyte-to-
target cell ratios. MG-21 gave better ADCC than 2B2.

TABLE 2

ADCC AGAINST M-2669 cl 13 MELANOMA CELLS WITH THREE DIFFERENT
RATIOS OF HUMAN LYMPHOCYTES PER TARGET CELL AND AT TWO DIFFERENT
ANTIBODY CONCENTRATIONS.

Number of lymphocytes/ target cell	Antibody*			
	2B2		MG-21	
	10 µg/ml	1 mg/ml	10 µg/ml	1 µg/ml
100	68	50	82	76
10	40	17	64	52
1	13	7	14	13

* Antibodies alone gave no cytotoxicity and lymphocytes alone
  gave ± 5% cytotoxicity.

We evaluated the ability of antibody 2B2 (10 µg/ml) and human lymphocytes (100 per target cell) to give ADCC against 5 different melanoma lines, four of which (M-2669 cl 13, M-2765, M-2568, and SK-MEL 28) strongly display the GD3 antigen and one of which (M-2634) expresses very little of it (if any); the M-2568 cells were isolated from tumors in nude mice. Lung carcinoma line CH27 was included as a negative control. M-2634 gave low ADCC (11%), while ADCC was high (65-82%) against the other four melanomas and CH27 cells were not affected. The ADCC effect observed in ^{51}Cr-release tests could be competitively inhibited by adding unlabelled cells from SK-MEL 28 or M-2586, but not by adding unlabelled CH27 cells.

The ADCC effector cells were not removed by incubation in plastic bottles followed by passage over a nylon wool column (data not shown), while ADCC reactivity disappeared after incubation of the effector cells with antibody Leu-11b and complement (Table 3).

TABLE 3

INHIBITION OF ADCC BY INCUBATION OF EFFECTOR CELLS FROM A NORMAL SUBJECT WITH ANTI-Leu 11b ANTIBODY AND COMPLEMENT.

Treatment of effector cells*	Antibody 10 µg/ml	% ADCC
None (culture medium)	MG-21	24
	None	3
Complement	MG-21	22
	None	3
Leu 11b + Complement	MG-21	2
	None	2

* Lymphocytes were treated as described under Materials and Methods.
M-2669 cl 13 cells were used as targets.

Anti-tumor effects in vivo. We investigated whether antibodies 2B2 or IF4 had any anti-tumor effect in nude mice transplanted with human melanoma; antibody 2B2, but not IF4, had been found to give ADCC with mouse effector cells (data not shown). Melanoma M-2586 was used as target, since it grows well in nude mice, can be used as target for 2B2-mediated ADCC, and can competitively inhibit ADCC against SK-MEL 28 cells. The mice were injected with a dose of antibody expected to give a blood concentration exceeding that needed for ADCC in vivo. Antibody 96.5 (anti-p97) was used in parallel, and a combination of all 3 antibodies was also included.

As shown in Table 4, antibody 2B2 suppressed the outgrowth of melanoma grafts so that only 1 of 10 injected sites had a detectable tumor 4 months after grafting, as compared to 19 of 20 sites in the control. The implanted tumor pieces had thus been rejected at all 10 sites in the 2B2 group except for one. Six months after grafting, 4 mice in the 2B2 group survived, tumor-free, while all the controls were dead with large (>15 mm diameter) tumors. Neither antibody 96.5 nor antibody IF4 inhibited tumor outgrowth. The group receiving a combination of antibodies 2B2, IF4, and 96.5 showed inhibition with 3 of 10 sites developing progressively growing tumors (16).

TABLE 4

ANTIBODY 2B2 INHIBITS THE OUTGROWTH OF HUMAN MELANOMA M-2568 IN NUDE MICE.§

Treatment	Number of sites with tumor/ total number of sites 4 months after transplantation of tumor*
Control (culture medium)	19/20
Antibody 2B2	1/10
Antibody IF4	10/10
Antibody 96.5	10/10
Combination (2B2,IF4,96.5)	3/10

§ Mice were transplanted bilaterally on the back with 1 x 1 mm tumor pieces. The next day, and for 5 more times, at 3-day intervals, they were injected intravenously with 1 mg antibody. There were 5 mice (10 "sites") per group except for the control, which had 10 mice (20 "sites").
* All mice were dead at 6 months after transplantation except for 4 of the 5 mice which got antibody 2B2 and 2 of the 5 mice which got the combination, which were all alive and tumor free.

Depressed ADCC reactivity with lymphocytes from cancer patients. Table 5 summarizes clinical data on melanoma patients, from which lymphocytes and sera were tested. Patient M-1 had a Stage I melanoma resected eight years previously and has since been followed without evidence of recurrent disease. Patient M-2 had a Stage I, Level IV, melanoma resected two months previously and also had been followed without evidence of recurrent disease. Both patients had no previous treatment other than surgical resection. These two patients showed ADCC of a degree close to that of controls. The other five patients had

Stage IV melanoma. Most of them had extensive disease, and, as indicated by their performance status, were debilitated. These patients had multiple prior therapies except for patient M-5. ADCC among these patients was very low (Table 6).

TABLE 5
CHARACTERISTICS OF MELANOMA PATIENTS DONATING
LYMPHOCYTES AND SERA.

Patient	Age	Sex	Stage	Performance status	Disease status when tested	Treatment when tested
M-1	55	M	I	100	None	None
M-2	62	M	I	100	None	None
M-3	67	F	IV	60	Current	Chemotherapy
M-4	65	F	IV	70	Current	Chemotherapy, corticosteroids
M-5	33	M	IV	60	Current	None
M-6	40	M	IV	60	Current	None
M-7	56	M	IV	70	Current	None

TABLE 6
ADCC WITH LYMPHOCYTES FROM NORMAL SUBJECTS OR MELANOMA PATIENTS
WHEN COMBINED WITH ANTIBODIES MG-21 AND 2B2 AND TESTED AGAINST
M-2669 cl 13 CELLS.

Lymphocyte donor Designation	% NK effect	% ADCC with antibody* 2B2	MG-21
Normal subject N-1	6	34	51
Melanoma patient M-3 (St. IV)	4	3	2
Normal subject N-2	5	17	32
Melanoma patient M-4 (St. IV)	1	4	5
Melanoma patient M-1 (St. I)	4	18	38
Normal subject N-3	6	38	55
Melanoma patient M-5 (St. IV)	3	5	7
Melanoma patient M-2 (St. I)	0	15	31
Normal subject N-4	7	29	NT
Melanoma patient M-6 (St. IV)	0	9	NT
Melanoma patient M-7 (St. IV)	0	3	NT

* % ADCC calculated as % cytotoxicity in the presence of both lymphocytes and antibody (50 µg/ml), as in footnote to Table 1. NT = not tested.

Lymphocytes incubated with T cell growth factor can be used as effector cells for ADCC. In view of the failure of lymphocytes from patients with disseminated melanoma (Table 6) or other forms of cancer (data not shown) to act as ADCC effector cells when combined with antibodies 2B2 or MG-21, we performed a preliminary experiment aiming at increasing lymphocyte reactivity by in vitro incubation with T cell growth factor (TCGF). As shown in Table 7, NK cell activity of lymphocytes from both a normal subject and two cancer patients substantially increased after incubation for 5 days with TCGF, and the TCGF-treated lymphocytes were able to act as effectors of ADCC.

TABLE 7
NK AND ADCC REACTIVITY OF LYMPHOCYTES INCUBATED IN VITRO WITH TCGF FOR 5 DAYS OR TESTED PRIOR TO INCUBATION. M-2669 CLONE 13 CELLS WERE USED AS TARGETS

Donor	Number per target cell	Antibody (10 µg/ml)	Untreated lymphocytes	TCGF-treated lymphocytes
N-4 (normal subject)	10	None	2	43
		mg-21	19	65
	1	None	0	9
		MG-21	2	17
P-1 (ca. prostat, Stage IV)	10	None	0	20
		MG-21	6	36
	1	None	0	4
		MG-21	3	7
B-1 (ca. breast, Stage II)	10	None	2	68
		MG-21	25	85
	1	None	2	29
		MG-21	11	55

Complement-dependent cytotoxicity. We studied whether antibodies 2B2 or MG-21 were cytotoxic to GD3-positive melanoma in the presence of human serum as a source of complement (16). Antibody MG-21 gave a strong cytotoxic effect with serum from normal healthy subjects, while antibody 2B2 was negative. CH27 lung carcinoma cells, which were used as controls, were not affected. Heat inactivation of the human serum abolished its complement activity (16).

Table 8 presents one of many similar experiments testing sera from melanoma patients, using sera from healthy human subjects as positive controls. As shown in the Table, MG-21 had a cytotoxic effect on melanoma cells in the presence of sera from either a Stage IV melanoma patient or a normal healthy subject.

TABLE 8
COMPLEMENT-DEPENDENT CYTOTOXICITY OF ANTIBODY MG-21 IN THE
PRESENCE OF SERUM FROM A NORMAL HUMAN SUBJECT ON A PATIENT WITH
STAGE IV MELANOMA AS TESTED AGAINST M-2669 CLONE 13 CELLS.

Serum donor	Antibody concentration μg/ml	% cytotoxicity
Normal	50	79*
	10	57*
	1	0
Melanoma M-7	50	83*
	10	64*
	1	0

* Percentage cytotoxicity statistically different from 0, $p < 0.01$.
no cytotoxicity was seen by antibody alone or by human serum
alone.

DISCUSSION

We have obtained three IgG3 antibodies which mediate
ADCC specific for a melanoma-associated GD3 antigen when
combined with human effector cells. The ADCC effect was
antigen specific, since cells lacking the GD3 antigen were
not killed, and since it could be competitively inhibited
by addition of antigen-positive tumor cells. One of our
antibodies, MG-21, was found to kill melanoma cells also in
the presence of human serum as a source of complement.
Another antibody, 2B2, which gives ADCC with both human and
mouse effector cells, inhibited the outgrowth of a human
melanoma in nude mice. Although most anti-tumor antibodies
previously tested by us and others lack these characteristics, an antibody to a proteoglycan antigen of melanoma
cells, as described by Schultz et al. (24), has an
anti-tumor effect which appears similar to that of 2B2.

Since antibody 2B2 was capable of destroying 1 mm
diameter tumor implants in nude mice, one may speculate
that it might destroy small melanoma implants (in the form
of micrometastases) also in man. If that is the case, 2B2
(and similar antibodies) may have therapeutic applications,
for example, in patients who have deeply penetrating
primary melanomas and, therefore, poor prognosis. As a
first step towards evaluating this clinically, one may
consider performing pilot studies in patients with advanced
metastatic disease (Stage IV), who are the patients
commonly chosen for initial testing of anti-cancer agents.
It is important, then, that lymphocytes from the Stage IV

melanoma patients tested served very poorly as effector cells for ADCC when combined with antibodies 2B2 or MG-21. This may relate to the depressed NK cell function commonly observed in cancer patients (25). It is difficult to determine the contribution (if any) of previous therapy to this depression. Only one patient with Stage IV disease had no previous treatment, and the treatments to which the the patients had been subjected (chemotherapy, cortico-steroids and/or radiotherapy) are all known to have immuno-suppressive properties. In view of the lack of ADCC reactivity of the untreated Stage IV patient we tend to believe, however, that lymphocyte activity is related to tumor burden.

If these data are extrapolated to the situation in vivo, infusion of antibodies 2B2 or MG-21 to patients with Stage IV melanoma would not be expected to induce anti-tumor activity based on ADCC (the antibodies might, of course, have an anti-tumor effect caused by some other mechanism). We suggest for consideration, therefore, the following three approaches towards tumor therapy with unmodified antibodies with properties similar to those we have described. First, one may confine treatment to patients whose lymphocytes have good effector activity in ADCC assays, which would most likely be patients with little tumor spread (like the two of our patients whose Stage I melanomas had been removed). Second, one may use antibodies (such as MG-21) which can utilize human complement. Third, one may bolster the NK (and K) cell reactivity of patient lymphocytes by treatment with some lymphokine, such as Interleukin 2 (26). The third approach is most attractive to us, since initial clinical trials on patients with little tumor spread are hard to both justify and evaluate, and since animal studies have shown that the in vivo effects of antibodies operating via complement-mediated cytotoxicity is often small, also against tumors which are highly sensitive to such antibodies in vitro (27). The preliminary data presented in Table 7 are encouraging, since they indicate that patient lymphocytes incubated with a T cell growth factor preparation (presumably containing Interleukin 2) can serve as effectors of ADCC.

ACKNOWLEDGMENTS

We thank Mr. Craig Bailey, Ms. Linda Katzenberger and Ms. Lucy Saldana for skillful technical assistance.

REFERENCES

1. Hellström KE, Hellström I. Monoclonal anti-melanoma antibodies and their possible clinical use. In: Baldwin RW, Byers VS (eds): "Monoclonal Antibodies for Tumour Detection and Drug Targeting," New York: Academic Press, in press.

2. Woodbury RG, Brown JP, Yeh M-Y, Hellström I, Hellström KE. (1980) Identification of a cell surface protein, p97, in human melanomas and certain other neoplasms. Proc Natl Acad Sci USA 77:2183.

3. Dippold WG, Lloyd KO, Li LTC, Ikeda H, Oettgen HF, Old LJ. (1980) Cell surface antigens of human malignant melanoma: Definition of six antigenic systems with mouse monoclonal antibodies. Proc Natl Acad Sci USA 77:6114.

4. Brown JP, Nishiyama K, Hellström I, Hellström KE. (1981) Structural characterization of human melanoma-associated antigen p97 using monoclonal antibodies. J Immunol 127:539.

5. Imai K, Wilson BS, Day NE, Ferrone S. (1981) Monoclonal antibodies to human melanoma cells: comparison of serological results of several laboratories and molecular profile of melnaoma-associated antigens. In: Hammerling GJ, Hammerling U, Kearney JF (eds): "Monoclonal Antibodies and T Cell Hybridomas," Amsterdam: Elsevier/North-Holland p 183.

6. Yeh M-Y, Hellström I, Abe K, Hakomori S, Hellström KE. (1982) A cell surface antigen which is present in the ganglioside fraction and shared by human melanomas. Int J Cancer 29:269.

7. Larson SM, Brown JP, Wright PW, Carrasquillo JA, Hellström I, Hellström KE (1983) Imaging of melanoma with ^{131}I-labelled monoclonal antibodies. J Nuclear Med 24:123.

8. Oldham RK, Foon KA, Morgan AC, Woodhouse CS, Schraff RS, Abrams PG, Fer M, Schoenberg CS, Farrell M, Kimball E, Sherwin SA. (1984) Monoclonal antibody therapy of malignant melanoma: In vivo localization in cutaneous

metastsis after intravenous administration. J Clin Oncol 2:1235.

9. Goodman GE, Beaumeir PL, Hellström I, Fernyhough B, Hellström KE. Phase I trial of murine monoclonal antibodies in patients with advanced melanoma. J Clin Oncol, in press.

10. Larson SM, Carrasquillo JA, Krohn KA, Brown JP, Mc-Guffin RW, Ferens JM, Graham MM, Hill LD, Beaumier PL, Hellström KE, Hellström I. (1983) Localization of p97 specific Fab fragments in human melanoma as a basis for radiotherapy. J Clin Invest 72:2101.

11. Carrasquillo JA, Krohn KA, Beaumier P, McGuffin RW, Brown JP, Hellström KE, Hellström I, Larson SM. (1984) Diagnosis and therapy of solid tumors with radiolabelled Fab. Cancer Treatment Reports 68:317.

12. Casellas P, Brown JP, Gros O, Gros P, Hellström I, Jansen FK, Poncelet P, Vidal H, Hellström KE. (1982) Human melanoma cells can be killed in vitro by an immunotoxin specific for melanoma-associated antigen p97. Int J Cancer 30:437.

13. Bumol TF, Wang QC, Reisfeld RA (1983) Monoclonal antibody and antibody-toxin conjugate to a cell surface proteoglycan of melanoma cells suppress in vivo tumor growth. Proc. Natl. Acad. Sci. U.S.A. 80:529.

14. Rowland GF, Axton CA, Baldwin RW, Brown JP, Corvalan JRF, Embleton MJ, Gore VA, Hellström I, Hellström KE, Jacobs E, Marsden CH. Pimm MV, Simmonds RG, Smith W. Anti-tumor properties of vindesine-monoclonal antibody conjugates. Cancer Immunol Immunothera, in press.

15. Nepom GT, Nelson KA, Holbeck SL, Hellström I, Hellström KE. (1984) Induction of immunity to a human tumor marker by in vivo administration of anti-idiotypic antibodies in mice. Proc Natl Acad Sci USA 81:2864.

16. Hellström I, Brankovan V, Hellström KE. IgG antibodies to a human melanoma-associated ganglioside antigen with strong anti-tumor activities. Proc Natl Acad Sci USA, in press.

17. Hellström I, Hellström KE, Yeh M-Y. (1981) Lymphocyte-dependent antibodies to antigen 3.1, a cell surface antigen expressed by a subgroup of human melanomas. Int J Cancer   27:281.

18. Nudelman E, Hakomori S, Kannagi R, Levery S, Yeh, M-Y, Hellström KE, Hellström I. (1982) Characterization of a human melanoma-associated ganglioside antigen defined by a monoclonal antibody. J Biol Chem   257:12752.

19. Garrigues HJ, Tilgen W, Hellström I, Franke W, Hellström KE. (1982) Detection of a human melanoma-associated antigen, p97, in histological sections of primary human melanoma. Int J Cancer 29:511.

20. Hellström I, Garriques HJ, Cabasco L, Mosely GH, Brown JP, Hellström KE. (1983) Studies of a high molecular weight human melanoma-associated antigen.   J Immunol 130:1467.

21. Cerrottini J-C, and Brunner KT. (1974) Cell-mediated cytotoxicity, allograft rejection, and tumor immunity. Adv Immunol 18:67.

22. Julius MH, Simpson E, Herzenberg LA. (1973) A rapid method for the isolation of functinal thymus-derived murine lymphocytes. Eur J Immunol 3:645.

23. Thompson JS, Goeken NE, Brown SA, Rhodes JL. (1982) Phenotype definition of human monocyte/macrophage subpopulations by monoclonal antibodies. II. Distinction of non-T, Non-B natural killer cells (NK) from antigen-presenting stimulating cells in the mixed lymphocyte response (MLR).   American Association for Clinical Histocomp. Testing, 8th Annual Meeting, p A23.

24. Schultz G, Bumol TF, Reisfeld RA (1983) Monoclonal-directed effector cells selectively lyse human melanoma cells in vitro and in vivo. Proc Natl Acad Sci USA 80:5407.

25. Herberman RB (ed) (1980): "Natural cell-mediated immunity against tumors," London: Academic Press.

26. Mule' JJ, Shu S, Schwarz SL, Rosenberg SA (1984) Adoptive immunotherapy of established pulmonary metastases with LAK cells and recombinant Interleukin-1. Science 225:1427.

27. Bernstein ID, Nowinski RC, Tam MR, McMaster B, Houston LL, Clark EA (1980) Monoclonal antibody therapy of mouse leukemia. In Kennett RH, McKearn TG, Bechtol KB (eds): "Monoclonal Antibodies," New York: Plenum Press, p 275.

Monoclonal Antibodies and Cancer Therapy, pages 165–172
© 1985 Alan R. Liss, Inc.

DESTRUCTION OF HUMAN TUMORS BY IgG2a MONOCLONAL
ANTIBODIES AND MACROPHAGES[1]

Dorothee Herlyn, Michael Lubeck, Zenon Steplewski,
and Hilary Koprowski

The Wistar Institute of Anatomy and Biology,
Philadelphia, Pennsylvania 19104

ABSTRACT   Ten murine monoclonal antibodies (MAbs) of
IgG2a isotype and one MAb of IgG3 isotype inhibited
growth of human tumors implanted in nude mice,
whereas MAbs of IgG1, IgG2b, IgM, and IgA isotypes were inefficient. The ability of IgG2a MAbs to
inhibit tumor growth in nude mice strongly correlated
with their reactivity in antibody-dependent
macrophage-mediated cytotoxicity (ADMC) assays. IgG2a
MAbs that were inactive in vivo were also unreactive
in these assays in vitro. The number of antibody
binding sites per tumor cell was significantly higher
for tumoricidal MAbs as compared to unreactive MAbs.
Based on the correlation between tumoricidal activities of MAbs in vivo, MAb isotype and reactivity
in ADMC assays in vitro, we have developed procedures
for selection early after fusion of hybridomas
secreting MAbs with tumoricidal potential in vivo.
In another approach to enhance the availability of
tumoricidal MAbs, we isolated hybridoma variant cells
that had switched from IgG1 to IgG2a MAb production
but that had retained the same idiotype.
    Analogous to murine macrophages, human macro-
phages were shown to lyse tumor targets in the presence of mouse IgG2a MAbs. The isolation of

[1]This work was supported by grants CA-25874,
CA-21124, and CA-10815 from the National Cancer Institute
and the National Institutes of Health.

macrophages with Fc receptors for mouse IgG2a MAbs
from human tumors further implicated these cells as
effector cells that mediated immunotherapeutic
effects of IgG2a MAb 17-1A administered to gastrointestinal cancer patients. ADMC reactivity of fresh
human peripheral blood monocytes was significantly
lower as compared to macrophages but could be
enhanced by treatment of monocytes with γ-interferon.
Murine IgG2a and IgG3 MAbs both bound to the same Fc
binding proteins (68-72,000 daltons) as human IgG1.

INTRODUCTION

The successful application of murine monoclonal
antibodies (MAbs) in the immunotherapy of human tumors
transplanted to mice (1-7) has encouraged the use of a
similar approach in the treatment of cancer patients
(8-12). In the present paper we summarize our studies on
the various factors that play a role in the tumoricidal
effects mediated by MAbs. These studies have greatly
enhanced the availability of MAbs with tumoricidal potential. The identification of the effector cell mediating
MAb-dependent tumor destruction has opened new approaches
to tumor therapy using MAbs in combination with poten-
tiators of effector mechanisms.

RESULTS

MAbs of IgG2a and IgG3 Isotype Inhibit Human Tumor Growth
in Nude Mice.

The effect of MAbs of various isotypes on growth of
human tumors transplanted to nude (nu/nu) mice was tested
as previously described (1). Nine MAbs of IgG2a isotype
and one MAb of IgG3 isotype inhibited tumor growth,
whereas 23 MAbs of other isotypes (IgG1, IgG2b, IgM, and
IgA) were found to be ineffective (3). IgG2a MAbs 17-1A
and GA-733, with binding specificity to tumors of the
gastrointestinal tract, effectively inhibited growth of
colon carcinomas in nude mice even when the MAbs were
first administered 6 to 7 days following tumor inoculation (3, 7).

Tumor Growth Inhibition by IgG2a and IgG3 MAbs in Nude
Mice Is Probably Mediated by Macrophages.

Complement depletion of nude mice by cobra venom
factor had no effect on tumor suppression by IgG2a MAb.
The role of T cells as effector cells was virtually excluded since the MAbs inhibited tumor growth in athymic
nude mice. The role of killer (K) cells as effector
cells was also unlikely, for although K cell activity in
adult nude mice is high, the MAb inhibited tumor growth
in 10- to 12-day-old nude mice, spleens of which showed
no K cell activity. Furthermore, treatment of adult nude
mice with anti-interferon serum, which suppresses K cell
activity, did not affect inhibition of tumor growth by
MAb. On the other hand, macrophages were strongly incri-
minated as effector cells because treatment of nude mice
with silica abolished the tumoricidal effect of MAb (3).
Murine peritoneal macrophages, elicited by thioglycolate
or stimulated by the $\beta(1-3)$ glucan lentinan, effectively
lysed human tumor cells in culture in the presence of
either IgG2a or IgG3 MAbs (3, 13, 14).

Inhibition of Human Tumor Growth by IgG2a MAbs Correlates
with Antibody Density on Tumor Cells.

Four of eight anti-melanoma MAbs inhibited growth of
these tumors in nude mice and all four antibodies reacted
in antibody-dependent macrophage-mediated cytotoxicity
(ADMC) assays in vitro. The MAbs that were inactive in
vivo were also unreactive in these assays in vitro. The
number of antibody binding sites per cell on the tumor
cell surface was significantly higher for tumoricidal
MAbs ($1.2-5.4 \times 10^6$) as compared to unreactive MAbs
($0.03-0.3 \times 10^6$). On the other hand, the percentage of
tumor cells binding the MAb and the binding affinity to
these cells were the same for the two groups of MAbs.
Also, tumoricidal and non-tumoricidal MAbs bound with
similar affinity and antibody density to Fc receptors on
macrophages. The importance of the number of antibody
sites on the tumor cell surface for tumor destruction by
MAbs was confirmed by the demonstration of tumoricidal
effects of mixtures of MAbs that were by themselves not
tumoricidal (6).

Selection of Human Tumor Growth-Inhibiting MAbs.

Hybridomas secreting IgG2a MAbs with binding specificities for human tumor cells were selected in radioimmunoassay (RIA), and then tested for reactivity in ADMC
assays. Using these procedures, we obtained two MAbs
that specifically inhibited the growth of colon carcinoma
in nude mice from a total of 1342 hybridoma cultures
obtained from mice immunized with tumor cells of the
gastrointestinal tract (7). In another approach to
enhance the availability of tumoricidal MAbs, we isolated
by cloning at limiting dilution (15) hybridoma variant
cells that have switched from IgG1 to IgG2a MAb production. In addition to the IgG2a-producing variant cells,
IgG2b-producing cells were also obtained. (These studies
were performed in collaboration with G. Spira and M.
Scharff, Albert Einstein College, New York, NY, and A.
Radbruch, University of Cologne, F.R.G.) The variant
immunoglobulins had retained the idiotype of the parental
IgG1 MAb as demonstrated with anti-idiotypic antisera and
exhibited the same binding specificity restricted to
gastrointestinal carcinomas. Furthermore, they bound
with similar affinities to the monosialoganglioside antigen expressed on these tumors. On the other hand, the
IgG2a variant MAb exhibited the highest ADMC reactivity
mediated by either human monocytes or murine macrophages,
and only the IgG2a MAb inhibited the growth of colorectal
carcinomas in nude mice (Table 1).

TABLE 1

IMMUNOLOGICAL PROPERTIES OF IgG1 MAb AND ITS
CLASS-SWITCH VARIANTS

Parameter studied	MAb		
	19-9-γ1	19-9-γ2b	19-9-γ2a
Antibody affinity[a] (X10^7 M^{-1})	~ 7.4	~ 9.7	~ 5.6
Binding specificity	GI[b] tumors	GI tumors	GI tumors
ADMC reactivity (% specific lysis) mediated by:[c]			
human monocytes	15.0	12.5	42.5
murine macrophages	53.3	23.3	63.3
Effect on colon tumor growth in nude mice	None	None	Inhibition

[a] Scatchard analysis (16) with tumor targets.
[b] GI = gastrointestinal
[c] For Methods, see refs. 3 and 17.

Interactions of IgG2a MAbs with Human Monocytes and Macrophages.

We have shown that IgG2a and IgG3 MAbs effectively lyse human tumor targets in conjunction with peripheral blood monocytes (13, 17). The ADMC reactivity of monocytes as well as the expression of Fc receptors for IgG2a MAbs was significantly increased following prolonged in vitro cultivation (17) or by treatment of monocytes with interferon-γ (100 U/ml). Human macrophages isolated from tumor tissues also exhibited ADMC reactivities. Competitive binding inhibition studies using ^{125}I-labeled murine IgG2a and IgG3 and human IgG1 antibodies indicated that all antibodies bind to the same Fc receptor (68-72,000 daltons) on human monocytes. Furthermore, the three types of antibodies showed equally high binding affinities for monocyte Fc receptors. (association contants: $2.4-13.9 \times 10^8$ M^{-1}).

DISCUSSION

Our studies on the tumoricidal effects of MAbs in experimental in vitro and in vivo models have important implications for the immunotherapeutic application of MAbs in cancer patients. The demonstration that MAbs of predominantly IgG2a isotype inhibit human tumor growth in nude mice has served to focus our investigations designed to obtain a large panel of MAbs for immunotherapy of human tumors. Thus, hybridoma cells secreting IgG2a MAbs with tumoricidal activity both in vitro and in vivo in nude mice could be easily selected either by RIA at an early time after fusion (7) or by isolation of hybridoma variant cells that have switched from IgG1 to IgG2a MAb production.

The identification of the macrophage as the cell mediating MAb-dependent tumor destruction in mice initiated our investigations on the interactions of human monocytes and macrophages with murine MAbs. Murine MAbs of IgG2a and IgG3 isotypes bound to the same Fc binding protein as human IgG1. In addition, murine IgG2a and IgG3 MAbs showed high affinity binding to monocyte Fc receptors comparable to that observed for the human IgG1 Fc receptor interaction. Interestingly, the binding affinity of murine IgG2a and IgG3 MAbs for human monocyte

Fc receptors exceeded the affinity reported for the
interaction of MAbs of these isotypes with the Fc receptors on murine macrophages (14, 18).

The immunotherapeutic efficacy of IgG2a anti-
colorectal carcinoma MAb 17-1A documented in some
patients with gastrointestinal cancers (11, 12) emphasizes the potential usefulness of IgG2a MAbs for immunotherapeutic approaches in cancer patients.

The activation for ADMC of murine macrophages by
lentinan (14) or human monocytes by interferon-γ treatment suggests other immunotherapeutic approaches
involving the combination of MAbs with these macrophage
activators.

REFERENCES

1. Herlyn D, Steplewski Z, Herlyn M, Koprowski H
    (1980). Inhibition of colorectal carcinoma tumor
    growth in nude mice by monoclonal antibody. Cancer
    Res 40:717.
2. Trowbridge IS, Domingo DL (1981). Anti-transferrin
    receptor monoclonal antibody and toxin-antibody con-
    jugates affect growth of human tumor cells. Nature
    294:171.
3. Herlyn D, Koprowski H (1982). IgG2a monoclonal anti-
    bodies inhibit human tumor growth through interac-
    tion with effector cells. Proc Natl Acad Sci USA
    79:4761.
4. Shouval D, Shafritz DA, Zurawski VR, Isselbacher KJ,
    Wands JR (1982). Immunotherapy in nude mice of human
    hepatoma using monoclonal antibodies against hepati-
    tis B virus. Nature 298:567.
5. Bumol TF, Wang QC, Reisfeld RA, Kaplan NO (1983).
    Monoclonal antibody and an antibody-toxin conjugate
    to a cell surface proteoglycan of melanoma cells
    suppress in vivo tumor growth. Proc Natl Acad Sci
    USA 80:529.
6. Herlyn D, Powe J, Ross AH, Herlyn M, Koprowski H
    (1985). Inhibition of human tumor growth by IgG2a
    monoclonal antibodies correlates with antibody den-
    sity on tumor cells. J Immunol, in press.

7. Herlyn D, Herlyn M, Ross AH, Ernst C, Atkinson B, Koprowski H (1984). Efficient selection of human tumor growth-inhibiting monoclonal antibodies. J Immunol Meth 73:157.

8. Nadler LM, Stashenko P, Hardy R, Kaplan WD, Button LN, Kufe DW, Antman KH, Schlossman SF (1980). Serotherapy of a patient with a monoclonal antibody directed against a human lymphoma-associated antigen. Cancer Res 40:3147.

9. Miller RA, Maloney DG, Warnke R, Levy R (1982). Treatment of B-cell lymphoma with monoclonal anti-idiotype antibody. N Engl J Med 306:517.

10. Dillman RO, Shawler DL, Sobol RE, Collins HA, Beau-Rega JC, Wormsley SB, Royston I (1982). Murine monoclonal antibody therapy in two patients with chronic lymphocytic leukemia. Blood 59:1036.

11. Sears HF, Mattis J, Herlyn D, Atkinson B, Ernst C, Steplewski Z, Koprowski H (1982). Phase I clinical trial of monoclonal antibody in treatment of gastrointestinal tumors. Lancet I:762.

12. Sears HF, Herlyn D, Steplewski Z, Koprowski H (1984). Effects of monoclonal antibody immunotherapy on patients with gastrointestinal adenocarcinoma. J Biol Resp Mod 3:138.

13. Herlyn D, Herlyn M, Steplewski Z, Koprowski H (1985). Monoclonal anti-human tumor antibodies of six isotypes in cytotoxic reactions with human and murine effector cells. Cell Immunol, in press.

14. Herlyn D, Kaneko Y, Aoki T, Powe J, Koprowski H (1985). Monoclonal antibody-dependent macrophage-mediated cytotoxicity against human tumors is stimulated by lentinan. GANN (Japan J. Cancer Res.), in press.

15. Müller CE, Rajewski K (1983). Isolation of immunoglobulin class switch variants from hybridoma lines secreting anti-idiotype antibodies by sequential sublining. J Immunol 131:877.

16. Scatchard G (1949). The attraction of proteins for small molecules and ions. Ann NY Acad Sci 51:660.

17. Steplewski Z, Lubeck MD, Koprowski H (1983). Human macrophages armed with murine immunoglobulin G2a antibodies to tumors destroy human cancer cells. Science 221:865.

18. Diamond B, Yelton DE (1981). A new Fc receptor on mouse macrophages binding IgG3. J Exp Med 153:514.

Monoclonal Antibodies and Cancer Therapy, pages 173–191
© **1985 Alan R. Liss, Inc.**

APPROACHES FOR IMMUNOTHERAPY OF MALIGNANT
MELANOMA WITH MONOCLONAL ANTIBODIES

Ralph A. Reisfeld
Gregor Schulz
David A. Cheresh

Scripps Clinic and Research Foundation
La Jolla, California 92037

ABSTRACT

Three antigens, a chondroitin sulfate proteoglycan, and disialogangliosides GD_2 and GD_3, are preferentially expressed on human melanoma cells and as such provide excellent targets for tumor destruction by specific monoclonal antibodies. This was demonstrated by effective destruction of established melanoma tumors in nude mice with injection of Mab 9.2.27 together with effector cells with NK activity. The proteoglycan antigen defined by Mabs 9.2.27 and 155.8 has distinct antigen epitopes on both the intact molecule of >400 KDa and on its 250 KDa core glycoprotein. Studies on biosynthesis suggest two pathways of intracellular transport being regulated in part by a low-pH mechanism in intra Golgi vesicles. Both ganglioside antigens were shown to be involved in binding of melanoma cells to substratum, and adhesion plaques remaining after removal of tumor cell monolayers from glass coverslips contained relatively large amounts of GD_2 and GD_3. The two ganglioside antigens also play a role in the attachment of melanoma cells to immobilized fibronectin and appear to interact mainly with the major cell attachment site of this molecule defined by a heptapeptide. Ganglioside GD_3 represents a particularly effective target for tumor cell killing both <u>in vitro</u> by complement-dependent cytotoxicity and ADCC and <u>in vivo</u> by suppressing melanoma tumor growth in nude mice.

INTRODUCTION

The accumulation of a large amount of information indicating that the neoplastic state is accompanied by cell surface changes has led to concerted efforts by an increasing number of investigators to characterize cell surface markers associated with human tumor cells (1). Although such efforts had been ongoing for over twenty years, it was really the discovery of Köhler and Milstein in 1975 (2) that somatic cell hybrids can produce monoclonal antibody which literally revolutionized research dealing with human tumor antigens. This was particularly true for cell surface antigens associated with human melanoma ever since the first report appeared in 1978 (3) which described the use of monoclonal antibody for their serological and functional characterization. In fact, since 1978 investigators working on human melanoma have increasingly pursued not only the serological characterization of a variety of melanoma-associated antigens with monoclonal antibodies but also used these reagents as effective probes to elucidate the structure and function of these tumor cell surface markers (1,4).

In this context, we describe here three antigens preferentially expressed on the surface of human melanoma tumor cells that serve as excellent targets for their destruction and are thus of potential interest for cancer immunotherapy. One of these antigens is a melanoma chondroitin sulfate proteoglycan (MPG) that is specifically recognized by Mab 9.2.27 and the other two are a GD_3 ganglioside and a GD_2 ganglioside recognized by Mabs MB3.6 and 126, respectively. The MPG was thoroughly characterized by a combination of biosynthetic and biochemical investigations using Mab 9.2.27 both as an immunological and molecular probe and was used as a target for effective melanoma cell destruction in vitro and in vivo. The GD_2 and GD_3 gangliosides, whose respective structures are known, were found to be localized in focal adhesion plaques at the interface of melanoma cells and their substratum. We will document here that gangliosides are effective targets for immunotherapy of melanoma since the monoclonal anti-GD_3 antibody MB3.6 proved effective for both in vitro and in vivo destruction of human melanoma tumor cells.

Molecular Characterization of MPG

The molecular structure of MPG is that of a non-cartilagenous type chondroitin sulfate protgeoglycan (CSP) as determined by biochemical and immunochemical analyses using Mab 9.2.27 (5,6). This antibody, as well as Mab 155.8, distinguishes distinct epitopes on both a > 400 KDa CSP and its 250 KDa core protein containing both N- and O-linked oligosaccharides as demonstrated by several lines of evidence (5,6,7).

First, the molecular profile of the molecules reacting with both monoclonal antibodies was clearly indicated when indirect immunoprecipitates obtained by reacting either 9.2.27 or 155.8 with detergent lysates of M21 melanoma cells, intrinsically labeled with [^{3}H] leucine, were analyzed by SDS-PAGE. Characteristic patterns obtained after digestion of the[^{3}H] -leucine labeled lysate with chondroitinase ABC showed only the 250 KDa component. In contrast, SDS-PAGE profiles obtained from immunoprecipitates of detergent lysates from $^{35}SO_4^{-2}$-labeled M21 cells revealed only a component of > 400 KDa, suggesting that the two antibodies each reacted with one sulfated and one non-sulfated component.

The proteoglycan nature of the molecule was further verified when chondroitinase ABC digestion of the same $^{35}SO_4^{-2}$-labeled lysate resulted in almost complete degradation of the sulfated component of > 450 KDa, leaving only a very faint band of 250 KDa. It is quite clear from these data that the sulfated > 400 KDa molecule, recognized by Mabs 9.2.27 and 155.8 is a chondroitin sulfate proteoglycan because of its susceptibility to digestion with chondroitinase ABC and its radiolabeling with $^{35}SO_4^{-2}$ (7).

The identity of the glycosaminoglycans (GAG) associated with the CSP recognized by the two monoclonal antibodies was established by alkaline/borohydride treatment of $^{35}SO_4^{-2}$-labeled immunoprecipitates and subsequent cellulose acetate electrophoresis. Using appropriate standards as controls, i.e. heparin, chondroitin sulfate A/C, chondroitin sulfate B, heparin sulfate and hyaluronic acid, it was shown that the O-linked GAG liberated by β-elimination were exclusively of the chondroitin sulfate A and/or C type (7).

Immunochemical Delineation of Two Distinct Antigenic
Determinants of MPG

Two separate lines of evidence indicated that Mabs
9.2.27 and 155.8 recognized separate and distinct
epitopes. First, sequential immunodepletion analysis of
155.8 and 9.2.27 indicated that 155.8 partially depletes
those molecules recognized by 9.2.27; however, in the
opposite direction, initial depletion with 9.2.27 removes
all molecules that can be recognized by 155.8. These
results combined with data obtained from a series of
binding studies with melanoma cells and tissue that
indicated Mab 155.8 to bind to a more limited extent than
9.2.27, suggest that either 155.8 recognizes a determinant
expressed in smaller numbers on the cell surface or that
there is a difference in affinity constants of the two
antibodies (7). Second, when a competitive binding ELISA
was used to assess whether Mab 155.8 could bind the same
epitope or one vicinal to the determinant defined by
9.2.27, Mab 155.8 was unable to competitively inhibit
peroxidase-conjugated 9.2.27 IgG to bind to its
determinant on M14 melanoma cells. Taken together, the
data from these experiments suggested that the 155.8
determinant is both distinct from and not immediately
proximal to that recognized by Mab 9.2.27 (7).
    Direct experimental evidence was obtained in addition
to that from chondroitin lyase ABC digestions which
suggested that the determinants recognized by Mabs 9.2.27
and 155.8 are expressed on the $>$400 KDa CSP as well as the
250 KDa glycoprotein. Specifically, we demonstrated that
Mabs 9.2.27 and 155.8 recognized the 400 KDa CSP in the
absence of the 250 KDa glycoprotein, clearly ruling out
that the CSP does not actually contain these specific
antigenic determinants, i.e. is simply complexed with the
250 KDa component and merely represents a "passenger" in
immunoprecipitates. Thus, after resolving the two
antigens extracted from melanoma cells by cesium chloride
density centrifugation in the presence of high salt and
detergents, we immunoprecipitated high density CSP alone
from fractions with a density of 1.487 g/liter as well as
the free 250 KDa glycoprotein from fractions with a
density of 1.317 g/liter (7). Further experiments clearly
showed identity of tryptic peptide maps of the CSP and the
250 KDa glycoprotein isolated from preparative SDS-PAGE.
Taken together, these data indicate that both the CSP and
the 250 KDa possess distinct antigenic determinants

recognized by Mabs 9.2.27 and 155.8 and also that the 250 KDa component is clearly the core glycoprotein of the CSP.

Biosynthesis of MPG

By using Mab 9.2.27 in a series of extensive pulse-chase analyses, it was shown that the biosynthesis of MPG proceeds through a 240 KDa component possessing N-linked, high mannose type oligosaccharides that decrease in size to 235 KDa after digestion with endo-β-N-acetylglucosaminidase H (5,6). Almost immediately following the processing of high mannose oligosaccharides to the complex type and addition of O-linked oligosaccharides, a core glycoprotein of 250 KDa is formed and synthesis of chondroitin Δ-di-4 and Δ-di-6 sulfated chains is initiated and these chains are elongated essentially as described for cartilage type proteoglycans (6). In fact, the overall structural organization of the non-cartilage type MPG was found to be quite similar to that of cartilage type proteoglycans which share extensive and characteristic post-translational modification, even though their core protein structures may differ considerably. In this regard, N-asparagine-linked "high mannose" type oligosaccharides are added to the core protein chain co-translationally within the rough endoplasmic reticulum. Such chains are then trimmed and terminally glycosylated with sialic acid to the "complex" form in Golgi-related vesicles. O-glycosylation occurs in the Golgi complex practically simultaneously with initiation and elongation of glycosaminoglycan chains. Finally, the maturation of the completely glycosylated proteoglycan is followed by its transport to the cell surface and exocytosis into the extracellular space (8).

In another study to be described elsewhere (9), we obtained evidence supportive for a hypothesis that compartments in the Golgi with acid pH facilitate regulation of proteoglycan synthesis for human melanoma cells by an effective low-pH mechanism that affects fusion and hence interaction of vesicular compartments in the Golgi apparatus. Apparently, such low-pH mechanisms are responsible for the delivery of mature core glycoprotein molecules to the site of glycosaminoglycan synthesis in Golgi-related vesicles. In addition, we found the addition of chondroitin sulfate side chains not to be required for expression of the 250 KDa core protein on the surface of human melanoma cells. Also, the exocytosis of such core proteins as well as intact MPG, once transported to the cell surface occurs apparently via enzymatic cleavage to an extracellular form with a core protein of 175 KDa.

Evaluation of MPG as a Target for Tumor Cell Destruction

A previous observation from our laboratory indicated that the growth of human melanoma tumors in nude BALB/c mice could be partially suppressed by the simultaneous injection of Mab 9.2.27 and splenocytes of BALB/c mice at the time of tumor cell inoculation (10). We assumed that this antibody-dependent suppression of tumor growth was caused by a cell-mediated mechanism and that at least some of the effector cells involved were those with NK activity since such cells evoke antibody-dependent cellular cytotoxicity (ADCC).

We summarize here some of the highlights of a study described in detail elsewhere (11) that examines this hypothesis. Several experiments were done to determine whether simultaneous injection of Mab 9.2.27 and cell populations with NK activity can cause the eradication of established melanoma tumors (mean volume 90 mm^3) in nude mice. Thus, BALB/c nude mice with 2-week old melanoma tumors received a single intravenous injection as follows: 400 ug 9.2.27 IgG; mononuclear BALB/c splenocytes (2 x 10^7); 2 x 10^7 mononuclear splenocytes and 400 ug 9.2.27 IgG. A group of tumor-bearing control mice received no injections. We observed that 7/10 animals injected simultaneously with splenocytes and Mab 9.2.27 were tumor-free four weeks after injection. All other animals treated with either antibody or splenocytes alone exhibited large tumors with the exception of one animal in the group that received only splenocytes. As illustrated in Fig. 1, mice that received only Mab 9.2.27 showed a mean tumor volume that was almost the same as that of control animals whereas tumors of mice that received only effector cells were ~50% smaller. Most interestingly, the mean tumor volume of mice that received 9.2.27 IgG together with effector cells was less than 10% of that of control tumors.

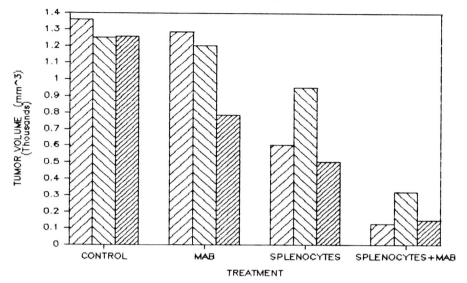

Figure 1:   Effect of Mononuclear Mouse Splenocytes and Mab 9.2.27 on Growth of Established Human Melanoma Tumors in Nude Mice.

Splenocytes were obtained from: 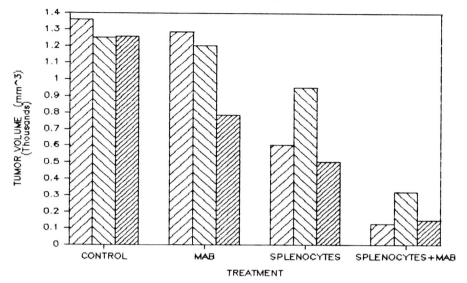 BALB/c mice; BALB/c nude mice bearing human melanoma tumors; BALB/c nude mice. Mean tumor size at onset of the experiment was 90 mm^3 at day 14 after tumor cell inoculation. Control: mice were only injected with tumor cells; MAB: all animals received one i.v. injection of 400 ug Mab 9.2.27; splenocytes: all animals received only one i.v. injection of 2 x 10^7 mononuclear splenocytes; splenocytes + Mab: all animals received simultaneously one i.v. injection of 2 x 10^7 splenocytes and 400 ug Mab 9.2.27. Data are given for results obtained 28 days after antibody and cell injection, i.e. 42 days after tumor inoculation.

Additional experiments were designed to determine whether the observed tumor eradication was possibly due to T cells present in the normal BALB/c splenocytes that are otherwise lacking in nude mice. Apparently, mature T cells are not involved in this phenomenon, since we found that in this case either source of mononuclear splenocytes injected together with Mab 9.2.27 was equally effective in eradicating established melanoma tumors. Mononuclear splenocytes from melanoma tumor bearing BALB/c nude mice also were almost equally effective as effector cells when obtained from either normal or nude mice of BALB/c origin.

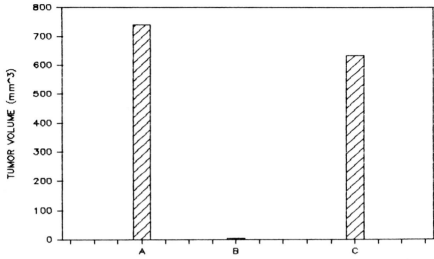

Figure 2:   Evidence for NK Cells as Effectors   in Suppression of Human Melanoma Tumor Growth.
Mean tumor size at the onset of the experiment was 90 mm^3.
A: C57BL/6 nude mice received one i.v. injection of 400 ug Mab 9.2.27; B: C57BL/6 nude mice received simultaneously one i.v. injection of 400 ug Mab 9.2.27 together with 2 x 10^7 splenocytes from C57BL/6 mice; C: C57BL/6 nude mice received the same treatment as in (B), but splenocytes injected were from C57BL/6 beige mice lacking NK cells.

Although mature T cells apparently did not play a major role in the type of tumor cell destruction observed in our experiment, several observations strongly suggested that cells with NK activity are the effector cells involved in this process. In this regard, splenocytes obtained from NK-deficient beige C57BL/6 mice were incapable of inducing tumor regression. Specifically, C57BL/6 nude mice with established human melanoma tumors were injected with 9.2.27 IgG, alone or together with splenocytes from NK-deficient C57BL/6 mice that carried the homozygous beige mutation. The results obtained are clearly illustrated by Fig. 2. None of ten mice that received normal C57BL/6 splenocytes and 9.2.27 IgG showed any tumor growth 4 weeks after injection. In contrast, 8/9 mice that received splenocytes from C57BL/6 bg/bg mice

showed large tumors (11). Since beige mice have low NK
activity (12), these data indicate that NK cells play a
key role in the eradication of established human melanoma
tumors in the nude mouse model system.

We determined whether Mab 9.2.27 and effector cells
with NK activity can lyse M21 human melanoma cells, since
it is well known that NK cells perform antibody-dependent
cell mediated cytolysis (ADCC) in vitro (12). For this
purpose, BALB/c mononuclear splenocytes, mixed with M21
melanoma cells were assayed for cytolytic activity in
^{51}Cr release assays, either in the absence or presence of
Mab 9.2.27. Effector cell lysed NK-sensitive YAC-1 target
cells or caused 25% cytolysis of melanoma cells in the
absence of Mab 9.2.27 as compared to 38% in the presence
of this antibody. In addition, removal of NK cells by
treatment of splenocytes with anti-asialo GM_1 markedly
reduced cytotoxicity, both in the absence and presence of
Mab 9.2.27. Effector cells treated in this manner also
failed to lyse YAC-1 target cells, indicating that NK
activity was eliminated by this treatment. Other
antibodies specific for murine NK cells, i.e. anti-Qa5 and
anti-NK1.1 (13,14) effectively abolished any cytolytic
effect of the effector splenocytes on M21 melanoma cells
and YAC-1 target cells. C57BL/6 effector cells were found
equally effective as BALB/c effector cells in mediating
cytotoxicity against M21 melanoma cells. Treatment of the
C57BL/6 effector cells with anti-Qa5 and anti-NK1.1, but
not with anti-Lyt 6.2, abolished their cytolytic activity
against YAC-1 and M21 cells, regardless of the presence of
Mab 9.2.27. Finally, C57BL/6 bg/bg effector cells that
have little if any NK activity failed to mediate any
efficient cytotoxicity in the ^{51}Cr release assay (11).

Our results thus strongly imply that NK cells play a
major role in antibody-dependent and antibody-independent
cytolysis of human melanoma cells. Furthermore, our in
vivo data also lead us to conclude that the cells chiefly
responsible for tumor elimination are most likely NK cells
since they are present in splenocytes of T cell-deficient
nude mice. This conclusion is further strengthened by the
fact that splenocytes were ineffective in suppressing
tumor growth when obtained either from NK-deficient beige
mice or from BALB/c mice treated with anti-asialo GM_1
antiserum, a treatment known to eliminate cells with NK
activity.

The fact that injection of Mab 9.2.27 by itself into tumor-bearing nude mice that have plenty of NK cells is insufficient to cause tumor rejection is also interesting if one considers eventual application of our regimen for the treatment of melanoma patients. At this time, we believe that antibody and effector cells have to be injected simultanenously so that the antibody can bind to the effectors, possibly via Fc receptors, and thereby "arm" them. It seems likely that this antibody effector cell interaction targets the effector cells to the tumor in a more effective way. It is, however, important to stress that the involvement of cells with NK activity in antibody-mediated tumor rejection in our studies does not at all preclude the participation of other cell types, e.g. neutrophils and macrophages which we also observed in preliminary experiments to be attracted to the tumor site, particularly at later stages of tumor destruction. It is also quite likely that the sequence of events in antibody-mediated tumor destruction may vary in different tumor systems. In this regard, we observed resistance of lung cancer cells to NK lysis in vitro (data not shown) and several reports have demonstrated that macrophages effectively mediate antibody-dependent cytotoxicity against colorectal tumor cells (15,16).

Although our nude mouse model with human melanoma tumors could be regarded as not optimally suited to predict the outcome of clinical studies, we conclude that the results from the experiments outlined here at least suggest that simultaneous injection of effector cells with a suitable monoclonal antibody specifically directed to a melanoma cell surface antigen may ultimately prove effective for tumor elimination in melanoma patients. Obviously, this contention remains to be proven by the results of clinical trials.

The Role of Disialogangliosides GD_2 and GD_3 in Interactions of Melanoma Cells with Substratum

Monoclonal antibodies 126 (IgM) and MB3.6 (IgG3) were used in a series of experiments designed to localize gangliosides GD_2 and GD_3 on the melanoma cell surface and to assess whether these molecules are found in focal adhesion plaques at the interface of cells and their substratum. In initial tests, we established the

ganglioside profile of ^{3}H-glucosamine labeled melanoma
cells and their substrate-attached materials.
Specifically, these experiments involved the treatment of
monolayers of human melanoma cells, grown on either
plastic tissue culture dishes or glass coverslips, with
phosphate-buffered saline (PBS) containing EDTA (1.4
mg/ml) and KCl (0.16 mg/ml) at room temperature for 5-10
minutes. Once microscopic examination indicated removal
of all cells, gangliosides were extracted with
chloroform/methanol from focal adhesion plaques as well as
intact melanoma cells, it was found by thin layer
chromatography of these extracts and antibody overlay with
Mabs 126 and MB3.6 and autoradiography that relatively
large amounts of GD_2 and GD_3 were present in both the
cells and their adhesion plaques. This was the case for
M21 melanoma cells whereas another melanoma cell line,
Melur, did produce large amounts of GD_3 but only minor
quantities of GD_2. At any rate, the gangliosides
deposited onto the substrate compared readily to those
associated with the melanoma cells themselves (17).

   The specificity of monoclonal antibodies 126 and
MB3.6 was indicated when each antibody reacted directly
with GD_2 and GD_3, respectively on TLC plates containing
total ganglioside extracts from either neuroblastoma or
melanoma cell lines. Mab 126 also specifically
immunostained authentic GD_2 which migrated in the
identical position on TLC as the GD_2 component detected by
the antibody in the gangliosides extract. The same was
true for Mab MB3.6 and GD_3 (17) which was visualized as a
doublet as observed previously (18), a phenomenon
apparently caused by the expression of identical sugar
moities on ceramides containing fatty acids of variable
length.

   The specificity of Mabs 126 and MB3.6 for ganglioside
GD_2 GalNacβ-4(NeuAcα2→8NeuAcα2→3)Gal β1→4Glc-ceramide
was further demonstrated by the specific inhibition
produced by this ganglioside standard in the binding of
Mab 126 to melanoma cells. In this same type of assay,
the binding of Mab MB3.6 to melanoma cells was
specifically inhibited only by the authentic ganglioside
GD_3 NeuAcβ2 → 8 NeuAcα2-3Galβ1-4Glc-ceramide (17). Since
the sole structural difference between these two
gangliosides is the terminal Gal Nac on GD_2, it appears
that the terminal sugars of these molecules play a

decisive role in the antigenic determinants defined by these antibodies.

Indirect immunofluorescence assays with Mabs 126 and MB3.6 clearly distinguished the topographic distribution of GD_2 and GD_3 when melanoma cells M21 and Melur were grown on glass coverslips.   Actually, as shown in Fig. 3, the immunofluorescence staining pattern of Mab 126 on Melur cells indicates that GD_2 is mainly associated with the plasma membrane. It is apparent from Fig. 3 that GD_2 is also localized in microspike projections emanating from the cell surface and extending toward other cells as well as the glass coverslip substratum. The topographical distribution of GD_3 on Melur cells is one of clusters recognized by Mab MB3.6 on the surface of > 90% of these cells. When stained with both antibodies, M21 melanoma cells also showed prominent surface staining of GD_2 (>100% positive) and > 80% positive for GD_3 (data not shown). Moreover, gangliosides GD_2 and GD_3 could be equally well localized with the two monoclonal antibodies by indirect immunofluorescence analysis of adhesion plaques that remained after melanoma cells M21 and Melur on glass coverslips had been removed by treatment with EDTA. Fig. 3 depicts typical adhesion plaques containing GD_2 localized by Mab 126. Similar data were obtained with Mab 3.6 specifically identifying GD_3 in adhesion plaques.   In contrast, Class I histocompatibility antigens could not be detected in these same adhesion plaques by Mab W6/32 that is known to react with the common framework determinants of these intrinsic membrane antigens (17).

The Role of Disialogangliosides GD_2 and GD_3 in Attachment of Melanoma Cells to Fibronectin.

Based on our data suggesting that disialogangliosides GD_2 and GD_3 are involved in the attachment of melanoma cells at the cell substrate interphase as well as reports from several investigators indicating that cell surface-associated gangliosides interact with fibronectin during cell adhesion, we proceeded with a follow-up study examining the binding of human melanoma cells to fibronectin. The highlights of this study, to be published elswhere (19), were that Mabs 126 and MB3.6 not only can inhibit the attachment of melanoma cells to fibronectin but specifically accomplish this via its

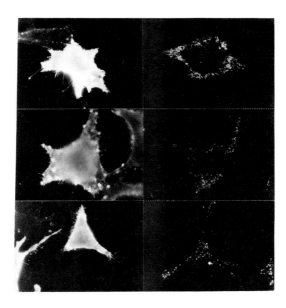

Figure 3:   Detection of GD_2 on human melanoma cells by indirect immunofluorescence. Melur melanoma cells (2 x 10^4) were grown on coverslips, fixed, incubated with Mab 126, and then stained by immunofluorescence (left panel). Adhesion plaques that appeared after removal of attached cells from the substrata by PBS, containing EDTA and KCl are shown in the right panel.

principal cell attachment site specified by a heptapeptide, glycyl-L-arginyl-glycyl-L-aspartyl-L-seryl-L-prolyl-L-cysteine (GRGDSPC) (20). This inhibition, which occurs mainly in the early phases of melanoma cell adhesion to immobilized fibronectin, is quite specific since it cannot be mediated by monoclonal antibodies directed against either protein or carbohydrate epitopes of such major melanoma cell surface antigens as HLA antigens, a chondroitin sulfate proteoglycan, a sialylated glycoprotein and a neutral glycolipid. It is also apparent from our studies that cell surface bound antibody does not interfere with cellular functions unrelated to the adhesion to fibronectin since melanoma cell adhesion to tissue culture treated plastic was not affected by pretreatment with Mabs 126 and MB3.6 (19). Of particular interest was the finding that addition of Mab MB3.6 to melanoma cells that were preattached to immobilized fibronectin caused significant cell rounding and detachment from the substrate, similar to that observed previously by Dippold et al. (21) with Mab R24 (IgG3) directed to GD_3. Cell viability remained high, i.e. > 95%, under these conditions and other Mabs such as 9.2.27 directed to MPG failed to produce this effect even when used at much higher concentrations than Mab 3.6 directed to GD_3. Also of interest, especially in view of recent reports indicating the existence of cell surface glycoprotein receptors for fibronectin (22,23,24), was our observation that melanoma cell attachment to fibronectin was partially sensitive to treatment with trypsin (19). These results taken together with our data indicating only partial inhibition of adhesion of melanoma cells to fibronectin by our anti-GD_2 and anti-GD_3 antibodies suggest that these gangliosides may act synergistically with glycoprotein receptors of fibronectin.

Our findings that disialogangliosides GD_2 and GD_3 represent major cell surface markers of human melanoma cells, their role in the interactions of cells with their substratum, their presence in focal adhesion plaques, and their involvement in adhesion of melanoma cells to fibronectin led us to evaluate the potential use of the anti-GD_3 antibody MB3.6 for immunotherapy of human melanoma. Although these investigations are as yet mainly preliminary and will be published in detail elsewhere, data obtained thus far clearly indicate Mab MB3.6 to be quite effective in melanoma tumor cell destruction in vitro and in vivo, either by mechanisms involving antibody-dependent cellular cytotoxicity (ADCC) and/or complement-mediated cytotoxicity. Specifically, Mab 3.6 could readily lyse (65-100%) a variety of human melanoma cell lines in the presence of human complement and also was effective in ADCC, inducing from 50-100% cytolysis with human peripheral blood leukocytes as effector cells obtained either from normal individuals or melanoma patients. Significantly, multiple intra-peritoneal injections of MB3.6 at dose levels ranging from 40-100 ug into athymic (nu/nu) mice that we initially injected subcutaneously with human melanoma cells either prevented the establishment of tumors or evoked the destruction of established tumors in the vast majority of the animals. These results, although preliminary, are sufficiently encouraging to develop optimal treatment modalities, possibly including the use of effector cells suitably "armed" with Mab MB3.6.

DISCUSSION

Combinations of immunochemical analyses, pulse-chase biosynthetic studies and enzymatic digestion experiments demonstrated that Mab 9.2.27 recognizes a non-cartilage chondroitin sulfate proteoglycan that is preferentially expressed on the surface of human melanoma cells. Furthermore, data from a number of experiments indicated that this antibody and Mab 155.8 recognize two distinct and separate antigenic determinants that are expressed on both the 250 KDa core glycoprotein and the intact > 400 KDa melanoma proteoglycan (MPG). Data from several experiments defined the chemical nature of the sulfated glycosaminoglycan side chains and direct evidence was obtained indicating that Mabs 9.2.27 and 155.8 recognize the MPG in the absence of the 250 KDa core glycoprotein. These results clearly rule out the possibility that the MPG does not contain the antigenic determinants recognized by the two Mabs and is complexed with the 250 KDa glycoprotein, i.e. representing merely a "passenger" in immunoprecipitates. Data from extensive pulse-chase analyses with Mab 9.2.27 can be interpreted to indicate that the biosynthesis of MPG proceeds through a 240 KDa component having N-linked, high mannose oligosaccharides which almost immediately after processing of these sugars to the complex type and addition of O-linked oligosaccharides forms a core glycoprotein of 250 KDa that proceeds to the intact proteoglycan after glycosamino-glycan chain initiation and elongation. Observations from a separate set of experiments designed to follow intracellular transport and cell surface expression of MPG and its core glycoprotein support the hypothesis that acidic compartments in the Golgi facilitate regular proteoglycan synthesis of human melanoma cells by an effective low-pH mechanism that affects vesicular interaction in the Golgi apparatus.

It is apparent from the data presented here that the MPG defined by Mab 9.2.27 represent an effective target for this antibody and simultaneously injected effector cells, i.e. mononuclear splenocytes with NK activity, to effectively destroy human melanoma tumors implanted into nude mice. It is even more encouraging that this can be achieved with relatively large established tumors by a single intravenous injection of effector cells and monoclonal antibody. With regard to the type of effector cells involved, we concentrated our efforts to assess whether cells with NK activity play an important role and we actually have shown this to be the case; however, we do not wish to imply at all that other effector cells, i.e. macrophages do not play a significant role in tumor destruction. We simply have not investigated the role of macrophages thus far even though others (15,16) have demonstrated that these cells effectively mediate ADCC against human colorectal tumor cells. As far as the usefulness of Mab 9.2.27 and patients' effector cells for therapy of human melanoma is concerned, it is only fair to caution that this will indeed require more experimental studies as well as a number of clinical trials. This is definitely the case even though the effectiveness of this very same antibody clone, given by our laboratory to investigators at the National Cancer Institute's Frederick Cancer Research Facility, was throughly evaluated in Phase I clinical trials, involving more than 20 patients with advanced stages of malignant melanoma and very heavy tumor burden. The studies indicated that although intravenous injection of the murine Mab 9.2.27 did not cause any serious health problems, it also failed to produce any significant reduction in tumor burden. One positive note was the excellent and specific localization of Mab 9.2.27 in tumor biopsies of the patients that had been treated. It should be pointed out that simultaneous injections of antibody and effector cells were never tested in these phase I clinical trials. However, one has to voice some caution concerning the application of this type of treatment in clinical trials since Mab 9.2.27, which does not fix complement but reacts in ADCC with murine effector cells (10,11) was somewhat less effective in this assay with human peripheral blood leukocytes. In fact, in our hands, this antibody evokes from 15-20% ADCC only with certain melanoma target cells and effector cells from some selected normal individuals.

In this regard, Mab MB3.6, directed to the disialoganglioside GD_3 which is preferentially expressed on many human melanoma cells seems a better candidate for immunotherapy than 9.2.27. Specifically, Mab MB3.6 is of IgG3 isotype, fixes complement, is active in ADCC, and proved indeed most effective in both of these in vitro reactions by quite effectively killing melanoma tumor cells. It is also a definite plus that MB3.6 effectively lyses cells in the presence of human complement and causes extensive cytolysis in ADCC with human peripheral blood leukocytes from either normal donors or melanoma patients. In fact, Mab MB3.6 injected without effector cells also appears to be more effective than 9.2.27 for inhibition of human melanoma tumor growth in nude mice and destruction of established tumors. Obviously, more experiments are required to definitely prove the efficacy of Mab MB3.6 in tumor cell destruction and the simultaneous injection of effector cells together with this antibody has still to be tested. Nevertheless, it appears certain that monoclonal antibodies to gangliosides preferentially expressed on human melanoma cells are excellent candidates to be critically evaluated for their efficacy in tumor immunotherapy in the very near future.

ACKNOWLEDGEMENTS

The authors wish to thank Ms. Lisa K. Staffileno, Diane Sander, and Regina Derango for excellent technical assistance. Special appreciation is extended to Ms. Bonnie Pratt Filiault for her excellent secretarial assistance.

This work was supported by a grant from the National Institutes of Health CA 28420. G.S. was supported by Deutsche Forschungsgemeinschaft Grant 1-3-Schu 512/1-1 and D.A.C. is supported by NIH Grant CA 07544.

This is Scripps Publication No. Imm-3826.

REFERENCES

1. Reisfeld RA, Harper JR, Bumol TF (1984). Human tumor antigens defined by monoclonal antibodies. In Atassi MZ (ed): "Critical Reviews in Immunlogy," Boca Raton: p 27.
2. Kohler G, Milstein C (1975). Continued cultures of fused cells secreting antibody of predefined specificity. Nature 256:495.
3. Koprowski H, Steplewski Z, Herlyn D, Herlyn M (1978). Study of antibodies against human melanoma produced by somatic cell hybrids. Proc Natl Acad Sci (USA) 75:3405.
4. Reisfeld RA (1985). Monoclonal antibodies as probes for the molecular structure and biological function of melanoma-associated antigens. In Sell S, Reisfeld RA (eds): "Cancer Markers III, " Clifton: Humana Press, in press.

5. Bumol TF, Reisfeld RA (1982). Unique glycoprotein-proteolycan complex defined by monoclonal antibody on human melanoma cells. Proc Natl Acad Sci (USA) 79:1245.

6. Bumol TF, Walker LE, Reisfeld RA (1984). Biosynthetic studies of proteoglycans in human melanoma cells with a monoclonal antibody to a core glycoprotein of chondroitin sulfate proteoglycans. J Biol Chem 259:12733.

7. Harper JR, Bumol TF, Reisfeld RA (1984). Characterization of monoclonal antibody 155.8 and partial characterization of its proteoglycan antigen on human melanoma cells. J Immunol 132:2096.

8. Hascall VC, Haskall GK (1981). Proteoglycans. In Hay ED (ed): "Cell Biology of Extracellular Matrix," New York: Plenum Press, p 39.

9. Harper JR, Reisfeld RA, Quaranta V (1985). Ammonium chloride modifies the expression of a human melanoma cell-asociated proteoglycan (MPG) and its core protein. Science, submitted.

10. Schulz G, Bumol TF, Reisfeld RA (1983). Monoclonal antibody directed effector cells selectively lyse human melanoma cells in vitro and in vivo. Proc Natl Acad Sci (USA) 80:5407.

11. Schulz G, Staffileno LK, Reisfeld RA, Dennert G (1985). Eradication of established human melanoma tumors in nude mice by antibody-directed effector cells. J Exp Med, submitted.

12. Herberman RB, ORtaldo JR (1981). Natural killer cells: Their role in defense against disease. Science 214:24.

13. Jacobsen JB, Hammerling GJ, Hammerling U, Koo GC (1980). Antigenic profile of human natural killer cells. J Immunol 125:1003.

14. Lotzova ES, Pollack S (1983). Prevention of rejection of allogeneic bone marrow transplants by NK1.1 antiserum. Transplantation 35:490.

15. Herlyn D, Koprowski H (1982). IgG2a monoclonal antibodies inhibit human tumor growth through interaction with effector cells. Proc Natl Acad. Sci (USA) 79:4761.

16. Steplewski Z, Lubeck MD, Koprowski H (1983). Human macrophages armed with murine immunoglobulin G2a antibodies to tumors destroy human cancer cells. Science 221:865.

17. Cheresh DA, Harper JR, Schulz G, Reisfeld RA (1984). Localization of the gangliosides GD_2 and GD_3 in adhesion plaques and on the surface of human melanoma cells (1984). Proc Natl Acad Sci (USA) 81:5767.

18. Cheresh DA, Varki AP, Varki NM, Stallcup WB, Levine J, Reisfeld RA (1984). A monoclonal antibody recognizes an O-acetylated sialic acid in a human melanoma-associated ganglioside. J Biol Chem 259:7453.

19. Cheresh DA, Pierschbacher MD, Herzig MA, Reisfeld RA (1985). Disialogangliosides GD_2 and GD_3 are involved in the binding of human melanoma cells to the cell attachment site of fibronectin. J Cell Biol, submitted.

20. Pierschbacher MD, Ruoslahti E (1984). Cell attachment activity of fibronectin can be duplicated by small synthetic fragments of the molecule. Nature 309:30.

21. Dippold WG, Knuth A, zum Bushenfelde KHM (1984). Inhibition of human melanoma cell growth in vitro by monoclonal anti-GD_3 ganglioside antibody. Cancer Res 44:806.

22. Oppenheimer-Marks N, Grinnell F (1984). Calcium ions protect cell-substratum adhesion receptors against proteolysis. Exp Cell Res 152:467.

23. Carter WG, Hakomori S (1981). A new cell surface detergent-insoluble glycoprotein matrix of human and hamster fibroblasts. J Biol Chem 256:6953.

24. Chapman AE (1984). Characterization of a 140 Kd cell surface glycoprotein involved in myoblast adhesion. J Cell Biochem 25:109.

Key Words: Immunotherapy, Melanoma, Molecular Structure, Biosynthesis, Proteoglycan Antigen, Ganglioside Antigens

Monoclonal Antibodies and Cancer Therapy, pages 193–203
© 1985 Alan R. Liss, Inc.

ANTIBODY-DEPENDENT CELLULAR CYTOTOXICITY (ADCC) AGAINST
HUMAN MELANOMA BY HUMAN EFFECTOR CELLS IN COOPERATION
WITH MOUSE MONOCLONAL ANTIBODIES

Ronald B. Herberman*
A. Charles Morgan*
Ralph Reisfeld+
David A. Cheresh+
John R. Ortaldo*

*Biological Therapeutics Branch
Biological Response Modifiers Program, DCT
National Cancer Institute
Frederick, Maryland 21701
and
+Scripps Clinic and Research Foundation
LaJolla, California 97037

ABSTRACT

Phase I clinical trials in patients with malignant
melanoma have been performed with the antimelanoma monoclonal antibody 9.2.27. Upon administration of greater
than 100 mg of antibody, coating of most tumor cells with
high levels of antibody could be consistently achieved.
However, administration of this antibody alone has had
no detectable effect on tumor size. In contrast, a Phase
I clinical trial in melanoma patients with a mouse monoclonal antibody against the GD3 ganglioside has shown
partial regressions of tumors in three of twelve patients.
Studies were, therefore, performed to compare the ability
of these monoclonal antibodies to mediate ADCC with human
effector cells. Purified large granular lymphocytes, with
high levels of NK activity, and purified monocytes were
used as effector cells, with or without pretreatment with
interferon or interleukin 2. MB3.6, a mouse monoclonal
antibody against the GD3 ganglioside, was shown to
induce high levels of ADCC activity upon interaction with
large granular lymphocytes but gave negative results with

monocytes. In contrast, the 9.2.27 monoclonal antibody gave low and less consistent levels of ADCC. Pretreatment of the effector cells with interferon α or interleukin 2 induced a substantial augmentation of ADCC activity with the anti-GD$_3$ antibody. Thus, it appears that large granular lymphocytes are the major effector cells in human peripheral blood for mediation of ADCC with mouse monoclonal antibodies and human tumor target cells. However, a variety of parameters appear to affect the results, including the levels of cytotoxic reactivity of the effector cells, the isotype and other characteristics of the monoclonal antibody and various properties of the target cell lines. Such parameters will need to be carefully evaluated before the promising results from experimental tumor models in mice can be translated into clinically applicable approaches.

Monoclonal antibodies against human tumor associated antigens have considerable potential for the therapy of human cancer. Most monoclonal antibodies, even if highly specific for cancer cells, will be expected to have therapeutic efficacy only when conjugated with toxic agents, e.g. radionuclides, toxins or chemotherapeutic agents. Some murine monoclonal antibodies have been shown to have antitumor effects against human tumors growing in nude mice (1) and clinical trials have been initiated in which a variety of murine monoclonal antibodies have been administered to cancer patients. In most of these clinical trials, little or no effects have been observed with the monoclonal antibodies administered by themselves (e.g. 2, 3). However, some antitumor effects have been observed in patients treated with monoclonal antibodies alone. For example, Houghton, et al. (4) have recently reported the preliminary results of a Phase I clinical trial in melanoma patients, utilizing the mouse monoclonal antibody R24, directed against the GD$_3$ ganglioside. Of twelve patients with metastatic melanoma treated with this antibody, clear partial regression of tumor was observed in three patients. A major challenge is to determine the basis for such positive results. Two main factors would seem to be essential for effective therapy by such monoclonal antibodies: 1) The administered antibodies need to be able to reach the site(s) of tumor growth and to react with most if not all of the tumor cells. 2) The antibodies would need to induce some toxic effects on the tumor cells,

either directly or more likely by interacting with host
components, e.g. complement or effector cells, to result
in cytolysis or growth inhibition.

One of the mouse monoclonal antibodies to human melanoma which has appeared promising in terms of its pattern
of specificity and potential for therapeutic use is 9.2.27,
an IgG2a antibody directed against a 250,000 molecular
weight proteoglycan on the surface of most melanoma cells
and undetectable on most normal or benign tissues (5).
The administration of the 9.2.27 soon after inoculation
of human melanoma cell lines into nude mice has resulted
in inhibition of tumor growth, and the ability of this
antibody to mediate antibody-dependent cellular cytotoxicity (ADCC) in cooperation with host effector cells
has been suggested to be a major component of its anti-
tumor efficacy (1). Recently, a Phase I clinical trial
has been performed with various amounts of 9.2.27, administered intravenously to patients with advanced stages of
melanoma (2). Doses of antibody in excess of 100 mg were
shown to effectively reach the tumor site and to bind to
the surface of most melanoma cells. However, no antitumor
effects were seen in this trial.

The present study was performed to explore one of
the possible factors which may have contributed to the
lack of therapeutic efficacy by this melanoma antibody
in patients with melanoma. In view of the ADCC observed
with 9.2.27 and mouse effector cells (1) and the potential
antitumor benefits to be achieved from such interactions,
we focused on whether this antibody could mediate ADCC
with human effector cells. For comparison, we performed
parallel studies with a rabbit antiserum against human
melanoma and MB3.6, a mouse IgG3 monoclonal antibody
directed against the GD_3 ganglioside (see Reisfeld, this
volume). Several mouse IgG3 monoclonal antibodies to
this glycolipid have been found to mediate strong ADCC,
and, as noted above, one such antibody, R24, has produced
major tumor regressions in a Phase I clinical trial.

Most of the studies were performed with the FeMex
Met II melanoma cell line developed by O. Fodstad, which
has been found to express high levels of the 250,000 dalton
antigen detected by 9.2.27 and which also has a high density of the GD_3 ganglioside. Peripheral blood mononuclear
leukocytes from all donors were tested against this cell
line in the presence of 9.2.27 or the other antibodies.
As shown in Table 1, 9.2.27 produced low levels of ADCC,

at least with the effector cells of some donors, and the
anti-GD$_3$ antibody produced substantially more. The strongest ADCC was observed with the rabbit antimelanoma antibody. To analyze the ADCC in more detail, we evaluated
the nature of the effector cells. Little information is
currently available about the nature of the human effector
cells which mediate ADCC in cooperation with mouse monoclonal antibodies. Herlyn, et al. (this volume) have
strongly suggested that macrophages are the predominant
effector cell for ADCC with mouse monoclonal antibodies;
but in general, K cells, a small subpopulation of lymphocytes which has recently been shown to be included within
the population of large granular lymphocytes (6), have
been shown to account for most ADCC activity between
conventional antisera and tumor target cells. To evaluate
this issue, peripheral blood mononuclear cells from normal
donors were separated by discontinuous peripheral density
gradient centrifugation into LGL-enriched and T cell-enriched fractions, and monocytes were obtained by adherence.
As shown in Table 1, cell populations enriched in LGL had

Table 1.   Antibody-Dependent Cellular Cytotoxicity (ADCC)
           with Anti-Melanoma Monoclonal Antibodies

| Effector Cells[b] | Lytic Units[a] vs. Fe Mex plus Antibody | | | |
	None	MB3.6	9.2.27	Rabbit
PBML	<1	8	2	34
LGL-enriched	21	136	<1	110
T cell-enriched	4	18	<1	39
Monocytes	<1	<1	<1	<1

[a] 6 hour ^{51}Cr release assay with various concentrations of
effector cells. A lytic unit was defined as the number
of effector cells required to give 30% cytotoxicity.
Shown is the number of lytic units per 10^7 effector
cells. The lytic units in the absence of antibody were
subtracted from the total cytotoxicity to give the
levels of ADCC shown here.

[b] Peripheral blood mononuclear leukocytes (PBML) were
separated, after removal of adherent cells on nylon
wool columns, by discontinuous Percoll density gradient
centrifugation. The low density fractions were highly
enriched in large granular lymphocytes (LGL) (>80%),
and the high density fractions were mainly T cells
(>90% OKT3[+] cells). Monocytes were isolated by adherence of PBML to plastic dishes.

high levels of ADCC activity with the anti-GD$_3$ antibody
and with the rabbit antiserum but had minimal effects with
9.2.27. The LGL in the absence of added antibodies also
showed substantial levels of cytotoxicity against the melanoma target cells. This observation fits with previous
findings that LGL account for most NK activity as well as
ADCC against tumor target cells (6). In contrast, monocytes
had no detectable ADCC activity. The T cell-enriched population had low levels of ADCC activity, but this seemed
attributable to contamination by some LGL, since the T cell-
enriched fraction also showed NK activity against K562
target cells, and more vigorous depletion of LGL resulted
in a complete loss of ADCC activity (data not shown).

It is of note that the ADCC observed occurred when
the monoclonal antibodies were added to the assay. The
incubation of target cells with monoclonal antibodies,
washing, and then addition of the coated targets to the
assay resulted in virtually no activity. This was surprising since these are the usual conditions for performing
ADCC experiments, and the rabbit antiserum was quite effective under such conditions. Studies are now in progress
to determine the basis for the apparent requirement for
the presence of the monoclonal antibody during the cytotoxic assay.

The levels of ADCC by LGL were found to vary considerably among normal donors (Table 2). Both the anti-
GD$_3$ monoclonal antibody and the rabbit antiserum induced

Table 2. Variation Among Normal Donors in Levels of LGL-
Mediated ADCC Against FeMex Melanoma Cells

LGL Donor	ADCC (% of non-antibody control in 6 hours)[a]		
	MB3.6	9.2.27	Rabbit
1	1,402	123	9,084
2	662	100	531
3	1,652	756	1,717
4	220	100	1,313
5	418	238	598
6	479	NT	3,721
7	864	NT	29,459

[a] Calculated as (lytic units in presence of antibody/lytic
units in absence of antibody) x 100.

ADCC with the cells from all of donors tested, but the
levels varied widely and there was no correlation between
the levels induced with each antibody. The 9.2.27 monoclonal antibody induced significant levels of ADCC with a
few donors, but the rest gave negative results. It is of
interest that there was no correlation between reactivity
with the 9.2.27 and the levels of ADCC induced by the other
antibodies, even the other monoclonal antibody, MB3.6.

To explore some of the parameters affecting levels of
ADCC activity, various antibodies were tested with LGL for
ADCC against several melanoma cell lines, in an 18 hour
as well as a short-term cytotoxicity assay. It seemed
possible that a 6 hour incubation period was insufficient
to obtain maximal levels of ADCC. As shown in Table 3,
the MB3.6 anti-GD3 antibody gave close to optimal levels
of ADCC against some cell lines after an incubation period
of six hours. However, with other targets (e.g. M10), high
levels of ADCC were seen only after the longer period of
incubation. The longer incubation period also brought out
more ADCC by the 9.2.27 monoclonal antibody and by the
rabbit antiserum.

NK and ADCC activities by human LGL have been shown to
be augmented substantially by pretreatment of the effector
cells with interferon (7). IL-2 has also been reported to
augment human NK activity (8), but has not been studied for

Table 3.   Effects of Length of Assay on ADCC by LGL vs.
           Human Melanoma Cell Lines

Antibody	Length of Assay (hrs)	Cytotoxicity (lytic units) vs:			
		FeMex	M10[a]	M16[a]	M21[a]
None	6	50	<1	<1	<1
MB3.6	6	694	<1	1	100
9.2.27	6	61	<1	<1	<1
Rabbit	6	4,497	<1	627	1,098
None	18	101	1	28	28
MB3.6	18	602	40	11	369
9.2.27	18	428	5	<1	12
Rabbit	18	30,200	16	1,025	NT

[a] Cell lines generously provided by Dr. D. Morton, UCLA.

its ability to augment ADCC activity. It was, therefore, of interest to determine whether the ADCC by monoclonal antibodies could be augmented by such pretreatments. As shown in Table 4, pretreatment of LGL with either recombinant IFN α or recombinant IL-2 induced substantial augmentation of NK activity against the melanoma target cell, whereas as previously observed (Ortaldo et al., manuscript in preparation), recombinant IFN γ induced only a modest degree of augmentation of NK activity. Pretreatment of the effector cells with either IL-2 or IFN α induced a substantial augmentation in ADCC activity with both the anti-GD3 antibody, considerably more than could be attributed to the addititive effects of cytokines and the antibodies. In contrast, interferon γ had more detectable ability to augment the ADCC induced by NB3.6. With the ADCC activity involving the other antibodies, more modest or no potentiating effects were seen upon pretreatment of the effector cells with any of the cytokines. With 9.2.27, significant augmentation of ADCC was only observed after pretreatment with IFN α. Under the conditions of these assays, the high levels of ADCC induced by the rabbit antiserum were not appreciably affected by pretreatment of the effector cells.

Table 4.   Augmentation of Monoclonal Antibody ADCC Against FeMex Melanoma Target Cells

Effector Cells[a]	Mean Lytic Units vs. FeMex Plus Antibody			
	None	MB3.6	9.2.27	Rabbit
LGL	8	38	12	294
LGL + r IL2 (1000 U)	51	197	54	219
LGL + r IFN α (1000 U)	61	195	100	297
LGL + r IFN γ (1000 U)	13	22	NT[b]	NT

[a] LGL were preincubated in medium alone or with IFN α for 2 hours or with IL-2 or IFN γ for 24 hours.
[b] Not tested

In the above studies, considerably stronger and more consistent ADCC activity was observed with the γ3 antibody to GD3 and with the γ2a antibody, 9.2.27. This was somewhat surprising since γ2a antibodies have been considered best for mediation of ADCC. To further evaluate the ability of human LGL to mediate ADCC by monoclonal

antibodies of various isotypes, studies were performed
with a series of monoclonal antibodies produced against
human colon carcinoma. Table 5 summarizes the initial
results from such studies. Each of the antibodies studied
induced some ADCC activity, but there was considerable
variation in these results, depending on the target cell
utilized. The γ3 antibody gave the highest levels of
ADCC against the SW1116 cell line, but each of the other
antibodies also induced ADCC against this target. In
contrast, some of the antibodies of other isotypes gave
ADCC against the other target cells, whereas the γ3 antibody gave negative results. In a more extensive recent
survey with more than 60 monoclonal antibodies against
human colon carcinoma, we have observed that most of the γ3
antibodies were quite active in inducing ADCC, whereas
antibodies of the other istotypes gave ADCC with substantially lower frequency.

Table 5. ADCC by Human LGL and MoAb of Various Isotypes

Antibodies vs. Colon Cancer	Isotype	ADCC (% of Control LU without Antibody)		
		LS180	SW1116	HT29
11-285	γ1	165[a]	383[a]	183[a]
2839	γ2a	136	219[a]	133
2945	γ2a	182[a]	167[a]	154[a]
586	γ3	144	553[a]	122
Rabbit		126	196[a]	262[a]

Significant ADCC above control without antibody.

A further issue in considering the possible role of
ADCC in therapeutic effects of monoclonal antibodies in
patients with cancer is the functional capabilities of the
patient's effector cells. We have, therefore, begun
studies to evaluate the ability of peripheral blood mononuclear cells from patients with melanoma to mediate ADCC
in cooperation with the various antimelanoma antibodies.
The results thus far have indicated that melanoma patients
have lower but detectable ADCC activity against melanoma
target cells and that such reactivity can be augmented
by pretreatment of the effector cells with interferon α

or IL-2. Such results are encouraging since they indicate
that therapeutic approaches with monoclonal antibodies
with the capability of mediating ADCC, perhaps in combination with interferon α or IL-2 treatment, may be useful in
malignant melanoma or other types of human cancer.

Based on the present results and previous studies, it
appears that many parameters may affect ADCC activity
against human tumor cells. First, the type of antibody
utilized appears to be quite important. Rabbit antisera
react against a wide array of target cells and appear to
usually induce higher levels of ADCC than mouse monoclonal
antibodies. With the murine monoclonal antibodies, the
isotype of IgG appears to be quite important. It is of
note that all of the anti-GD3 antibodies which have been
effective in ADCC have the IgG3 isotype. However, in
other antigen systems, IgG2a and other isotypes have also
been shown to be effective for inducing ADCC. From our
recent survey with antibodies to colon cancer, it appears
that the γ3 antibodies may be particularly effective for
mediating ADCC, and this may account for the strong ADCC
activity observed with the anti-GD3 antibodies. However,
the molecular nature of the antigen detected by the antibodies and the position of the antigen in the surface membrane may also play critical roles. It is quite possible
that the GD3 ganglioside is particularly well situated
in the membrane for effective interactions with antibodies
and effector cells, whereas other antigens such as the
250,000 dalton proteoglycan recognized by 9.2.27 may not
have a configuration in the membrane which is optimal for
ADCC. The density of the antigens on the target cells
also plays an important role in ADCC, with cells with high
density being much more likely to be suitable targets for
ADCC. As demonstrated in the present study, the effector
cells mediating ADCC and their levels of reactivity have
an important influence on the results with the antibodies
and target cells studied here. LGL appeared to account
for virtually all of the observed ADCC activity, whereas
monocytes had no detectable activity. These results are
in contrast with those of Herlyn, et al. (elsewhere in
this volume). The reason for these divergent results is
not clear. On the one hand, it is possible that the anti-
body-antigen system which they have studied is sufficiently
different to allow ADCC by monocytes rather than LGL.
Alternatively, the methods utilized for obtaining the
effector cells and performing the assays appear to be

substantially different and may have strongly influenced the results. It should be noted that they only detected reactivity by human monocytes after they were cultured in vitro for a prolonged period of time and purified populations of LGL have not been evaluated in their test system. The levels of ADCC reactivity of the donors' effector cells also have been shown to have a major influence on the results. The reactivity of various normal adult donors has been shown to vary considerably. The basis for such variation in ADCC activity is not clear. That may be due to a variety of factors, including the levels of activation of the effector cells for cytotoxic activity and the levels of Fc_γ receptor expression. Because of the ability of cytokines such as interferon α and IL-2 to strongly augment the cytotoxic reactivity LGL, such pretreatment of the effector cells appears quite useful for optimal detection of ADCC reactivity. The type of interaction of the antibody with the effector and target cells also seems to have an important influence on the induction of ADCC. For classical ADCC with conventional antisera, coating of the target cells with the antibodies has generally been optimal. In contrast, in the present studies with murine monoclonal antibodies, the presence of the antibody in the medium during the assay seemed to be required. Finally, the length of the cytotoxicity assay has been found to have a significant influence on the levels of ADCC observed at least with certain target cells. Assays of 18 to 24 hours have given more uniformly positive results than the usual four to six hour assays. However, it should be noted that the longer term assays have more problems with high background levels of isotope release and, therefore, it remains preferable to perform short term assays when the particular antibody-target cell combination is effective under such conditions.

The present study demonstrates that substantial ADCC against human tumor cells can be observed upon interaction between large granular lymphocytes and various mouse monoclonal antibodies. Although considerably more studies are needed to develop optimal procedures for producing ADCC, and to adequately understand the parameters determining effective ADCC activity, the results provide encouragement for ADCC-related therapeutic approaches for cancer patients.

REFERENCES

1. Bumol TF, Wang QC, Reisfeld RA, and Kaplan NO. Mono-
    clonal antibody and an antibody-toxin conjugate to a
    cell surface proteglycan of melanoma cells suppress
    in vivo tumor growth. Proc Natl Acad Sci (USA)
    80:529-533, 1983.
2. Oldham RK, Foon KA, Morgan AC, Woodhouse CS, Schroff
    RW, Abrams PG Fer M, Schoenberger CS, Farrell M,
    Kimball E and Sherwin SA. Monoclonal antibody therapy
    of malignant melanoma: in vivo localization in cutan-
    eous metastasis after intravenous administration.
    J Clin Oncol, in press.
3. Foon KA, Schroff RW, Bunn PA, Mayer D, Abrams PG, Fer
    M, Ochs J, Bottino GC, Sherwin SA, Carlo DJ, Herberman
    RB, and Oldham RK. Effects of monoclonal antibody
    therapy in patients with chronic lymphocytic leukemia.
    Blood 64:1085-1093, 1984.
4. Houghton AN, Mintzer D, Cordon-Cardo C, Welt S, Fleigel
    B, Vanhan S, Carswell E, Melamed MR, Oettgen HF, and
    Old LJ. Mouse monoclonal IgG3 antibody detecting GD3
    ganglioside: A phase I trial in patients with malignant
    melanoma. Proc Natl Acad Sci (USA), in press.
5. Morgan AC, Galloway DR, and Reisfeld RA. Production
    and characterization of monoclonal antibody to a mela-
    noma-specific glycoprotein. Hybridoma 1:27-30, 1981.
6. Timonen T, Ortaldo JR, and Herberman RB. Character-
    istics of human large granular lymphocytes and rela-
    tionship to natural killer and K cells. J Exp Med
    153:569-582, 1981.
7. Herberman RB, Ortaldo JR, and Bonnard GD. Augmentation
    by interferon of human natural and antibody-dependent
    cell mediated cytotoxicity. Nature 277-221-223, 1979.
8. Domzig W, Stadler BM, and Herberman RB. Interleukin-2
    dependence of human natural killer (NK) cell activity.
    J Immunol 130:1970-1973, 1983.

V. DRUG-ANTIBODY CONJUGATES

Monoclonal Antibodies and Cancer Therapy, pages 207–214
© 1985 Alan R. Liss, Inc.

EFFECT OF MONOCLONAL ANTIBODY-DRUG CONJUGATES ON THE
IN VIVO GROWTH OF HUMAN TUMORS ESTABLISHED IN NUDE MICE

Nissi M. Varki
Ralph A. Reisfeld
Leslie E. Walker

Department of Immunology
Scripps Clinic and Research Foundation
La Jolla, California 92037

ABSTRACT

Methotrexate was covalently conjugated (15 moles
drug/mole antibody) to monoclonal antibody KS1/4 which is
directed to a 40,000 M_r glycoprotein expressed on
adenocarcinoma of the lung. The monoclonal antibody and the
monoclonal antibody-drug conjugate were then tested both in
vitro and in vivo for their ability to suppress or kill the
adenocarcinoma of the lung cell line UCLA-P3 either in
culture or established in nude mice. In vitro the antibody
had no effect while the antibody-drug conjugate did
effectively kill tumor cells. However, in vitro unconjugated
methotrexate was significantly more effective than the
antibody-drug conjugate. In vivo the antibody-drug conjugate
was much more efficient in suppressing tumor growth than
either unconjugated drug or unconjugated antibody. These
observations suggest that monoclonal antibodies are capable
of effectively directing drugs to tumors and that the
released drug is still potent enough to suppress the growth
of established tumors.

INTRODUCTION

The use of antibodies in cancer therapy was first postulated by Ehrlich in 1906 when he predicted that antibodies armed with toxic substances would serve as "magic bullets" to kill tumor cells. The advent of monoclonal antibody technology and the enhanced understanding of tumorogenisis has made testing of this hypothesis feasible. While the results with polyclonal antibody-drug conjuguates (for a review, see Arnon and Sela)(1) appeared to be quite encouraging, limitations due to the availability and specificity of the polyclonal antibody restricted their usefulness. More recently, Garnett (3) and this volume monoclonal antibodies have been used as carriers of drugs. We report here the use of monoclonal antibody-drug conjugates in the therapy of human lung tumor established in nude mice. The monoclonal antibody used is designated KS1/4 and has been shown to bind highly specifically to adenocarcinomas. The drug conjugated is the folate antagonist methotrexate.

MATERIALS AND METHODS

Monoclonal Antibody

Monoclonal antibody KS1/4 was produced as previously described (4). The monoclonal antibody was purified from ascites fluid by chromatography on an Affigel Blue DEAE column (BioRad Laboratories, Richmond, CA). Elution was by a step gradient of sodium chloride. Monoclonal antibody KS1/4 (IgG2a) was eluted with 50 mM NaCl in 20 mM Tris pH 8.0. The purified antibody was judged to be greater than 90% homogenous by SDS-PAGE analysis.

Conjugation of Methotrexate to Monoclonal Antibodies

Methotrexate (Lederle, Pearl River, NY) 5 mg in 0.5 ml of normal saline mixed with 10 mg of EDAC and allowed to react for 15 min at room temperature. Monoclonal antibody KS1/4 (10 mg) in 1 ml of saline was then added and the reaction was continued for 1 hr. The free and conjugated drug were then separated by gel filtration on a 1 cm x 20 cm P-6 gel filtration column. As measured spectrophotometrically at 410 nm, the conjugation ratio was typically 10-15 moles of methotrexate per mole of antibody.

Growth of UCLA-P3 Adenocarcinoma of the Lung Tumor Cells in Nude Mice.

UCLA-P3 cells (10^6) were injected subcutaneously onto the back of female athymic (nu/nu) mice and allowed to establish for 3 days prior to the initiation of treatment with monoclonal antibody or monoclonal antibody drug conjugate. The tumors were approximately 100 mm^3 and all of the mice developed tumors.

Treatment with Monoclonal Antibodies or Monoclonal Antibody-Drug Conjugates.

Tumor-bearing mice were injected interperitoneally with either 0.5 mg of monoclonal antibody, 0.5 mg of monoclonal antibody-methotrexate conjugate, the equivalent amount of free methotrexate as was conjugated to the antibody or normal saline. The mice were treated every third day and the tumor volume measured prior to treatment.

RESULTS

Specificity of Monoclonal Antibodies KS1/4 and KS1/9

The specificity of monoclonal antibody KS1/4 is shown in Table 1. Immunoperoxidase staining of fresh frozen normal and tumor tissues with monoclonal antibody KS1/4 demonstrates that the antibody binds to adenocarcinomas of the lung, colon, breast, and stomach and squamous carcinomas of the lung, but not to melanomas. Reaction of monoclonal antibody KS1/4 with normal tissues is minimal. A faint reaction was occasionally detected with monoclonal antibody KS1/4 on proximal tubules of the kidney and bronchiolar lining epithelium. Monoclonal antibody KS1/4 did, however, react strongly with fetal lung, kidney, and colon, suggesting that the antigen may be fetal in origin.

Table 1

Reactivity of MoAbs by Immunoperoxidase Staining of Tissues

Tumors (no. of specimens tested)	KS1/4
Adenocarcinoma	
Lung (6)	+[a]
Colon (3)	+
Stomach (1)	+
Breast (1)	+
Pancreas (1)	+
Epidermoid carcinoma, lung (3)	+
Small-cell carcinoma, lung (6)	+
Melanoma (4)	–
Normal	
Spleen (3)	–
Liver (3)	–
Colon (3)	–
Kidney (3)	±
Lung bronchioles (3)	±
Lung alveoli (3)	±
Pancreas (3)	±
Brain (3)	±
Fetal Tissues	
Lung	+
Kidney	+
Colon	+

Nature of the Antigens Reactive with KS1/4

Monoclonal antibody KS1/4 has been shown to react with a 40,000 M_r glycoprotein that is probably an integral membrane protein and is not shed in any significant amount into tissue culture media (4). The location of this antigen has been established to be on the cell surface of lung tumor cells by immunofluorescence staining of live UCLA-P3 adenocarcinoma of the lung cells. Furthermore, this 40,000 M_r antigen appears to contain at least one phosphate residue as detected by indirect immunoprecipitation with monoclonal antibody KS1/4 and ^{32}P-labeled tumor cell extracts.

In Vitro Effect of Monoclonal   Antibody KS1/4 and KS1/4-
Methotrexate Conjugate

The monoclonal antibody and its drug conjugate were
tested for their ability to inhibit the growth of
adenocarcinoma of the lung cells, UCLA-P3, in vitro. Cells
were incubated with the indicated concentrations of KS1/4,
KS1/4-methotrexate conjugate, or methotrexate for 24 hours.
Following this incubation, the cells were pulsed for 4 hr
with ^{3}H-thymidine and the incorporation determined by liquid
scintillation counting. The results are shown in Figure 1.
The monoclonal antibody, KS1/4, did not inhibit the tumor
cells while both the antibody drug conjugate as well as free
methotrexate were very effective in inhibiting their growth.
These results indicate that in vitro the free drug is
significantly more effective than the antibody-drug
conjugate.

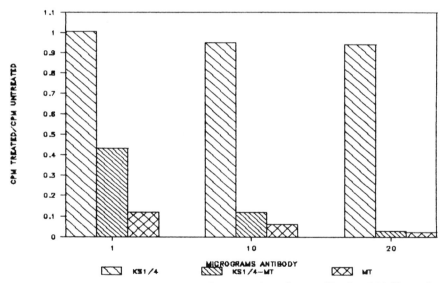

Figure 1: Effect in vitro of monoclonal antibody KS1/4 and
KS1/4-methotrexate
Adenocarcinomas of the lung cells, UCLA-P3, were
cultured for 4 hours in the presence of the indicated amounts
of KS1/4, KS1/4-methotrexate conjugate or free methotrexate
equivalent to the amount of methotrexate conjugated to KS1/4.
^{3}H-thymidine was added to the cultures and 24 hours later,
the incorporation of thymidine was measured by liquid
scintillation counting. The results are expressed as a
ratio of counts incorporated without treatment divided by
counts incorporated following treatment.

Treatment of Human Lung Tumors Established in Nude Mice

Monoclonal antibody KS1/4 alone and conjugated with methotrexate were used to treat UCLA-P3 adenocarcinoma fo the lung cells established in athymic (nu/nu) mice. The tumor cells (10^6) were injected subcutaneously and allowed to establish for three days prior to the start of therapy. The tumor-bearing mice (6/group) were then treated bi-weekly with 0.5 mg of either KS1/4, KS1/4-methotrexate conjugate, the equivalent concentration of methotrexate as was present on the conjugate (15 ug) or saline. The results are shown in Figure 2. In contrast to the results obtained in vitro, the antibody-drug conjugate KS1/4-methotrexate, was a much more effective suppressor of tumor growth than either the monoclonal antibody alone or free methotrexate.

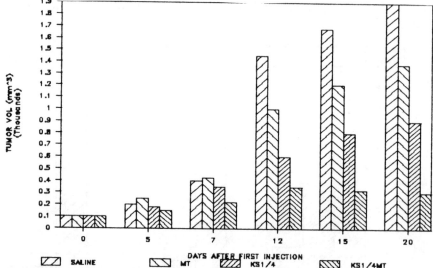

Figure 2. Effect in vivo of monoclonal antibody KS1/4 and KS1/4-methotrexate.

Adenocarcinoma of the lung cells, UCLA-P3, were transplanted on the backs of nude mice and allowed to establish for 3 days. Saline, KS1/4 (0.5 mg), KS1/4-methotrexate (0.5 mg) or free methotrexate at a concentration equivalent to the methotrexate concentration on the conjugate was injected bi-weekly. Tumor volume was measured on the indicated days.

DISCUSSION

We have demonstrated that a monoclonal antibody can be used to effectively deliver a drug to human lung tumors established in nude mice in concentrations sufficient to suppress tumor growth to an extent greater than that observed with either the monoclonal antibody or the drug alone.

While other investigators (2,3) have found it necessary to conjugate to antibodies molecules such as dextran or albumin as the actual carrier of drugs, this was not found to be necessary with monoclonal antibody KS1/4. Presumably, this is the case because the monoclonal antibody KS1/4 is remarkably stable to conjugation, i.e. an extreme number of drug molecules can be attached to each molecule of antibody with little loss of reactivity. The conjugated KS1/4 monoclonal antibody (15 moles drug/mole antibody) still retains 75% of its initial binding activity as determined by ELISA on UCLA-P3 tumor cells. Additionally, the cell surface density of the antigen detected by monoclonal antibody KS1/4 is high relative to other reported tumor markers. This density is comparable to Class I histocompatibility antigens as measured by the binding of monoclonal antibody W6/32 which is directed to a determinant expressed on all Class I histocompatibility antigens. Thus, the effectiveness of the KS1/4-methotrexate conjugate is probably due to relatively large quantities of drug delivered to the tumor site by the monoclonal antibody.

It is surprising that the KS1/4-methotrexate conjugate is less effective than free methotrexate in vitro yet is much more effective than the free drug in vivo. In vitro the free methotrexate is probably more effective because, unlike the KS1/4-methotrexate conjugate, its entry into the tumor cell is not restricted by a limited number of binding sites and it does not have to be enzymatically released as would the antibody-drug conjugate. Undoubtedly, in vivo, however, the antibody-drug conjugate is more effective due to the antibody's ability to "home" the drug to the tumor site which results in a high local concentration of the drug.

The tumor suppressive activity of the unconjugated antibody is potentially the result of either the recruitment of effector cells which, in turn, destroy the tumor or the activation of complement (human) but, at least in the initial trial, very poor in directing effector cells. Whether this is the mechanism responsible for the in vivo effect of the antibody is questionable, however, given the relatively low effect of the complement in a nude mouse and the depressed ability of monoclonal antibody KS1/4 to active mouse complement.

In conclusion, while we have shown that a monoclonal antibody directly conjugated with the drug methotrexate is capable in suppressing the growth of a human lung tumor established in nude mice, a number of questions remain unanswered. We are currently attempting to determine the kinetics of internalization by the antibody-drug complex and compare that to unconjugated antibody. This reaction is probably the rate-limiting processing the effectiveness of antibody-drug conjugates and thus potentially the optimization either using other monoclonal antibodies, drugs, or conjugation technology may greatly enhance the efficiency of antibody-drug conjugate therapy. Further, we are attempting to determine the nature of the drug once it is enzymatically released from the antibody. It is critical for effective cell killing that the drug be rapidly released and that the freed drug retain as closely as possible full activity. If these two processes can indeed be optimized, the usefulness of antibody-drug conjugate chemotherapy may be improved to the extent such that it becomes clinically beneficial.

REFERENCES

1.   Ehrlich P (1960). "Chemotherapy" Proc. 17th Int. Congress Med. In: F. Himmellweit (ed) The Collection of Papers of Paul Ehrlich. Pergamon Press, London.

2.   Arnon R, Sela M (1982) In vitro and in vivo efficacy of conjugates of daunomycin with anti-tumor antibodies. Immuno Rev 62:5-35.

3.   Garnett MC, Embleton MJ, Jcobs E, Baldwin RW (1983) Preparation and properties of a drug-carrier-antibody conjugate showing selective antibody directed cytotoxicity in vitro. Int J Cancer 31:661-670.

4.   Varki NM, Reisfeld RA, Walker LE (1984) Antigens associated with a human lung adenocarcinoma defined by monoclonal antibodies. Canc Res 44:681-687.

Monoclonal Antibodies and Cancer Therapy, pages 215–231
© 1985 Alan R. Liss, Inc.

DESIGN AND THERAPEUTIC EVALUATION OF MONOCLONAL ANTIBODY
791T/36-METHOTREXATE CONJUGATES

Robert W. Baldwin[1], Lindy Durrant[1], M.J.Embleton[1],
M.Garnett[1], M.V.Pimm[1], R.A.Robins[1], J.D.Hardcastle[2],
N.Armitage[2] and K.Ballantyne[2]

[1] Cancer Research Campaign Laboratories and
[2] Department of Surgery, University Hospital, University of
Nottingham, NG7 2RD, U.K.

ABSTRACT Methotrexate (MTX) has been conjugated to monoclonal antibody 791T/36 directly (MTX-791T/36) or indirectly using human serum albumin (HSA) as a carrier for
MTX (MTX-HSA-791T/36). With MTX-791T/36 conjugates, the
degree of antibody substitution was limited since substitution ratios greater than 4:1 resulted in loss of
antibody reactivity. Higher substitution ratios were
achieved using HSA as a carrier for MTX, products containing 38 MTX residues/antibody molecule retaining antibody reactivity. MTX-antibody conjugates were cytotoxic
in vitro for osteogenic sarcoma 791T cells as assessed
by post incubation labelling of tumor cells with [75]Se-
selenomethionine or by inhibition of colony formation.
Directly linked MTX-791T/36 conjugates were less cytotoxic than free drug, but conjugates prepared using
MTX-HSA were as active or more so than free MTX. MTX-
HSA-791T/36 conjugates also displayed specificity for
osteogenic sarcoma 791T cells compared with bladder
carcinoma T24 cells which express much lower levels of
the 791T/36 antibody defined-antigen. In vivo trials
against 791T xenografts in immunodeprived mice demonstrated that treatment with conjugate suppressed tumor
growth. With the treatment regimen selected (twice
weekly intraperitoneal injection), MTX-HSA-791T/36 was
about twice as effective as free drug without displaying
any significant toxicity.
MTX-antibody conjugates were cytotoxic for colon tumor
cells using cell lines developed from primary colon
tumors, whereas the tumors were resistant to free MTX.
This indicates that antibody mediated events contribute

to MTX entry into tumor cells so that antibody conjugates
may be effective with tumors insensitive to free MTX.
Monoclonal antibody 791T/36 localizes in colorectal carcinomas, this being demonstrated by gamma camera imaging
of patients injected with [131] I- and [111] In-labelled preparations. Furthermore, flow cytometry tests showed that
tumor cells derived from regional lymph node and liver
metastases in colorectal cancer patients bind 791T/36
antibody. These observations suggest that MTX-791T/36
antibody conjugates may have potential in the treatment
of colorectal cancer.

INTRODUCTION

Monoclonal antibodies which react with antigens associated with malignant cells offer new approaches for targeting
anti-cancer agents. This may increase their therapeutic index
either by improving the localization of agents in tumors,
especially metastatic deposits, or by minimizing toxic responses in normal tissues, this being a major limitation in
conventional cancer chemotherapy. The design and development
of antibody conjugates with anti-tumor agents will be considered with respect to monoclonal antibody 791T/36 (isotype
IgG2b) produced by a hybridoma obtained following fusion of
splenocytes from a mouse immunized against human osteogenic
sarcoma 791T cells and murine myeloma P3NSI (1). This
antibody reacts with target cells derived from human
osteogenic sarcomas, but not with normal fibroblasts from
cultures derived from donors of positive tumors including the
donor of 791T. Primary and metastatic osteogenic sarcomas
also react with 791T/36 antibody as demonstrated by immunoperoxidase staining of surgically derived tumor specimens (2).
In vivo localization of monoclonal antibody 791T/36 in
osteogenic sarcomas has also been demonstrated by gamma camera
imaging of patients receiving [131] I-labelled antibody (3).
This antibody also localizes in colorectal and ovarian cancers
and [131] I iodine or [111] In-indium preparations have been used to
detect primary, recurrent and metastatic lesions by gamma
camera imaging (4-6).
Conjugates have been prepared by linking monoclonal
antibody 791T/36 to a range of agents including vindesine (7)
methotrexate (8) and daunomycin (9) and also to interferon α
as a method for targeting immunomodulating agents (10). These
developments are reviewed by considering the design and
evaluation of methotrexate-791T/36 antibody conjugates.

Methotrexate-791T/36 Antibody Conjugates

Methotrexate (MTX) has been selected as one of the anti-neoplastic agents for conjugating to monoclonal antibody 791T/36 in view of its clinical usage. Also it is highly cytotoxic for osteogenic sarcoma 791T cells, 50 percent inhibition of growth in culture (IC50) being produced at a concentration of 1×10^{-8} M (8).

Conjugates containing MTX directly linked to antibody were prepared using the N-hydroxysuccinimide ester of MTX (8). This was prepared by incubating equimolar quantities of MTX, N-hydroxysuccinimide and dicyclohexyl carbodiimide in dimethylformamide. Substituted 791T/36 was then prepared by reacting the MTX ester with antibody in aqueous medium, yielding products with an average molar substitution ratio in the range 2 to 3. Higher substitution ratios invariably resulted in an unacceptable loss of antibody reactivity.

Conjugates have also been prepared with human serum albumin (HSA) as a carrier for MTX, using a three-step conjugation procedure (8). Firstly MTX-substituted HSA was prepared by reacting an excess of MTX and ethylcarbodiimide with HSA and unwanted polymerized MTX-HSA products removed by size exclusion chromatography. Secondly iodoacetyl-substituted 791T/36 antibody was produced by reacting a 3 to 4-fold molar excess of N-hydroxysuccinimidyl iodoacetate with antibody. Finally MTX-HSA conjugate was treated with dithiothreitol to reduce free sulphydryl groups (available in oxidized unreactive form) and reacted with iodoacetyl-substituted 791T/36 antibody. Reaction products were then separated by size exclusion chromatography to remove polymerized products to yield conjugates in the molecular weight range 200,000 to 400,000 daltons.

Characterization of Antibody Conjugates

a)   Antibody Reactivity.   A flow cytometry technique has been developed for the assessment of antibody binding activity in antibody conjugates (11). Antibody conjugate is mixed with fluorochrome labelled antibody, and the mixture is then allowed to compete for binding to tumor cells under conditions where the antibody is in excess. At equilibrium, the relative amounts of labelled and unlabelled antibody bound per tumor cell is estimated by a quantitative fluorescence measurement. The degree of competitive binding of antibody conjugate will reflect both quantitative and qualitative changes in antibody binding activity caused by the conjugation procedure.

For these assays, 791T/36 was directly labelled with fluorescein isothiocyanate (FITC-791T/36), and its binding activity to 791T tumor cells measured using a FACS IV cell sorter. Titration of labelled antibody established that saturation of the binding sites of 791T tumor cells was obtained when 1μg of FITC-791T/36 was mixed with 2 x 10^5 cells. It was also found that with this level of FITC791T/36, the tumor cell/antibody mixture could be analysed without washing the target cells. This allows the analysis of competition experiments directly at equilibrium (11).

To establish that the fluorescein isothiocyanate labelling of the 791T/36 antibody had not damaged its binding activity, competition assays using unlabelled antibody were performed. As shown in Table 1, the reduction in binding to 791T cells of FITC-791T/36 by unlabelled 791T/36 is very close to the expected reduction. For example, a mixture of 1μg FITC-791T/36 and 2μg unlabelled antibody would be expected to give a 66% reduction in fluorescence compared to 1μg FITC791T/36 alone, if the labelled and unlabelled antibodies were binding equally well. The measured reduction was 65%, and reductions close to the expected values were observed for the other combinations tested (Table 1).

TABLE 1
COMPETITIVE INHIBITION OF FITC-791T/36
ANTIBODY BINDING TO 791T CELLS.

Unlabelled 791T/36 Added to FITC 791T/36	Expected Reduction in Binding	Mean Fluorescence Intensity	Percent Reduction
-	-	935	-
4	80	197	79
2	66	328	65
1	50	493	47
0.5	33	661	29
0.25	20	771	18

a 791T tumor cells incubated with 791T/36 antibody (1ug/2 x 10^5 cells) labelled with FITC with or without added unlabelled 791T/36 antibody for four hours. Cells were then analysed by flow cytometry.
b Fluorescence intensity expressed in arbitary units calculated from mean fluorescence channel number.

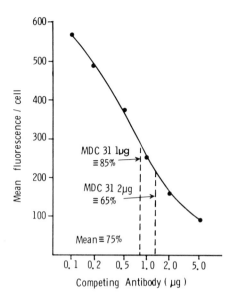

FIGURE 1. Competition of binding of FITC-labelled antibody with 791T cells by unconjugated 791T/36 antibody and a methotrexate conjugate (MDC31).

When evaluating antibody conjugates, comparison is usually made between the conjugate and an unlabelled antibody preparation. This is illustrated in Figure 1, where a standard curve was constructed using unlabelled antibody, concentrations ranging from 0.1 to 5.0μg, competing with 1μg of FITC-791T/36. A methotrexate-791T/36 conjugate (MDC 31; molar substitution ratio 2.7:1) was tested at the equivalent of 1 and 2μg antibody. This antibody conjugate competed almost as well as unlabelled antibody, with a mean retention of activity of 75%. Tests with other conjugates of methotrexate directly linked to 791T/36 have shown that there is severe loss of antibody activity when more than 4 methotrexate residues are linked per 791T/36 antibody molecule. Conjugates prepared using human serum albumin as a carrier for methotrexate and containing 23 to 38 moles methotrexate per mole antibody retained 28 to 32% of the reactivity of unsubstituted antibody in competition assays (Table 2).
b. In Vitro Cytotoxicity. The in vitro cytotoxicity of MTX-791T/36 conjugates was measured by incubating target tumor cells with a range of concentrations of conjugate in micro-

titre plates for 24 hours and measuring tumor cell survival by post-incubation labelling with ^{75}Se-selenomethionine (7). The reactivity of conjugates was then assessed from the dose-response curve and expressed as IC50 doses, this being the level of conjugate required to produce a 50 percent inhibition of tumor cell survival.

TABLE 2

CHARACTERISTICS OF METHOTREXATE-791T/36 MONOCLONAL ANTIBODY CONJUGATES

Preparation	MTX substitution MTX:791T/36	Antibody reactivity[a] Percent
MTX-791T/36		
MDC26	2.5:1	36
MDC29	1.9:1	68
MDC31	2.7:1	75
MTX-HSA-791T/36		
MT1	32:1	28
MT7	27:1	36
MT11	23:1	32
MT17	38:1	32

[a] Determined by competition binding assay in which binding of FITC-labelled 791T/36 antibody to tumor cell is measured by flow cytometry (see 11 for details).

Directly linked MTX-791T/36 conjugates were tested against osteogenic sarcoma 791T cells which express approximately 6×10^5-791T/36 antibody binding sites/cell and bladder carcinoma T24 cells which express of the order of 10^4 binding sites/cell. These conjugates were cytotoxic for both these MTX-sensitive cell lines, but with reduced activity when compared to that of free drug (Table 3).

MTX-791T/36 conjugates were also tested against colon carcinoma C168 and C170 and colon adenoma C146 derived cell lines using a 48 hour incubation procedure. As shown in Figure 2 these cell lines developed in collaboration with the Department of Surgery, University Hospital, Nottingham, from primary tumors express the 791T/36-defined antigen. These tests were carried out with FITC-791T/36 antibody under saturating conditions so that the number of antibodies bound/cell could be determined. This indicated that the colon tumor-derived cells bound between 1.68 x 10^5 and 2.85 x 10^5 antibody molecules/cell compared with a value of 6 x 10^5 for osteogenic sarcoma 791T cells (11).

The colon tumor-derived cell lines were resistant to free MTX (Table 4). In comparison MTX-791T/36 conjugates were cytotoxic for all three colon tumor cell lines (IC50 63 to 170 ng/ml). This is particularly relevant with respect to the application of MTX-antibody conjugates for the treatment of colorectal cancer and implies that entry of MTX into cells is effected through antibody mediated interactions.

Conjugates in which the level of MTX substitution was increased through the use of an HSA carrier (Table 2) were more cytotoxic against osteogenic sarcoma 791T cells, the reactivity now being comparable to that of free MTX (Table 3). Furthermore with these conjugates, it was possible to demonstrate discrimination in their cytotoxicity for osteogenic sarcoma 791T and bladder carcinoma T24 cells, this being related to the level of binding of 791T/36 antibody.

TABLE 3

CYTOTOXICITY OF METHOTREXATE-791T/36 ANTIBODY CONJUGATES

Reagent	Cytotoxicity (IC50[a] ng/ml) against	
	Osteogenic Sarcoma 791T	Bladder Carcinoma T24
Direct Conjugate		
MTX-791T/36 (MDC27)	204.0	112.0
MTX	6.6	2.5
MTX-791T/36 (MDC30)	178.0	178.0
MTX	6.0	5.0
MTX-791T/36 (MDC31)	70.8	ND
MTX	12.6	ND
HSA-Carrier Conjugate		
MTX-HSA-791T/36 (MT5)	18.6	251.0
MTX	6.2	6.3
MTX-HSA-791T/36 (MT17)	2.4	316.0
MTX	4.8	6.0
MTX-HSA-791T/36 (MT18)	50.0	ND
MTX	10.0	

[a] IC50 - concentration in terms of MTX in culture medium producing 50 percent inhibition of tumor cell survival as estimated by ^{75}Se-selenomethionine uptake.

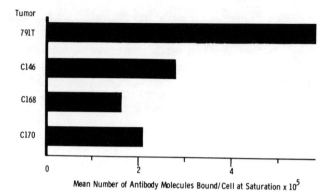

Figure 2. Binding of 791T/36 antibody to osteosarcoma
791T cells and colon tumor determined by flow cytometry.

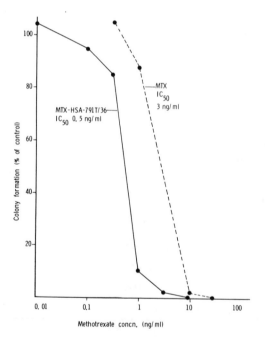

Figure 3. Cytotoxicity of MTX-HSA-791T/36 conjugate
against 791T osteogenic sarcoma cells as measured by colony
inhibition assay. Conjugate concentration is expressed as
a percentage of the number of colonies formed in growth
medium controls.

c. Clonogenic Assay. The cytotoxic potential of MTX and MTX-/36 antibody conjugates for osteogenic sarcoma 791T cells was also assessed using a clonogenic assay in which tumor cells were incubated together with reagent for 5 to 7 days and then tumor colonies counted. As shown in Figure 3 MTX-HSA-791T/36 was more effective than free MTX, the dose in terms to MTX to produce 50 percent inhibition of colony formation being 0.5 ng/ml and 3 ng/ml respectively for conjugate and free drug.

Therapeutic Activity of Methotrexate-791T/36 Antibody Conjugates

The therapeutic potential of methotrexate-791T/36 antibody conjugates has been evaluated initially against osteogenic sarcoma 791T xenografts in mice immunodeprived by thymectomy, and whole body irradiation (^{60}Co γ-irradiation 9Gy) with cytosine arabinoside protection. One test, illustrated in Figure 4 compares the subcutaneous growth of 791T xenografts in mice treated with MTX or MTX-HSA-791T/36.

TABLE 4
CYTOTOXICITY OF METHOTREXATE-791T/36
CONJUGATES AGAINST TUMOR CELLS.

Target Cell[a]	Cytotoxicity (IC50[b] ng/ml):	
	MTX	MTX-791T/36
Osteogenic Sarcoma		
791T	12	90
Colon Tumour		
C146	1000	63
C168	8000	400
C170	1800	170

[a] Colon tumor cell lines generated from primary tumors express the 791T/36-defined antigen (Figure 2).
[b] IC50. Concentration in terms of MTX in culture medium producing 50 percent inhibition of tumor cell survival as estimated by ^{75}Se-selenomethionine uptake following tumor cell:MTX or conjugate incubation for 48 hours.

Mice were treated twice weekly starting 4 days after tumor
cell inoculation with a total dose of 17.5 mg/kg body weight
of free or conjugated MTX. Considerable toxicity was observed
following treatment with free MTX resulting in 6/10 mice
dying. Tumors developed in 3 of the remaining 4 survivors.
In comparison, no toxic deaths were observed in MTX-HSA-
791T/36 treated mice and only 4/10 developed tumors. The
growth curves (Fig.4) indicate that tumors initially developed
in all mice but then regressed in 6/10 mice treated with
MTX-HSA791T/36, so that by day 32 there was a marked therapeutic response compared to tumor growth in untreated
controls. In further trials 791T xenografted mice were again
treated twice weekly with MTX or MTX-HSA-791T/36 conjugate,
and growth inhibition assessed by comparison of tumor weight
following termination of experiments after 40 days. These
trials summarized in Figure 5 indicate that the conjugates
were therapeutically more effective than free MTX. This can
be assessed from the dose of MTX required to produce 50 percent inhibition of tumor growth which for MTX-HSA-791T/36 was
17mg/kg body weight and for free drug 33mg/kg body weight.

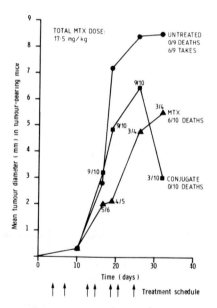

Figure 4. Therapy of 791T tumor xenografts with
MTX-HSA-791T/36 or free MTX.

The maximum dose of MTX-HSA-791T/36 (as MTX) so far tested was 20mg/kg, this being equivalent to 200mg/kg of antibody with this conjugate administered in 10 divided doses over 5 weeks. In this respect immunopharmokinetic studies (12) with ^{125}I-labelled 791T/36 antibody have demonstrated that single doses of the order of 100mg/kg intervals are required to saturate 791T xenografts. Therefore it should be feasible to increase the therapeutic response against 791T xenografts providing the dose of MTX delivered in the conjugate does not result in toxic responses.

Localization of 791T/36 Monoclonal Antibody in Primary and Metastatic Colorectal Cancers

One of the objectives in designing methotrexate-791T/36 antibody conjugates is to evaluate their potential in the treatment of colorectal cancer. This approach is based upon trials where colorectal cancers have been detected following gamma camera imaging of patients injected with ^{131}I or ^{111}In-labelled 791T/36 antibody (4,5,13). Since it is proposed that

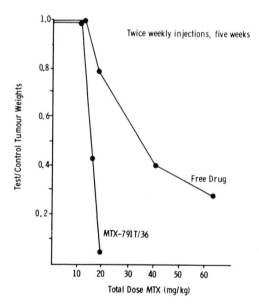

Figure 5.   Influence of MTX-HSA-791T/36 conjugate on growth of 791T xenografts (dose response studies).

MTX-conjugates may be used to treat metastatic deposits of colorectal cancer, tests have been carried out to demonstrate 791T/36 antibody binding to these tumors. For this purpose, cells from primary colon carcinomas and liver and/or lymph node metastases, brought into suspension by collagenase treatment, were reacted with 791T/36 monoclonal antibody as well as a range of other murine monoclonal antibodies. Cell bound antibody was then detected with FITC-labelled rabbit anti-mouse Ig and analysed by FACS IV flow cytometry, using appropriate gating procedures to select tumor cell populations. One example of this approach (Figure 6) indicates that 791T/36 antibody reacts with tumor cells derived from a primary colon carcinoma and from liver and lymph node metastases from the same patient. The tests summarized in Figure 6 also indicate that the reactivity of 791T/36 antibody was as intense as that observed with an anti-CEA monoclonal antibody (C194/2). The most intense binding reaction with the primary and lymph node metastasis-derived tumor cells was with monoclonal antibody C14/1/46/10 which reacts with Y hapten associated with colon carcinomas (14). In this test the reactivity of C14-antibody with tumor cells derived from the liver metastasis was significantly lower than that with tumor cells from the primary and draining lymph node metastasis (Figure 6). This heterogeneity in antigen expression in tumor cells from primary and metastatic lesions has been observed

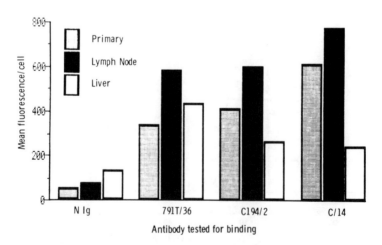

Figure 6. Binding of 791T/36 Monoclonal antibody to primary and metastatic colon carcinoma cells. (Flow cytometric tests).

with other antibodies including anti-CEA antibodies (cf C194/2 test, Figure 6).

Localization of ^{125}I-labelled 791T/36 in Colon Carcinoma Xenografts

791T/36 antibody reacts with target cells from colon tumor cell lines derived from soft agar colonies established from primary tumors (Figure 2). Furthermore, colon tumor cells continue to express the 791T/36 antibody defined antigen when they are grown as xenografts in athymic or immunodeprived mice.

To confirm that radiolabelled 791T/36 antibody localizes in colon carcinomas developing as xenografts in athymic nude mice, groups of mice with established xenografts were injected intraperitoneally with a mixture of ^{131}I-791T/36 and ^{125}I-normal mouse IgG2b. Mice were killed after 4 days, and blood tumor and visceral organs counted for radioactivity. There was preferential accumulation of ^{131}I-791T/36 in all three xenograft lines. For example, as shown in Figure 7, with colon carcinoma C170 xenografts, the tissue to blood ratio of ^{131}I in the tumor was 2.2:1, compared to a maximum of 0.45:1 for any of the normal organs. ^{125}I-normal IgG2b levels in tumor tissue were comparable to those of all normal organs. A localization index, calculated as the ratio of tumor:blood

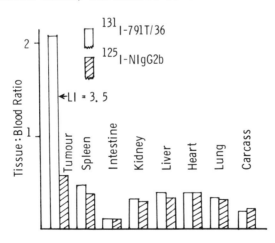

Figure 7. Localisation of ^{131}I-labelled 791T/36 monoclonal antibodies in colon carcinoma C170 xenografts.

ratio of ^{131}I-antibody to tumor:blood ratio of ^{125}I-normal
IgG2b was 3.5. Similar results were obtained with xenografts
of C168 and C146 colon tumors, with localization indices of
2.45 and 2.95 respectively.

DISCUSSION

These investigations with methotrexate-791T/36 antibody
conjugates demonstrate the feasibility of constructing conjugates which retain, to some degree, both anti-tumor and
antibody-cell binding reactivities. The degree of antibody
substitution which can be achieved without significantly
reducing target cell binding is restricted, with 791T/36 antibody, this being of the order of 4 methotrexate residues/
antibody molecule. Direct conjugation of daunomycin to
791T/36 antibody by reaction of antibody with a 25 molar
excess of 14-bromo daunomycin similarly indicated that conjugates with drug:antibody molar ratios of the order of 3 to 4
retained antibody reactivity (9). Also drug antibody molar
ratios of 6:1 could be achieved following reaction of desa-
cetylvinblastine azide with antibody without causing loss of
antibody reactivity (15). These examples indicate that only
limited amounts of agent can be directly linked to antibody
791T/36 and this was the experience when other monoclonal
antibodies were linked to vindesine (15). One approach
explored to increase the drug carrying capacity of 791T/36
antibody has been to link human serum albumin-MTX conjugates
to antibody. This procedure allowed a 10-fold increase in the
MTX:antibody ratio and these conjugates demonstrated specific
cytotoxicity for target cells expressing the 791T/36 antibody
defined antigen (Table 3).

The in vivo trials with 791T xenografts in immunodeprived
mice indicate that MTX-HSA-791T/36 conjugates suppress tumor
growth, the response being superior to that obtained with free
methotrexate (Figure 5). In these trials, MTX-conjugate was
administered intraperitoneally twice weekly, this treatment
protocol being based upon immunopharmokinetic studies on the
organ distribution of ^{125}I-labelled 791T/36 antibody in tumor
791T xenografted mice (12). In these studies, it was shown
that maximum levels of antibody in tumor occurred 3 to 4 days
after injection and then tumor localized antibody persisted
for at least 8 days. Further trials are being carried out,
therefore, to optimize treatment schedules. Dose-response
studies are also required since the maximum dose of MTX-HSA-
791T/36 conjugates so far tested was 20mg/kg body weight (as

MTX). This must then be related to the overall toxicity of the conjugate in comparison with free drug (Figure 4).

Although monoclonal antibody 791T/36 was generated against osteogenic sarcoma cells, it localizes in a range of human tumors including colorectal carcinoma (4,5,13) and ovarian tumors (6). In the colorectal cancer series, localization of 791T/36 has been demonstrated following gamma camera imaging of patients injected with ^{131}I- and ^{111}In-labelled preparations (4,5,13). Analysis of tissue levels of radioactivity in surgically resected specimens from patients injected with radioisotope labelled 791T/36 antibody also demonstrated that the levels in tumor tissue were at least two to three fold higher than in adjacent normal colonic tissue. This reflected specific binding of antibody since ^{123}I-labelled normal mouse IgG2b did not localize in colorectal cancer (5) and the colon carcinoma-associated antigen binding ^{131}I-labelled 791T/36 was identified as a 72,000 dalton glycoprotein with characteristics comparable with those of the product isolated from 791T cells (16). Consistent with these clinical studies, colon carcinoma cells derived from primary and metastatic tumors bind FITC-labelled 791T/36 antibody (Figure 2). Cultured cell lines and xenografts have been established from resected colon tumors which also react with 791T/36.

In vitro studies have established that colon tumor cells are susceptible to cytotoxic attack by methotrexate-791T/36 antibody conjugates even though these tumors were MTX-insensitive. Furthermore ^{131}I-labelled 791T/36 antibody localized in these colon tumor xenografts. Therapeutic trials of 791T/36-antibody conjugates with colon tumors are currently in progress to establish whether, like 791T xenografts, they are susceptible to MTX-linked conjugates. In this respect conjugates of Ricin A-chain (RTA) with 791T/36 antibody and anti-CEA monoclonal antibodies have been prepared which are highly cytotoxic for colon carcinoma cells. It will be possible, therefore, to treat colon carcinomas with cocktails of antibody conjugates. The feasibility of this approach has already been demonstrated in trials with colon carcinoma xenografts showing localization of 791T/36 antibody and an anti-CEA monoclonal antibody when administered simultaneously.

ACKNOWLEDGEMENTS

This work was funded by the Cancer Research Campaign, London, U.K.

REFERENCES

1. Embleton MJ, Gunn B, Byers VS, Baldwin RW (1981). Anti-tumour reactions of monoclonal antibody against a human osteogenic sarcoma cell line. Br J Cancer 43:582.
2. Roth JA, Restropo C, Scuderi P, Baldwin RW, Reichert CM, Hosoi S (1984). Analysis of antigenic expression by primary and autologous metastatic sarcomas using mono-clonal antibodies. Cancer Res 44:5320.
3. Farrands PA, Perkins A, Sully L, Hopkins JS, Pimm MV, Baldwin RW, Hardcastle JD (1983). Localisation of human osteosarcoma by anti-tumour monoclonal antibody (791T/36). J Bone & Joint Surg 65:638.
4. Farrands PA, Perkins AC, Pimm MV, Hardy JG, Baldwin RW, Hardcastle JD (1982). Radioimmunodetection of human colorectal cancers using an anti-tumour monoclonal anti-body. Lancet ii:397.
5. Armitage NC, Perkins AC, Pimm MV, Farrands PA, Baldwin RW, Hardcastle JD (1984). The localisation of an anti-tumour monoclonal antibody (791T/36) in gastrointestinal tumours. Br J Surg 71:407.
6. Symonds EM, Perkins AC, Pimm MV, Baldwin RW, Hardy JG, Williams DA (1984). Clinical implications for immuno-scintigraphy in patients with ovarian malignancy. Br J Obs & Gynae In press.
7. Embleton MJ, Rowland GF, Simmonds RG, Jacobs E, Marsden CH, Baldwin RW (1983). Selective cytotoxicity against human tumour cells by a vindesine-monoclonal antibody conjugate. Br J Cancer 47:43.
8. Garnett MC, Embleton MJ, Jacobs E, Baldwin RW (1983). Preparation and properties of a drug-carrier-antibody conjugate showing selective antibody-directed cytotoxi-city in vitro. Int J Cancer 31:661.
9. Gallego J, Price MR, Baldwin RW (1984). Preparation of four daunomycin-monoclonal antibody 791T/36 conjugates with anti-tumour activity. Int J Cancer 33:737.
10. Pelham JM, Gray JD, Flannery GR, Pimm MV, Baldwin RW (1983). Interferon conjugation to human osteogenic sarcoma monoclonal antibody 791T/36. Cancer Immunol Immunother 15:210.
11. Roe R, Robins RA, Laxton RR, Baldwin RW (1984). Kinetics of divalent monoclonal antibody binding to tumour cell surface antigens using flow cytometry: standardization and mathematical analysis. Molecular Immunol 22:11

12. Pimm MV, Baldwin RW (1984). Quantitative evaluation of the localization of a monoclonal antibody (791T/36) in human osteogenic sarcoma xenografts. Europ J Cancer 20:515.

13. Armitage NC, Perkins AC, Pimm MV, Baldwin RW, Hardcastle JD (1984). Indium-111, a superior radiolabel for the imaging of colorectal cancer using the antitumour monoclonal antibody 791T/36. Nucl Med Comm In press.

14. Brown A, Ellis IO, Embleton MJ, Baldwin RW, Turner DR, Hardcastle JD (1984). Immunohistochemical localization of Y hapten and the structurally related H type 2 blood group antigen on large bowel tumours and normal adult tissues. Int J Cancer 33:727.

15. Rowland GF, Simmonds RG, Corvalan JRF, Baldwin RW, Brown JP, Embleton MJ, Ford CHJ, Hellstrom KE, Hellstrom I, Kemshead JT, Newman CE, Woodhouse CS (1983). Monoclonal antibodies for targeted therapy with vindesine. In Peeters H (ed): "Protides of the Biological Fluids" Oxford: Pergamon Press, p 375.

16. Price MR, Pimm MV, Page CM, Armitage NC, Hardcastle JD, Baldwin RW (1984). Immunolocalization of the murine monoclonal antibody, 791T/36 within primary human colorectal carcinomas and identification of the target antigen. Br J Cancer 49:809.

Monoclonal Antibodies and Cancer Therapy, pages 233–236
© 1985 Alan R. Liss, Inc.

LOCALIZATION AND BIODISTRIBUTION STUDIES OF A
MONOCLONAL ANTIBODY IN PATIENTS WITH MELANOMA

P.G. Abrams, A.C. Morgan, R.W. Schroff, C.S.
Woodhouse, J. Carrasquillo, H.C. Stevenson,
M.F. Fer, R.K. Oldham and K.A. Foon
          BRMP, NCI, Frederick, MD 21701
          Present address: NeoRx Corporation,
          410 West Harrison St., Seattle, WA 98119

ABSTRACT. Monoclonal antibody (MA) 9.2.27 recognizes a 250K glycoprotein/proteoglycan that is
expressed by >90% of malignant melanomas. Doses
from 1-500mg were administered to patients to assess safety, localization in tumor nodules, the
degree of saturation of available binding sites
on tumor cells, pharmacokinetics, and antiglobulin and immune complex formation. Preliminary
biodistribution studies with 111-indium labeled
9.2.27 demonstrated localization in tumor
nodules as small as 5 X 5 mm but substantial
uptake by the RES. We conclude that MA 9.2.27
by intravenous infusion is safe, localizes to
both subcutaneous and visceral melanoma metastases, and can be given in sufficient doses
(200-500) to saturate all available binding
sites on tumors. These data and preclinical
studies indicate that the antibody is a good
candidate for immunotoxin development.
Introduction. Because of the accessibility of
subcutaneous nodules, malignant melanoma is an
ideal system to study parameters important for
in vivo use of monoclonal antibodies including
localization and antigen saturation of tumors
plus safety, efficacy, pharmacokinetics, and
host immune responses. MA 9.2.27 (1), IgG2a,
recognizes a 250 Kd. glycoprotein/proteoglycan
expressed by >90% of human melanomas, and binds

to occasional cells of human vascular endothelium, sebaceous glands and the basal layer of skin, but to no other normal human tissue; the 250 Kd antigen does not circulate in serum in levels detectable by 9.2.27. Pre-clinical studies had previously demonstrated selective localization of MA 9.2.27 in antigen positive melanoma xenografts in athymic mice (2). For these reasons, this antibody appeared to be an attractive candidate for these studies.

Initial study plan. The initial phase of the study focused upon safety, tumor localization and immunologic response of the host to the infused immunoglobulin (3). Patients received 1, 10, 50, 100 and 200mg of MA 9.2.27 twice weekly; biopsies of subcutaneous nodules were performed 24-96 hours after a dose and assessed by flow cytometry to determine the percentage of cells binding MA 9.2.27 and the percentage of the antigen binding sites taken up by the antibody, and by immunoperoxidase staining of cryostat sections to determine the pattern of antibody binding within the nodule. Serum was analyzed for levels of murine Ig, human anti-mouse antibodies and immune complexes.

Administration of MA 9.2.27 by this schedule was safe. All patients developed fevers, the highest 103° C., but these were well tolerated, caused no serious discomfort and permitted outpatient therapy. One patient developed a serum sickness like syndrome that responded promptly to systemic steriods. Mouse Ig levels (tested 2, 4, 6, 12 and 24 hrs) were higher with increasing doses. Antiglobulin responses were usually rapid (within 2 weeks), occurred in 1/3 of the patients, were primarily IgG and, with one exception, were cross-reactive with most murine IgGs; most importantly, however, it did not inhibit localization of the antibody on tumor cells (5). There were no clinical antitumor responses.

Analysis of resected subcutaneous tumor nodules (4) demonstrated detectable murine Ig specifically bound to tumor cells at doses of 50mg or higher, with more cells stained at greater intensities with higher doses. By flow cytometry, we showed that 100% of the tumor cells bound antibody at doses of 200mg or higher, but increased flourescence intensity when excess 9.2.27 was added in vitro indicated that 100% saturation of antigen binding sites was not achieved in all cases.

Immunoperoxidase staining of cryostat sections revealed perivascular binding at the 50mg dose with staining in more distant (i.e., more hypoxic) areas with increasing doses.

Second study phase. A few patients received dose escalations to 500mg. Saturation of all antigen binding sites, a logical endpoint for dose escalation studies with monoclonal antibodies, was achieved in some patients. Achievement of this endpoint is also critical because: i) it establishes the basis for optimal immunoconjugate delivery; ii) it ensures that cells furthest from vessels, that are more hypoxic and more resistant to most forms of therapy, receive the maximum doses; and iii) it decreases chances for selecting of a resistant clone due to suboptimal conjugate delivery.

Third study phase. To determine an optimal MA 9.2.27 delivery schedule, patients received 500mg as a single dose, or in 5 equal daily divided doses, with a 4 week interval to allow all residual antibody to be cleared from the tumor nodules. Both schedules produced saturation in some patients, but the first dose, regardless of the schedule, was generally better than the second due, in 3 cases, to the development of anti-murine antibodies by the host during the interval.

Fourth study phase. 1mg of MA 9.2.27 was chelated to 5 mCi 111-Indium using diethylenetriaminepentaacetic acid (DTPA) (Hybritech, Inc. La Jolla, CA) and administered to patients either alone, or with the addition of 50mg of unconjugated 9.2.27. Serum half-life of the labeled and unlabeled antibody was approximately 30 hours. The latter dose was superior for imaging tumors, detecting masses as small as 5 X 5mm, and occult metastases. There was, however, substantial uptake of tracer by the RES. In vitro studies at 37° C revealed gradual loss of the 111-indium from the chelate. The degree to which

RES uptake is due to the properties of 111-Indium is unknown; administration of 111-In colloid reproduced the biodistribution of 111-In/ 9.2.27 except for splenic and tumor uptake with the latter. Comparisons to antibody labeled with iodine by current techniques may not be valid due to the abundance of hepatic dehalogenases that may lead to underestimation of the percentage of the dose in the liver.

Future directions. MA 9.2.27 was safe, localized in melanoma tumor nodules selectively, and could bind all available sites in these nodules at doses of 200-500mg. MA 9.2.27/111-indium revealed visceral tumor localization but also substantial RES uptake. Future studies will employ different isotopes (e.g., 99m-Tc). This antibody appears to be a good candidate for immunoconjugate development, and has been successfully employed in that setting in animal models (Morgan et al., infra).

References.

1. Morgan AC, Jr., Galloway DR, Reisfeld RA. 1981. Production and characterization of a monoclonal antibody to a melanoma-specific glycoprotein. Hybridoma 1:27.
2. Hwang KM, Morgan AC, Jr., Fodstad O, Oldham RK. 1984. Radiolocalization of xenografted human malignant melanoma by a monoclonal antibody (9.2.27) to a melanoma associated antigen. Cancer Res. In press.
3. Oldham RK, Foon KA, Morgan AC, Jr., Woodhouse CA, Schroff RW, Abrams PG, Fer MF, Schoenberger CS, Farrell MM, Kimball ES, and Sherwin SA. 1984. Monoclonal antibody therapy of malignant melanoma: In vivo localization in cutaneous metastases after intravenous administration. J. Clin.Oncology 2:1235.
4. Schroff RW, Foon KA, Beatty SM, Oldham RK and Morgan AC, Jr. 1985. Human anti-murine immunoglobulin responses in patients receiving monoclonal antibody therapy. Cancer Res. 45:879.
5. Schroff RW, Woodhouse CS, Foon KA, Oldham RK, Morgan AC, Jr. 1984. Intratumor localization of monoclonal antibody in patients with malignant melanoma treated with antibody to a 250 Kd. melanoma-associated antigen. JNCI. In press.

Monoclonal Antibodies and Cancer Therapy, pages 237–241
© **1985 Alan R. Liss, Inc.**

PARAMETERS AFFECTING THE UTILITY OF MONOCLONAL
ANTIBODIES AS CARRIERS OF DRUGS, TOXINS
AND RADIOISOTOPES

Alton C. Morgan, Jr.*
Robert W. Schroff*
John W. Pearson
Gowsala Pavanasasivam*

Biological Therapeutics Branch
Biological Response Modifiers Program, DCT
National Cancer Institute
Frederick, Maryland 21701

*Present address: Neo Rx Corp., 410 W. Harrison Street,
Seattle, Washington 98119

ABSTRACT

Monoclonal antibodies conjugated with toxins, drugs,
or radioisotopes offer a great hope for the development of
cancer-selective cytotoxic reagents. Results in in vivo
models have pointed to some of the limitations of
monoclonal-antibody-directed therapy but at the same time
have given us better insight into the most important questions to be emphasized in the future.

INTRODUCTION

In order to assess the numerous variables associated
with optimizing monoclonal antibody therapy, conjugates
have been examined both in in vitro cell culture systems
and to a lesser degree in animal models, primarily murine.
For the most part, in vivo animal model results have not
proven as impressive as in vitro results would have
predicted (1). In this report we will address two major
parameters, antibody delivery and tumor burden, that
affect the utility of monoclonal antibodies as carriers of
toxins, drugs, or radioisotopes in vivo based on our
experience with monoclonal antibody to a human melanoma
associated antigen 9.2.27 (2), and the D3 antibody to LIO
hepatocellular carcinoma in guinea pigs (3).

CONJUGATE DELIVERY

The question of delivery or localization to tumors
has been primarily addressed with radiolabeled antibodies.
Biodistribution with unconjugated antibody may not be predictive of the in vivo behavior of drug or toxin conjugates. With this proviso, radiolabeled antibody studies
have demonstrated that only a relatively small proportion
of the total administered antibody actually localizes to
the tumor.

Most antibody, administered by the intravenous
route, remains in the circulation or is taken up by the
reticuloendothelial system (RES) organs - lungs, liver,
and spleen [reviewed by Goldenberg (4)]. We have compared
murine monoclonal antibody localization and biodistribution in nude mice and in a heterologous species, guinea
pigs. The pattern of biodistribution of the same antibody
was significantly different in the two species. RES organ
and kidney accumulation of the two murine monoclonals, was
dramatically increased in the heterologous species
compared to the homologous species, nude mice. This nonspecific uptake in guinea pigs increased with increasing
doses of labeled antibody. These distinctions may reflect
a host response to homologous vs heterologous antibody and
analogously, clinical application of murine monoclonals
may have considerably greater problems of biodistribution
than those predicted by studies in nude mice.

The fate of antibody, once bound to tumor cells, is
an important parameter for immunoconjugate studies. In
contrast to lymphoid antigens which undergo rapid modulation when bound by antibody, many antigens of solid tumors
show little modulation (4). Even though there is no
detectable modulation, there can be major differences in
the rate of in vivo turnover. In the two solid tumor
systems we have studied, the D3 antibody in L10 tumors
shows a rapid accretion (maximum at 24 hr.), and then an
equally rapid loss, similar to the rate of loss from
normal organs. In contrast, the 9.2.27 antibody shows a
slower rate of accretion in human melanoma, a steady state
period for up to 5 days, then a gradual loss. These
properties affect the quality of tumor imaging. The
localization and turnover of antibody may also affect
radiotherapy with α- or β-emitting isotope conjugates, but
seems to have little effect on the efficacy of toxin
conjugates. Both antibodies, when conjugated to toxins,

have shown therapeutic effects against established palpable tumors (3,7). Though low antigen density has not been thought to be a limitation for toxin conjugate therapy, for other types of conjugates with drug and therapeutic isotopes, high antigen density should enhance localization, and thus, efficacy. Data from our own radiolabeled antibody studies with 9.2.27 indicate that antibody localization is dependent on antigen density. In comparing human melanoma tumor of different antigen density (8), both the percent of the input dose adsorbed into the tumor and the specific activity (cpm/gram tumor tissue) were higher in a high antigen density tumor than in an intermediate antigene-xpression tumor. These results indicate that the degree of antigen expression in vivo is an important parameter for localization and potentially for the toxic effect of immunoconjugates.

TUMOR BURDEN

For evaluation of therapeutic efficacy of conju-gates, investigations have utilized, for the most part, animal models in which the tumor burden has been limited and the tumors not established (e.g. 9,10). When tumor burden has been increased or the therapeutic regimen delayed until several days after injection of the tumor inoculum, the effect of conjugates on tumor growth has been minimal (1). The lack of success of conjugates against larger tumor burdens may be due to rapid in vivo turnover of antibody, antigenic heterogeneity, or simply to administration of insufficient conjugates. Based on our own studies with trace-labeled 9.2.27, gelonin conju-gates localized 8-fold less and ricin conjugates 15-fold less well than unconjugated antibody. The decreased localization can be accounted for by the greatly shortened serum half-life of conjugates which have a T 1/2 of 6 hr. vs 36 hr. with unconjugated antibody. Thus approximately 0.01% or less of the conjugate dose reached the tumor site in a small, palpable tumor. A potential solution to dealing with increased tumor burden is to increase the amount of conjugate injected, assuming that toxicity would not be limiting, or to increase tumor localization by inhibiting non-antigen-specific uptake. A third attrac-tive alternative is to utilize models in which therapy can be directed at established microscopic metastases. We have treated guinea pigs bearing primary tumors and microscopic lymph node disease with abrin-A-chain conjugate of D3 and found we could inhibit the onset and subsequent growth of lymph node metastases (3).

Another approach that has already been successfully used is combining immunoconjugate therapy with "debulking" therapies like radiation or chemotherapy. Employed in a murine chronic lymphocytic leukemia model, the combination of radiation, splenectomy, and conjugate therapy resulted in cures (10). This approach could be further extrapolated to the use of combinations of immunoconjugates or to combining different toxic agents within the same conjugate. The latter approach could conceivably combine toxins, such as intact ricin or abrin, which internalize well, with drugs which may not internalize well. It is hoped that future in vivo animal model studies will identify new combinations of agents which act in a synergistic fashion and that the efficacy of these combinations of agents can be enhanced by conjugation to specific antibody.

REFERENCES

1. Blythman, HE, Casellas, P, Gros, P, Jansen, FK, Palucci, F, Pau, B, and Vidal, H. Immunotoxins. Hybrid molecules of monoclonal antibodies and a toxin subunit specifically kill tumor cells. Nature 290: 145-146, 1981.
2. Morgan, AC, Jr, Gallowa, DR, and Reisfeld, RA. Production and characterization of monoclonal antibody to a melanoma-specific glycoprotein. Hybridoma 1:27-36, 1981.
3. Hwang, KM, Foon, KA, Cheung, PH, Pearson, JW, and Oldham, RK. Selective antitumor effect of a potent immunoconjugate composed of the A chain of abrin and a monoclonal antibody to a hepatoma associated antigen. Cancer Res., in press.
4. Goldenberg, DM. Tumor imaging with monoclonal antibodies. J. Nucl. Med. 24:360-362, 1983.
5. Schroff, RW, Farrell, MM, Klein, RA, Oldham, RK, and Foon, KA. T65 antigen modulation in a phase I monoclonal antibody trial with chronic lymphocytic leukemia patients. J. Immunol., in press.

6. Hellstrom, I, Brown, JP, and Hellstrom, KE. Melanoma associated antigen P-97 continues to be expressed after prolonged exposure of cells to specific antibody. Int. J. Cancer 31:553-556, 1983.

7. Morgan, AC, Jr, Pavanasasivam, G, Hwang, KM, Woodhouse, CS, Schroff, RW, Foon, KA, and Oldham, RK. Preclinical and clinical evaluation of a monoclonal antibody to a human melanoma associated antigen. In: Protides of the Biological Fluids, XXXII Annual Colloquium. H. Peeters (Ed.). Elsevier/North Holland Press, Amsterdam, in press.

8. Hwang, KN, Morgan, AC, Jr, Fodstad, Ø, and Oldham, RK. Radiolocalization of xenografted human malignant melanoma by a monoclonal antibody (9.2.27) to a melanoma associated antigen. Cancer Res., in press.

Monoclonal Antibodies and Cancer Therapy, pages 243–256
© **1985 Alan R. Liss, Inc.**

MONOCLONAL ANTIBODIES FOR IMMUNOTARGETING
OF DRUGS IN CANCER THERAPY

Ruth Arnon,[1] Bilha Schechter,[1] and
Meir Wilchek,[2]

Departments of Chemical Immunology[1] and Biophysics[2]
The Weizmann Institute of Science, Rehovot, Israel

ABSTRACT In the following we describe the results
achieved in our laboratory by using monoclonal
antibodies as carriers of drugs for the purpose of
immunotargeting. In tumor systems for which polyclonal
antibodies had been previously obtained, and similarly
investigated, a comparison between them and the
respective monoclonal antibodies is made. Chemotherapeutic drugs such as daunomycin, adriamycin,
methotrexate and cis platinum were bound to the
monoclonal antibodies and the various drug conjugates
were evaluated for their efficacy in vitro and in
vivo. All the conjugates retained the full
pharmalogical activity of the drug and were at least
as effective in vitro, as their corresponding free
drugs. As for the antibody activity - the drug
conjugates with the monoclonal antibodies usually
maintained their original antigen-binding capacity.
Consequently, for most tumor systems, including a rat
hepatoma, mouse lung carcinoma (3LL), and neuroblastoma lines, an in vitro specific cytotoxicity
towards the tumor cells to which the antibody was
directed was demonstrated. In their in vivo efficacy,
the drug conjugates were also of beneficial effect,
although a more extensive variability among various
tumor systems was observed.

INTRODUCTION

Chemotherapy constitutes a major therapeutic approach for the treatment of cancer, with some advantage in comparison to surgery and radiotherapy, since it can be used effectively for disseminated as well as localized cancer. Its major drawback, however, is that agents effective in killing neoplastic cells usually have detrimental effects on normal cells, particularly the rapidly proliferating ones of the gastrointestinal tract and bone marrow. As a consequence, cancer chemotherapy is ultimately limited by the toxicity of the drugs to normal tissues, especially when employed in high dosages.

One possible approach aimed at overcoming this limitation is by employing affinity chemotherapy, namely, by attaching the anti-tumor drug to a carrier that would target it to the cancerous cell, and thus selectively increase its local concentration, while the systemic concentration would be maintained low. In this way the selectivity of the drug toxicity for the tumour cells might be enhanced. The carrier can be any molecule with an affinity for certain tumor - specific component, either a surface receptor or a defined antigen. It is still open to question whether genuinely tumor specific antigens do exist. However, without going too deeply into this problem, it is clear that antibodies, either polyclonal or monoclonal, can be prepared that can distinguish between tumor cells and normal ones in a selective fashion, and may thus serve as adequate carriers by virtue of this selectivity.

Therapy by antibodies against tumor associated antigens alone or by antibodies and complement, has in general not been too successful, with the exception of one reported case (1) in which a cancer patient was cured using monoclonal antibody against its own tumor. However, although anti-tumor antibodies as such may not provide an effective means of treatment, their combination with anti-cancer drugs could be helpful, provided that the conjugate retains both antibody and drug activities.

In our studies we attempted to use conjugates, in which drugs were linked chemically to the antibody carrier, for immunotargeting in several experimental tumor systems. We have attached drugs such as daunomycin, adriamycin, cytosine arabinoside, 5 fluorouridine and methotrexate to various antitumor directed antibodies, usually via a polymeric "bridge" or "handle". In addition, we have used derivatives in which platinum salt was complexed to the antibodies, in an attempt to construct cis-platinum structure on antibody conjugates. As for the antibodies - to be suitable as drug carriers they have to be highly specific, and to possess high binding affinity and avidity towards the tumor target cell. When conservative polyclonal antibodies are employed, exhaustive absorption by normal tissue is necessary to ensure the required specificity. With monoclonal antibodies it is possible to obtain monospecific reagents against tumor cells by direct screeing procedures. But, polyclonal antibodies often show higher avidity to the tumor cells due to their simultaneous reactivity with many antigenic determinants. Their polyclonality also makes them less sensitive to loss of antibody activity during to the drug-binding procedures. We have, therefore, engaged antibodies of both polyclonal and monoclonal nature. Some of our studies will be described in the following, with emphasis on our most recent results.

METHODS

The Preparation of Antibodies

Polyclonal antibodies against whole cells or against tumor associated antigens were prepared by immunizing either rabbits, goats or mice, and subsequent adsorption of the antisera with normal tissues and cells of the relevant mouse strain (2, 3). In most cases the IgG fraction of the antiserum was used, but when possible, the antibodies were affinity purified on immunoadsorbents consisting of fixed tumor cells.

Hybridomas were prepared by fusing spleen cells of immunized mouse or rat cells with NS1 or NSO myeloma cells (4). For the preparation of antibodies against whole tumor cells adoptive transfers of immune spleen cells preceeded the hybridization; the immune spleen cells were transferred into irradiated recipients which received an additional antigenic challenge (5). Antibodies against purified surface antigens were prepared by direct fusion to the myeloma cells.

The screening for antibody activity was performed by solid phase radioimmunoassay with whole tumor cells (6), which were attached to the walls of a soft microtiter plate by drying followed by formaldehyde fixation. The antibody-containing supernatants were then assayed indirectly using ^{125}I-labeled second antibody. For the detection of antibodies

against tumor associated antigens, reverse solid phase radioimmunoassay was used. For that purpose the second antibody was
bound to the wells of the microtiter plates, reacted with the
antibody-containing supernatant and detected by the use of
^{125}I-labeled antigen.

Drug Conjugation Procedures

Daunomycin was linked to antibodies via dextran-T10 (M.W.
10000). The dextran, oxidized by sodium periodate (2, 7)
was reacted first with daunomycin and then with the antibodies.
The coupling, most probably Schiff base formation between the
aldehyde groups on the oxidized dextran and the amino groups
on the drug and the antibody, was stabilized by partial
reduction with sodium borohydride (8). Adriamycin was bound
via a bridge of carboxymethyldextran hydrazide (9), utilizing
the carbonyl side chain group on the drug rather than the
aminosugar (10). The antibody was attached to the dextran
hydrazide derivative by cross linking with glutaraldehyde.
Recently we have attached adriamycin to monoclonal anti-Thy
1.1 antibodies via periodate-oxidized dextran T40 (M.W.40000),
similarly to the method of coupling of daunomycin. This conjugate was stable at neutral pH without any reduction process.
Methotrexate was attached via a copolymer of glutamic acid
and lysine (Glu:Lys 4.7:1, M.W. 18,700) by two steps with water
soluble carbodiimide (11). Platinum was complexed to the
antibodies by direct interaction with the Pt salt K_2PtCL_4 (12).
In more recent experiments complexing of Pt to antibodies via
polymeric bridges was also attempted. The extent of drug binding in the different conjugates varied from 25-50 mol/mol when
antibodies of the IgG class were employed, to 250-500 mol/mol
for IgM antibodies.

Determination of Biological Activity

The conjugates were evaluated for the pharmacological
activity of the drug as well as for the antibody activity.
The pharmacological activity was usually assessed in vitro
primarily by the inhibition of cellular RNA or DNA synthesis
in the various cells, as manifested by the incorporation of
^{3}H uridine, ^{3}H thymidine or ^{3}H deoxuridine, respectively,or
by the inhibition of protein synthesis as manifested by incorporation of radioactively labeled leucine. The antibody
activity was measured for each system according to their

specificity, usually by binding capacity to the intact tumor
cells or isolated antigen therefrom.

The specific cytotoxicity of the conjugates was evaluated
in vitro by allowing them to attach to the target cell during
a short incubation, after which the cells were washed to
remove unbound drug conjugates, and further incubated in
culture medium for assessment of residual drug effect (13).

Therapeutic effectivity of the conjugates in vivo was
assessed in mice or rats in which the tumor cells were previously transplanted. The conjugates were administered at various doses, routes and schedule, and their effect estimated
according to the tumor development and prolongation of survival.

RESULTS

Studies with the Yac Lymphoma

In our early experiments with this tumor system (2) we
used daunomycin conjugates with polyclonal affinity purified
antibodies that were prepared in goats against membrane antigen obtained from the tumor cells by papain digestion. These
antibodies were specific towards Yac cells as determined by
complement-mediated cytotoxicity, but were nevertheless able
to bind to normal splenocytes as well. In therapy studies the
daunomycin-dextran-anti Yac conjugates did show some beneficial
effect (2). We therefore envisaged that antibodies with higher
specificity might improve the efficacy of the drug-antibody
conjugate. Monoclonal antibodies were prepared for this purpose, by hybridization of spleen cells from (BALB/c x A/J) F1
mice immunized with whole tumor cells. These antibodies
designated KH_{3-4}, which were of the IgM class, bound to Yac
cells 10-50 fold better than to normal spleen cells and did
not react with normal thymocytes or with lymph node cells.
The effectivity of the KH_{3-4} dextran-daunomycin conjugate
(containing 500 mol of daunomycin per mol antibody) was tested
in vivo and compared to the polyclonal goat anti-Yac conjugate described above. In this experiment (Table 1) the tumor
which was transplanted subcutaneously was quite sensitive to
daunomycin, and a dose of 12 mg/kg of the free drug led to 60%
long-term survival. The drug conjugate with the purified
polyclonal goat anti-Yac antibodies was very effective and
when used in the same dose, it led to 100% long-term survival.
However, the daunomycin conjugate of the more specific monoclonal antibody was less effective, and only at a higher drug

dose (25 mg/kg), at which a non-specific Ig-drug conjugate was similarly beneficial. The reason for the lower efficacy of this monoclonal antibody as compared to the polyclonal one is not clear. It could be due to its IgM nature, or to a lower avidity to the tumor cells.

Table 1

THE IN VIVO[a] EFFECT OF DAUNOMYCIN   CONJUGATES WITH MONOCLONAL AND POLYCLONAL ANTI-YAC ANTIBODIES.

Treatment[b]	Drug (mg/kg)	Antibody (mg/kg)	Median (days)	% Survival
PBS	-	-	24	0
Daunomycin	12	-		60
	17	-		60
Dau-dex-KH$_{3-4}$[c]	12.5	100	23	20
	22	250		80
Dau-dex-X63[d]	12.5	75	25	20
	22	250		80
Dau + KH$_{3-4}$	12.5	250	28	0
Dau-dex-G anti-Yac(Ab)[e]	12.5	50		100
Dau + G anti-Yac(Ab)	12.5	100		60
G anti-Yac (Ab)	-	100	23	20

[a] YAC cells, 10^5 in 0.5 ml PBS were injected subcutaneously into male A/J mice (10 weeks old).
[b] Treatment was given i.v. on day 3.
[c] KH$_{3-4}$ anti-YAC monoclonal antibody, of the IgM class.
[d] X63, normal IgG produced by the NS-1 myeloma.
[e] G anti-YAC (Ab), purified goat anti-YAC antibodies.

Studies with Neuroblastoma

Our studies were concerned with both human neuroblastoma cell line LA-N-I that was developed by Seeger, and a mouse neuroblastoma N 115, originally developed by Nirenberg (14). Both neuroblastomas express specific surface differentiation antigens, Thy-1 and Thy1.1, respectively, against which appropriate monoclonal antibodies were prepared. In the case of the human cell line only in vitro studies were performed whereas with the N 115 the availability of the mouse model enabled some in vivo experiments.

The mouse hybridoma against the LA-N-I was developed by Seeger et al (15) and the monoclonal antibody was characterized as anti-Thy-1. A conjugate of adriamycin with this antibody, which was shown to retain the activities of both the drug and the antibody (9) was evaluated for its in vitro activity on the tumor cells by measuring the effect on the cell cycle traverse. The results are shown in Table 2.

TABLE 2

EFFECT OF ADRIAMYCIN CONJUGATED TO 390 MONOCLONAL
ANTIBODY ON NEUROBLASTOMA CELL CYCLE

Treatment	Time in Culture (hr)	Percentage of cells in:		
		G_1	S	G_2
Anti-Thy-1	24	$42.1^\pm10.9$	$42.9^\pm12.6$	$14.9^\pm2.9$
	48	$38.4^\pm9.4$	$46.2^\pm10.8$	$18.9^\pm7.4$
Adriamycin	24	$51.1^\pm4$	$29.7^\pm5$	$19.2^\pm2$
	48	$56.1^\pm9.2$	$12.4^\pm6.6$	$31.5^\pm8.1$
Adriamycin-anti-Thy-1	24	$36.1^\pm2$	$36.4^\pm4.1$	$27.6^\pm6.8$
	48	$46.4^\pm6.1$	$16.9^\pm6.1$	$37.6^\pm4.1$

NOTE: Neuroblastoma cells, 10^5/well in 100μl. were incubated with anti-Thy-1 adriamycin and adriamycin-antibody conjugate. After the appropriate incubation time, the cells from three wells for each treatment were removed and subjected to DNA distribution studies.

The normal distribution of DNA in neuroblastoma cells after periods of 24 and 48 hr was not altered by the anti-Thy-1 antibody alone - the cells were almost evenly divided between G_1 and S phases and 15-19% were in G_2+M. Treatment with adriamycin caused some retardation in G_1, a reduction S phase and an accumulation of cells in G_2 which probably interferes with subsequent cell mitosis. The adriamycin-anti-Thy-1 treatment of log phase, non synchronized cells caused a similar reduction in S phase and mainly an even higher accumumation in G_2 phase than that caused by the free drug. These effects further increased after 48 hr incubation, and might imply that the adriamycin-antibody conjugate is a better cytotoxic agent than the free drug.

The mouse neuroblastoma maintained as a cell line N115 can be effected to grow in male A/J mice either subcutaneously (by s.c. injection) or as metastatic nodules mostly in the lungs (by i.v. injection). None of the drugs we tested was effective against the s.c tumor, hence the immunotargeting experiments were performed on the metatastic tumor. The antibody employed was an anti Thy 1.1 mouse monoclonal antibody (16) belonging to the IgM class. Its conjugate with adriamycin, via dextran T10, was evaluated for its therapeutic effect in vivo on the development of tumor and survival of the mice. The results of one experiment, as depicted in Fig.1, demonstrate a favorable effect of the specific antibody conjugate as compared to the controls. The free adriamycin had a slight effect at a low dose (300 μg/mouse) but was toxic at a higher concentration (375 μg/mouse). The conjugate with dextran alone could be employed at a higher dose (650 μg/mouse) where it was toxic to some of the mice, but those that survived benefited from the treatment.

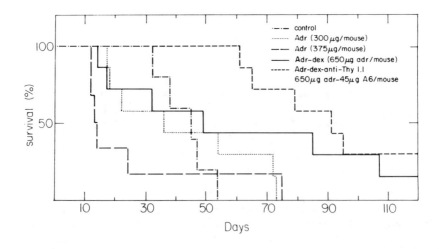

FIGURE 1.   Chemotherapeutic effect of adriamycin-antibody conjugate on lung metastasis in mice preinjected i.v. with 5x10^5 neuroblastoma N115 cells. Treatment at day 5 with a single dose of the drug conjugate or other controls.

Studies with Lewis Lung Carcinoma (3LL).

    This tumor which is maintained in mice as a local tumor, with later development of lung metastases (17) is quite resistant to chemotherapy by various cytotoxic drugs such as daunomycin, adriamycin or methotrexate, although these drugs are effective against the tumor cells in vitro. We have pre-pared monoclonal antibodies (denoted 6B) against this tumor, that showed strong anti lung-tissue reactivity and were con-sequently capable of effective homing, with specific accumu-lation factor of approximately 30 in the metastatic lungs of tumor-bearing mice (15). We hoped that as a result of this homing, the efficacy of drug conjugates of this antibody will be increased. However, experiments with conjugates of either daunomycin, adriamycin or methotrexate were disappointing and did not lead to a significant therapeutic effect.
    The only promising results with this tumor system were obtained with antibody-platinum complexes. We have previously shown that platinum salts can be complexed to antibody mole-cules either directly (12) or via dextran amine (dextran-ethylen diamine derivative). In such complexes a cis-platinum-like structure is most probably obtained, and they retain both the pharmacological and antibody activities (18). The in vitro activity of dextran amine-antibodies complexes with the mono-clonal anti 3LL antibodies is shown in Fig. 2.

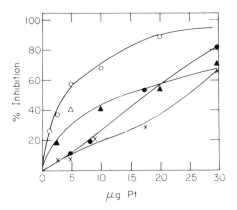

    FIGURE 2. Inhibition of DNA synthesis in 3LL cells
(5 x 10^4) by : Pt-dextran amine-anti 3LL monoclonal antibodies
(o), Pt-dextran amine normal Ig ( ), Pt-dextranamine (x)
and K_2Pt Cl_4 (o). Cultures were incubated for 21 hr at 37°c.

The results demonstrate the advantageous effect of the relevant complex as compared to the various controls of the free platinum salt or its complexes with dextran amine alone, or a derivative of normal immunoglobulin. Figure 3 demonstrates the therapeutic activity of the relevant platinum antibody complex in vivo on the tumor development and prolongation of survival of mice transplanted with the 3LL tumor. The beneficial effect of the complexes is compared to that of cis-Pt, which is highly toxic at a higher dose (300 μg/ mouse), and at a lower dose (100 μg/mouse) is ineffective.

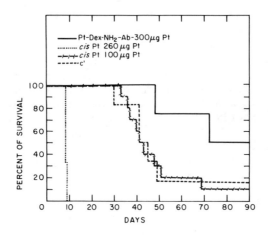

FIGURE 3. Chemotherapeutic effect of Pt-dextran amine-anti-3LL monoclonal antibody complex on mice bearing 3LL tumor. Mice were treated i.v. one day after tumor injection with a single dose of the respective reagent.

Studies with Rat Hepatoma

Rat hepatoma (AH 66) is an α-fetoprotein (AFP)-producing hepatoma maintained in Donryu rats. In the case of this tumor system we evaluated (18) drug conjugates of both polyclonal (horse) and monoclonal (mouse) antibodies that were prepared by immunization with rat AFP. Daunomycin was linked via dextran T10 to both types of antibodies. The drug activity in different preparations of the conjugates, as determined by the inhibition of ^{3}H-thymidine incorporation, amounted to 60-100% of the free drug activity. The antibody binding activity was also fully sustained in the conjugates, as determined by their reaction with ^{125}I-labeled antigen. In their specific cytotoxicity towards the hepatoma cells in vitro the conjugates of dauno-mycin with the horse anti-AFP and the monoclonal antibodies were also of similar activity, both demonstrating higher effi-cacy than free daunomycin.

To evaluate the chemotherapeutic effectivity of the con-jugates, they were injected into tumor-bearing rats. Each rat was treated 5 times from the third day after tumor injection, on alternate days, with i.v. administered conjugate solution. As shown in Fig. 4 treatment with the specific antibody-drug conjugates led to a remarkable life prolongation as well as to 60% long-term survival. In this case as well, a close simil-arity was observed between the efficacy of the drug conjugates of the monoclonal antibody and that of the conventional poly-clonal antibody.

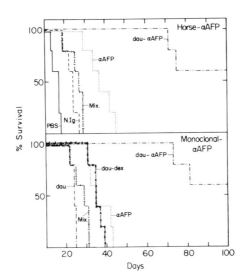

FIGURE 4. The therapeutic effectivity of daunomycin-anti-body-conjugates on rats preinjected with AH66 hepatoma (10^5 cells). Treatments were given i.v. at days 3, 5, 7, 9 and 11 after tumor cells injection, at a dose of 200 μg daunomycin and 2 mg antibody per injection.

DISCUSSION

The problem we addressed ourselves to in this paper is the potential use of drug-antibody conjugates for targeted immunochemotherapy for the treatment of cancer. In this approach the prerequisite is that the conjugates will retain the activities of both the antibody and the drug. This prerequisite was indeed fulfilled and in most cases very high in vitro activity of the conjugates was observed towards the specific tumor cell recognized by the antibodies. In the in vivo studies the situation was somewhat more complex, with wider variability between the results obtained for different tumors, probably due to different parameters.

For example, in the case of mouse lung carcinoma (3LL), conjugates of the polyclonal and even more so of the monoclonal antibody (directed to lung-associated antigen) exhibited efficient homing to the metastasized lungs. However, the resultant high drug concentration at the tumor site did not overcome the intrinsic ineffectivity of drugs such as daunomycin, adriamycin or methotrexate against this tumor in vivo. Only complexes of platinum with the specific antibodies proved of some benefit. In a mouse T lymphoma (Yac), conjugates of both polyclonal and monoclonal antibodies had a beneficial effect, leading to prolongation of life as well as to long-term survival. However, in this case, the monoclonal antibodies were less effective drug carriers than the polyclonal purified goat antibodies. This could stem from the IgM nature of these particular antibodies, from their low avidity, or from the paucity of the specific antigenic determinants on the surface of the tumor cell. In the studies on a rat hepatoma, both monoclonal and horse polyclonal antibodies against rat AFP were available, which had similar binding affinities for either the isolated immunogen or the whole tumor cell. In this case, drug-antibody conjugates of either kind were effective in vitro and in vivo, indicating that both types of antibodies worked equally well as drug carriers for efficient therapeutic effect in tumor bearing rats. The high efficacy of the monoclonal antibodies in this system is not surprising in view of the abundance of AFP on the hepatoma cell surface, which facilitates the immunotargeting.

The main conclusions from these studies are that antibodies may indeed serve as carriers for anti-cancer drugs for the purpose of immunotargeting. The monoclonal antibodies have both advantages and disadvantages over the polyclonal ones. They are advantageous since they can be readily obtained by immunization with the whole tumor cells, including neoplasms

which do not bear a known tumor marker; they can also be prepared from naturally existing antibody-producing peripheral
blood lymphocytes by in vitro culturing procedures, thus leading
to human-human hybridomas; they are uniformly specific, and if
directed against an abundant antigen - may show very high
efficiency. Their uniformity can be of a disadvantage if they
are directed towards a scarce antigen on the tumor cell, or if
the drug-binding modification leads to a loss of their reactivity. In such cases, polyclonal antibodies may be superior.
It is thus apparent that both polyclonal and monoclonal antibodies should be considered in future efforts towards
immunotargeted chemotherapy.

REFERENCES

1. Miller RA, Moloney DG, Warnke BS, Levy R. (1982). Treat-
    ment of B-cell lymphoma with monoclonal anti-idiotype
    antibody New Eng J Med 306:517.
2. Hurwitz E, Maron R, Bernstein A, Wilchek M, Sela M, Arnon
    R, (1978). The effect in vivo of chemotherapeutic drug-
    antibody conjugates in two murine experimental systems.
    Int J Cancer 21:747.
3. Hurwitz E, Schechter B, Arnon R, Sela M, (1979). Binding
    of anti-tumor immunoglobulins and their daunomycin con-
    jugates to a tumor and its metastasis. In vitro and in
    vivo studies with Lewis lung carcinoma. Int J Cancer
    24:461.
4. Eshhar Z, Ofarim M, Waks T, (1980). Generation of hybrid-
    omas secreting murine reaginic antibodies of anti-DNP
    specificity. J Immunol 124:775.
5. Hadas E, Hurwitz E, Eshhar Z, (1984). Identification of
    a surface antigen, common to murine Lewis lung carcinoma
    by monoclonal antibodies. Int J Cancer 33:369.
6. Huang J C -C, Berczi I, Froese G, Tsay H M, Sehon A H,
    (1975). Microradioimmunoassay for antibodies to
    tumor-associated antigens. J Nat Cancer Inst 55:879.
7. Bernstein A, Hurwitz E, Maron R, Arnon R, Sela M, Wilchek
    M, (1978), Higher anti-tumor efficacy of daunomycin when
    linked to dextran: In vivo and in vitro studies. J Natl
    Cancer Inst 60:379.
8. Arnon R, Hurwitz E, (1983). Antibody and polymer drug
    conjugates. In "Targeted Drugs" (ed. E P Goldberg) Wiley
    N Y. P.23.
9. Hurwitz E, Arnon R, Sahar E, Danon Y, (1983). A conjugate
    of adriamycin and monoclonal antibodies to Thy-1 antigen

inhibits human neuroblastoma cells in vitro. Annual N Y Acad Sci 417:125.

10. Hurwitz E, Wilchek M, Pitha J, (1980). Soluble macromole cules as carriers for daunomycin. J App Biochem 2:25.

11. Arnon R, Sela M, (1982). In vitro and in vivo efficacy of conjugates of daunomycin with anti-tumor antibodies. Immunol Rev 62:5.

12. Hurwitz E, Kashi R, Wilchek M, (1982). Platinum-complexed anti-tumor immunoglobulins that specifically inhibit DNA synthesis of mouse tumor cells. J Nat Cancer Inst 69:47.

13. Levi R, Hurwitz E, Maron R, Arnon R, Sela M, (1975). The specific cytotoxic effects of daunomycin conjugated to anti-tumor antibodies. Cancer Res 35:1182.

14. Mano T, Richelson E, Nirenberg M, (1972). Neurotransmitter synthesis of Neuroblastoma clones PNAS. 69:258.

15. Seeger R C, Danon Y L, Rayner S A, Hoover F, (1982). Definition of a Thy-1 determinant on human neuroblastoma, glioma, sarcoma and teratoma cells with a monoclonal antibody. J Immunol 128:983.

16. Marshak-Rothstein A, Fink P, Gridley T, Raulet D.H, Bevan M J, Gefter M L, (1979). Properties and application of monoclonal antibodies directed against determinants of the Thy-1 locus. J Immunol 122:2491.

17. Sugiura K, Stock C C, (1955). Studies in tumor spectrum. III. The effect of phosphoramide on the growth of a variety of mouse and rat tumors. Cancer Res 15:38.

18. Tsukada Y, Hurwitz E, Kashi R, Sela M, Hibi N, Hara A, Hirai H, (1982). Chemotherapy by intravenous administration of conjugates of daunomycin with monoclonal and conventional anti-rat α-fetaprotein antibodies.

Monoclonal Antibodies and Cancer Therapy, pages 257–259
© 1985 Alan R. Liss, Inc.

WORKSHOP SUMMARY: MONOCLONAL ANTIBODY
CONJUGATES WITH DRUGS OR TOXINS

Thomas F. Bumol

Department of Immunology
Lilly Research Laboratories
Lilly Corporate Center
Indianapolis, Indiana 46285.

This workshop examined in detail several approaches by
different investigators for the application of drug or
toxin conjugates of monoclonal antibodies (moab) for ex
vivo or in vivo cancer therapy. T. Bumol introduced this
topic with comments on practical considerations for
monoclonal antibody conjugate cancer therapy in terms of
several theoretical problems with the approach. These
potential problems included: 1) insufficient drug
density/delivery for drug-moab conjugates for tumor cell
kill, 2) nonspecific innocent bystander toxicities that may
be monoclonal antibody directed, 3) rapid catabolism
resulting in poor pharmacokinetics, 4) target tumor cell
antigenic heterogeneity, and 5) host anti-immunoglobulin or
anti-drug/toxin responses. In addition, it was discussed
that optimal drug targeting must also involve efficient
endocytosis and release of drugs and toxin subunits from
the conjugate to intracellular sites of action such as the
nucleus or cytoplasm.
    Several investigators then summarized their efforts in
developing therapeutic monoclonal antibody toxin or drug
conjugates. Additional information on these presentations
can be found in abstracts by the authors listed in the
Journal of Cellular Biochemistry, Supplement 9A, 1985.
    J. Fulton described his experiments on developing a
more potent ricin A chain-antibody conjugate by enhancing
this conjugate's toxicity in a synergistic fashion by a
second conjugate containing ricin B chain. Utilizing
conjugation procedures with Ellman's reagent he described a
number of in vitro toxicity experiments exploring the use
of Fab fragment conjugates in this fashion. He
demonstrated that univalent Fab ricin A chain-antibody
conjugates could be enhanced ten-fold in specific toxicity
by a corresponding ricin B chain-antibody conjugate thus
establishing that the synergy response was unaffected by

antibody valency in the conjugate. These developments
suggested that an in vivo strategy utilizing the synergy
approach could be feasible with the potential advantages of
Fab fragment catabolism.

A. E. Frankel summarized a number of efforts on the
development of breast cancer monoclonal antibody-toxin
conjugates. The analysis of 124 hybridomas defining breast
tumor antigens was presented indicating that 50 antibodies
defined tumor associated antigens. An extensive effort
examining the in vitro specific toxicity of toxin
conjugates to these antibodies was presented including
toxins such as ricin A chain, pokeweed antiviral protein,
diphtheria toxin and others. In addition, A. E. Frankel
announced the successful recent conjugation of a monoclonal
antibody to a recombinant ricin A chain. These studies
demonstrated that antibodies having a high KA and a high
antigenic copy number on the target cell surface were more
effective immunotoxin conjugates in vitro. Frankel then
mentioned that several active immunotoxins were tested in
xenograft/nude mouse efficacy experiments and the data
suggested that effective doses for tumor growth suppression
(50-80% suppression) also demonstrated some toxicities. He
stressed that effective immunotherapy with toxin conjugated
monoclonal antibodies will have to have improved
pharmacokinetics with more favorable tumor localization in
vivo and altered catabolic pathways. The advent of
recombinant toxins and the potential for genetically
engineered antibodies suggested several future directions.

K. Matthay then described her studies combining
monoclonal antibodies with drug containing liposomes for an
alternative means of antibody directed drug targeting. In
a model murine T cell leukemia system, she demonstrated the
delivery and cytotoxicity in vitro of antibody-protein
A-liposomes containing a poorly transported derivative of
methotrexate; methotrexate-γ-aspartate. While the ensuing
discussion suggested that this technology might not offer a
realistic in vivo therapy, the application of this
technique to ex vivo removal of unwanted cells from bone
marrow remains an interesting possibility.

T. Bumol next presented a summary of drug targeting
studies examining a conjugate of a monoclonal antibody
defining a human adenocarcinoma associated antigen and a
derivative of vinblastine. Specific antibody directed
vinca associated mitotic blocks could be demonstrated in
vitro versus a human lung adenocarcinoma cell line
indicating cytoplasmic localization of the drug. In vivo

experiments in a xenograft model demonstrated a
dose-dependent suppression of tumor growth in monoclonal
antibody-drug conjugate treated nude mice and preliminary
toxicology experiments in mice suggest that these
conjugates do not have the toxicities observed with free
drug. Staggered I.V. treatment protocols with drug and
toxin conjugates (ricin A and pokeweed antiviral protein)
of the same antibody revealed efficacy with the
drug-conjugates but poor tumor suppression of
toxin-conjugates. It was again stressed in this workshop
that detailed pharmacokinetic experiments were necessary to
optimize immunotherapy protocols of conjugated antibodies.
It was suggested that conjugation of antibodies with low
molecular weight drugs might result in a conjugate with
decreased catabolism in vivo compared to toxin conjugates.
Further experiments establishing the efficacy of drug
conjugated monoclonal antibodies on more established tumors
and in metastasis models as well as the toxicology in
animal species more sensitive to vinca alkaloids such as
nonhuman primates were stated to be in progress.

        T. Bumol concluded the workshop by stating that an
overall goal of these types of monoclonal antibody
conjugate studies would be to demonstrate increase in the
therapeutic index of oncolytic drugs and perhaps add novel
agents such as protein toxins or highly toxic synthetic
drugs to site directed cancer therapy.

VI. TOXIN-ANTIBODY CONJUGATES

Monoclonal Antibodies and Cancer Therapy, pages 263–274
© **1985 Alan R. Liss, Inc.**

POTENTIATION OF CYTOTOXICITY INDUCED BY IMMUNOTOXINS

Pierre Casellas, Hildur E. Blythman, Bernard J.P. Bourrié,
X. Canat, Dominique Carrière, Guy Laurent and F.K. Jansen

Department of Immunology
Centre de Recherche Clin Midy (Groupe Sanofi)
34082 MONTPELLIER CEDEX FRANCE

ABSTRACT   Immunotoxins (ITs) are hybrid molecules
designed for a more selective therapy of cancer,
which combine an antibody preferentially directed
against tumour cells and the A-chain of the toxin
ricin. Although a majority of them are highly and
selectively cytotoxic to their target cells in vitro,
only some of them gave rise to a therapeutic effect
in animal models. In vitro kinetics studies suggested
the importance of a rapid mode of action for in vivo
efficacy, which is not the property of all IT. Ways
of accelerating and potentiating such conjugates are
proposed. Lysosomotropic amines such as ammonium
chloride, chloroquine, methylamine and carboxylic
ionophores such as monensin, which are known to
interfere with the uptake of certain macromolecules,
strongly increased the rate of protein synthesis
inhibition by all ITs tested and increased 4-to
50 000-fold the sensitivity of cells to the IT.
Enhancement in the inactivation rate was as much as
7- to 10-fold when either of these compounds was
added, generating kinetics comparable to those of
ricin. Whereas the in vivo use of these activations
is still under research, their in vitro use rise to
a six orders of magnitude the cytoreduction of
leukemic cells and thus is directly applicable to
clinical situations such as bone marrow transplantation.

INTRODUCTION

Immunotoxins (ITs) have been described in the literature since 1980 (1, 6), patented in 1978 (7). They are conjugates between subunits specifically directed against target cells to increase the antibody mediated cytotoxicity. Thus ITs combine the potential of the most powerful toxins with the specificity of selected antibodies. The results obtained with these reagents demonstrated the expected specific in vitro cytotoxicity since more than 99.9% of target cells were eliminated, whereas cells not expressing the relevant antigens were unaffected. However, despite these encouraging data, ITs are far less toxic than the parent toxin ricin and in in vivo experiments, complete eradication of tumor cells in animal models has not been possible with IT treatment. In recent studies, we (8) and others (9, 11) have pointed out that the rate of cell killing induced by ITs, is extremely slow and this may account for the relative ineffectiveness of the ITs in vivo. However, since the kinetics of cell killing by ITs has so far been inadequately studied, a more detailed examination is warranted.

We show here from a kinetic analysis of a number of ITs that the time required to kill target cells can vary within a wide range depending on the model used and that two variables affect the rate of cell killing : the number of IT molecules bound per cell and the class of the antibody moiety. In addition, the previously described enhancement of target cell killing in the presence of ammonium chloride (8) is here extended to include a variety of lysosomotropic amines and a group of carboxylic ionophores. These compounds which improved both activity and specificity of ITs could have important therapeutic implications.

RESULTS AND DISCUSSION

I) Importance of the Kinetics of Cytotoxicity Induced by Immunotoxins.

    To understand why the IT is not potent enough for in vivo therapy, we studied the efficacy of IT in terms of kinetics of cytotoxicity and compared it to that of ricin, since ricin is more potent that IT. Figure 1 summarizes the kinetics of action of ricin and three different ITs.

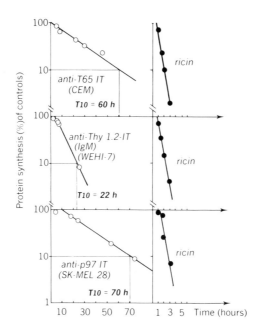

FIGURE 1.   Kinetics of inhibition of protein synthesis induced by ricin and immunotoxins

The cells were treated with ricin or ITs at a dose which saturated receptor or antigen sites, and protein synthesis was measured at various times. The time required to reduce protein synthesis by a factor of 10 is the T10 value and used to compare the kinetics. Even when all antigen sites are satured by ITs the time required for IT to affect cells is typically between 20 and 70 hours. The T10 value was 22 hrs with the IT directed against the Thy 1.2 antigen on the mouse W-7 cells. It was 60 hours with the anti-T65 IT on CEM cells and even longer T10 of 70 h was obtained with IT recognizing the human melanoma associated antigen P97 on the human melanoma SK-Mel28 cells. It can be seen from these curves that in each case the complete eradication of the target cells would require an extremely long period of several days or even weeks. This could explain the low in vivo anti-tumor effect.

In contrast ricin showed a fast inactivation rate with a T10 value in the range of 1 to 2 hours only. We therefore examined if the differences between ricin and ITs could be explained by differences in number of molecules bound per cell. We found, from binding analyses, that at the doses tested in figure 1 the number of A-chain molecules bound per cell was between 2×10^6 and 7×10^6 with ricin on WEHI-7 and on CEM cells, respectively, whereas it was 1.5×10^6 with the anti-Thy 1.2 IT (IgM) on WEHI-7 cells, 4×10^4 with the anti-T65 IT on CEM cells and 4.5×10^5 with the anti-p97 IT on SK-MEL 28. In order to compare the ability of the bound toxin and ITs to intoxicate cells we performed kinetic experiments at concentrations ensuring an identical number of A-chain molecules bound per cell. The results are given in table 1. Although the rate of protein synthesis inactivation induced by ricin slightly decreased when the number of ricin molecules bound per cell diminished, ricin induced 30-fold and 12-fold faster inactivation rates compared to anti-T65 IT and anti-Thy 1.2 IT (IgM), respectively, demonstrating the higher efficacy of ricin versus ITs. However, the differences between the two toxins could vary dramatically with the IT examined, as illustrated with the anti-Thy 1.2 IT (IgG). The rate of protein synthesis inactivation induced by anti-Thy 1.2 IT (IgG) on WEHI-7 cells was only 2.3-fold longer than that obtained with ricin (Table 1).

TABLE 1
KINETICS OF CYTOTOXICITY INDUCED BY ITs AND RICIN
AT COMPARABLE AMOUNT OF A-CHAIN MOLECULE BOUND PER CELL.

CELL LINE	TOXIN	A-CHAIN MOLECULES BOUND PER CELL	T_{10} HOURS
CEM	Ricin	4×10^4	2
	Anti-T65 IT	4×10^4	60
WEHI-7	Ricin	1.5×10^6	1.7
	Anti-Thy 1.2 IT (IgM)	1.5×10^6	20
	Ant-Thy 1.2 It (IgG)	1.5×10^6	4

    In addition, this example demonstrated the impor-
tance of the antibody moiety class for the IT efficacy
since the simple substitution of the anti-Thy 1.2 IgM by
an IgG of same specificity improved by a factor of 5 the
rate of cell killing measured under comparable conditions.
This anti-Thy 1.2 IT assembled with a rat IgG2c antibody
which displayed fast cytotoxicity kinetics was evaluated
in vivo (figure 2). Fifteen thousand Thy-1.2 positive
murine lymphoma T2 cells were injected i.v. into congenic
Thy 1.2 negative BL 1.1 mice. Twenty four hours later
mice were treated with a PBS buffer or antibody alone for
controls or with 200 microgrammes of IT. On day 160, 80%
of animals survived when treated with IT while all controls
were dead at day 22 or 38. These good results stroongly
suggested that, in addition to a selective effect, rapid
kinetics of toxicity is essential for any succesful in vivo
therapy.

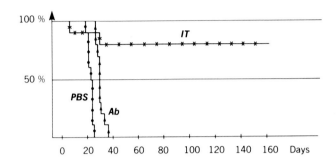

FIGURE 2.   Survival of BL 1.1 mice after treatment
            with an anti-Thy 1.2 (IgG) IT.

II) Influence of Lysosomotropic Amines and Monensin on
    the Rate of the Protein Synthesis Inhibition Induced
    by ITs.

     We studied, with an electron microscope, the process
of internalization and intracellular transport of an IT
presenting a slow inactivation rate. We chose the anti-
T65 IT and examined it on the CEM cell line. This IT was
absorbed on particles of colloïdal gold. This procedure
did not alter signilicantly the binding capacity of the
IT as well as the specific cytotoxicity on the target
cell. After 1 h at 4° C IT was bound to the plasma membrane as shown in figure 3. When cells were transferred
to 37° C, the ligands were internalized into the cell.
After 15 min the tagged IT was observed in endocytic
vacuoles and also in tubular structures near the Golgi
region and then quickly discharged within lysosomes. This
suggested that IT could be degraded in his compartment.
We have already described that lysosomotropic amines such
as NH4Cl or chloroquine which disturb the acidification
of lysosomes strongly enhanced the speed of action of ITs.
We recently found another class of compounds which also
possess similar properties : the carboxylic ionophores.

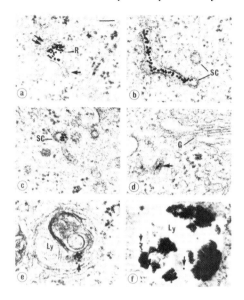

FIGURE 3. Intracellular transport of IT-Au
          in CEM cells:
a.   Receptosome labelled with colloidal gold,
b.c. IT-Au in tubular structures,
d.   IT-Au in tubular elements of the Golgi system,
e.   Lysosome labelled with IT-Au,
f.   Reacting positively with the detection of acid
     phosphatase.

     When the humam T leukemia CEM cells were treated with
the anti-T65 in concert with 10mM NH4Cl a 10-fold increase
in the rate was observed. With Monensin a higher accel-
eration was obtained. The advantage of monensin is that it
was much more potent than NH4Cl. In the presence of
20 - 50nM Monensin the T10 value was only 2.5 h which is
very close to that of ricin ; the second advantage is that
by acting catalytically it was effective with a minuscule
amount ; this should have a major consequence for in vivo
applications. Other carboxylic ionophores such as Nigericin
or Lasalocid also act as activators like monensin (12).

We studied the fate of anti-T65 IT in the presence of monensin on CEM cells. Observations made under the electron microscope showed that, as we noted previously with NH4Cl, monensin did not interfere with the internalization process of the anti-T65 IT tagged with gold particles. The number of gold particles per cell internalized, measured at various time intervals, was similar if the activator was present or not. In contrast, in the presence of monensin, the intracellular distribution of IT was profoundly changed. We noted an almost total absence of the IT in the lysosomes but an accumulation of IT in a large non-lysosomal compartment developed from endocytic vacuoles or receptosomes. In this organelles, the ligand is usually bound to the membrane suggesting the presence of intact ligand/receptor complexes. Therefore monensin, as NH4Cl, could enhance the IT activity by preventing ITs degradation by lysosomal enzymes (13).

III) Influence of Lysosomotropic Amines and Carboxylic
     Ionophores on the Cytotoxicity of ITs.

Although the activation mechanism is not completely understood this effect is of considerable practical interest because such compounds led also to an important activation of the IT in the dose-response curve. Figure 4 shows the specific activity of the anti-T65 IT on CEM cells. In the presence of NH4Cl the potency of the IT showed a 50-fold increase while on the other hand the non-specific toxicity was not affected. As a consequence the preferential enhancement of IT resulted in an increase in the specificity factor. It reaches 2.5×10^5 instead of 8×10^3. In the presence of monensin the potency of the IT was even higher. The IC50 was as low as 4.10^{-14} M. At this dose only 10 molecules of IT were bound per cell. This indicated that the utilisation of IT with an activator and especially monensin could attack cells whose target antigen expression is very low. In the presence of monensin the IC50 for A-chain or an unrelated IT was also increased, however this enhancement was largely inferior to that obtained with the specific IT, therefore the specificity factor was also improved in this case.

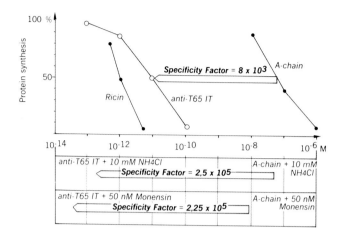

FIGURE 4. Effect of NH4Cl and monensin on the specificity factor of IT.

We examined the efficacy of activated IT in a highly
sensitive clonogenic assay (Table 2). CEM cells were
treated with the anti-T65 IT at a dose of 10^{-8} M. The
number of surviving cells decreased by one log with IT
treatment. When cells were treated with IT plus 10mM NH4Cl
more dramatic results were obtained with four logs of cytoreduction. In contrast, treatment of cells with an unrelated IT with or without NH4Cl was not toxic.

However when a higher IT dose was administered the
number of surviving cells were not diminished. We isolated
the clones and cultured them for analysis. The quantitative
determination of the expression of the T65 antigen on the
cell surface showed that they express no detectable T65
molecule whereas before treatment they expressed a mean
of 20 000 molecules per cell. The possibility that the
original cell line could contain an undetectable number of
negative cells was examined by cloning experiments. The CEM
line was cloned and we derived a subclone cell line (CEM1)
possessing the same average T65 expression as the original
CEM line. Treatment of this subclone (CEM1) with IT, under
the same conditions as before, resulted in a complete

eradication of cells from one million treated cells. This
demonstrates that the limit of IT efficacy in the previous
experiment was due to the presence of some negative cells,
and that all cells expressing the target antigen at a
sufficient number could be eliminated with at least a 6 log
efficacy factor (14).

These findings show that IT could be of great value
for marrow purging of leukemic cells or T mature lymphocytes in view of autologous or allogenic bone marrow
transplants. In this aspect the anti-T65 IT is of particular interest because the treatment of human bone marrow
with the anti-T65 IT up to 10^{-8} M was not toxic on the
multilineage hematopoietic progenitors CFU-GEMM (14,15).

TABLE 2

EFFICACY OF ACTIVATED IT IN A SENSITIVE CLONOGENIC ASSAY

CELLS	IT (10^{-8} M)	NH_4Cl (10 mM)	LOG KILL
CEM	—	—	0
CEM	anti-CEA	+	0
CEM	anti-T65	—	1
CEM	anti-T65	+	4
CEM$_1$	anti-T65	+	>6

On mature T-cells, which are less sensitive to the IT
than malignant cells 2 to 3 logs could be depleted after
IT treatment. On this basis patients undergoing marrow
transplantation for various malignant blood diseases
received, from histocompatible siblings, marrow pretreated
with anti T65 IT. All patients engrafted. The hematological
recovery was normal in all patients. Surprisingly, the
efficacy of bone marrow purging carried out in clinical
conditions was found dramatically reduced in 3 out of the
7 evaluable patients. In only four patients an effective
cytoreduction of more than 95% was achieved. Among them no
severe GVH was found while on the other hand the two
patients grafted with T-cell undepleted bone marrow
developed grade IV GVH.

The lack of reproductibility in the clinical trials has been found to be related to the ficoll fraction containing red blood cells which could inhibit the activator NH4Cl. Consequently we pursue our clinical investigation using ficoll fractionated bone marrow.

To summarize: the ITs which possess the properties of specificity and cytotoxicity need to have an improved kinetics of action, which is essential for tumor therapy. We showed that two possibilities exist to ameliorate the kinetics: 1) the selection of antibody/antigen systems which mediate rapid toxicity, 2) the use of an activator. This alternative which could be useful today for ex vivo treatment has to be explored in vivo. The utilisation of lysosomotropic amines in vivo seems very difficult considering the fairly high concentration required. In contrast, the carboxilic ionophores seem to be good candidates. The low concentrations required make it probable that these drugs may be useful in vivo.

REFERENCES

1. Gilliland DG, Steplewski Z, Collier RJ, Mitchell KF, Chang TH, Koprowski H (1980). Proc Natl Acad Sci USA 77:4539.
2. Jansen FK, Blythman HE, Carrière D, Casellas P, Diaz JR, Paolucci F, Pau B, Poncelet P, Richer G, Salhi SL, Vidal H, Voisin GA (1980). Immunol Lett 2:97.
3. Krolick KA, Villemez C, Isakson P, UHR JW, Vitetta ES (1980). Proc Natl Acad Sci USA 77:5419.
4. Masuho Y, Hara T (1980). Gann 71:759.
5. Miyazaki H, Beppu M, Terao T, Osawa T (1980). Gann 71:766.
6. Raso V, Griffin T (1980). J of Immunol 125:2610.
7. French patent (1978) N° 2437 213.
8. Casellas P, Brown JP, Gros O, Gros P, Hellström I, Jansen FK, Poncelet P, Roncucci R, Vidal H, Hellström KE (1982). Int J Cancer 30:437-443.
9. Trowbridge IS, Domingo DL (1981). Nature (Lond.) 294: 171-173.
10. Youle RJ, Neville DM Jr. (1982). J Biol Chem 257:1598-1601.
11. Raso V, Ritz J, Basale M, Schlossman ST (1982). Cancer Res 42:457-464.
12. Casellas P, Bourrie BJP, Gros P, Jansen FK (1984). J Biol Chem 259:9359-9364.

13. Carrière D, Casellas P, Richer G, Gros P, Jansen FK
     (1985). Exp Cell Res (in press).
14. Casellas P, Canat X, Fauser AA, Gros O, Laurent G,
     Poncelet P, Jansen FK (1985). Blood (in press).
15. Douay L, Gorin NC, Lopez M, Casellas P, Liance MC,
     Jansen FK, Voisin GA, Baillou C, Laporte B (1985).
     Cancer Res (in press).

Monoclonal Antibodies and Cancer Therapy, pages 275–286
© 1985 Alan R. Liss, Inc.

INHIBITION OF HUMAN PERIPHERAL BLOOD T-CELLS BY IMMUNOTOXINS CONTAINING POKEWEED ANTIVIRAL PROTEIN[1]

S. Ramakrishnan[2], F. M. Uckun,[*] and L. L. Houston[2]

Department of Biochemistry
University of Kansas
Lawrence, Kansas 66045

[*]Department of Therapeutic Radiology
University of Minnesota,
Minneapolis, Minnesota 55455

ABSTRACT   Immunotoxins containing pokeweed antiviral protein (PAP) and antibodies directed against 3A1 antigen on human T-cells or human transferrin receptor were shown to be highly cytotoxic against target cells.   3A1-PAP at moderate concentrations was not cytotoxic to human bone marrow stem cells.   Chloroquine, but not leucine methyl ester, potentiated cytotoxicity of 3A1-PAP.

INTRODUCTION

Immunotoxins (1) are potentially useful in a variety of diseases, but most investigations have been centered around their use to treat cancer. They have been used successfully on cells grown in culture and against tumor challenges in vivo (1), but their use in vivo is likely to encounter many more problems than their use ex vivo. Bone marrow transplantation is one of the most obvious applications of immunotoxins because cells can be treated

[1]This work was supported by a grant (CA 29889) from the National Cancer Institute.

[2]Present address: Cetus Corporation, 1400 Fifty-Third Street, Emeryville, CA 94608

outside the body, circumventing problems associated with delivering the immunotoxin through the blood to the site of the tumor.

Pokeweed antiviral protein conjugated to monoclonal antibodies forms a highly specific immunotoxin (2-5). Because pokeweed antiviral protein is an enzyme, internalization of only a few molecules into the cytoplasm proves lethal to the cell. Pokeweed antiviral protein exists in three different forms: PAP from spring leaves of Phytolacca americana, PAP-II from late summer leaves, and PAP-S from the seeds of the plant. The plant is widely distributed and is easily identifiable. The three species of the protein have about the same molecular weight (29,000) and all inhibit the activity of eucaryotic ribosomes (6,7) with about the same efficiency. Unlike ricin, PAP does not bind to cell surface receptors.

For this work, two immunotoxins were synthesized by conjugating PAP to two monoclonal antibodies: one, 3A1, is directed against CD 7(T, p41) surface antigen that is present in all T-ALL cells; the other, 5E9-11, is directed against the transferrin receptor which is expressed on many highly proliferative cells. The immunotoxins were tested i) for their ability to inhibit the mitogen-induced proliferation of normal human peripheral blood T-cells and human leukemic T-cells, and ii) the effect of lysosomotropic agents such as chloroquine and leucine methyl ester on the immunotoxin mediated cytotoxicity. If immunotoxins are to be used in bone marrow transplantation therapy, they must be shown not to affect significantly the growth of normal progenitor cells. Therefore, the effect of the immunotoxins on normal human bone marrow cells was also assayed.

MATERIALS AND METHODS

Antibodies: Hybridoma cell lines T3-3A1 (ATCC No. HB-2) and 5E9-11 (ATCC No. HB01) produce IgG1 (kappa) antibody. Both antibodies were purified from ascites fluid by sodium sulfate precipitation (16% w/v) followed by ion exchange chromatography on a DEAE-Affigel Blue column (2).

Test cells: HSB-2 cells, a T-cell line derived from human lymphoblastic leukemia, were grown in RPMI 1640 containing 20% fetal calf serum, 2 mM glutamine, 50 μM sodium pyruvate and 50 μM mercaptoethanol at 37°C in 5% carbon dioxide. Bone marrow cells and peripheral blood samples were obtained after informed consent from healthy volunteer donors. Mononuclear cells were isolated by a single-step centrifugation on Ficoll (5%)-sodium diatrizoate (9%) gradient (Histopaque, Sigma Chemical Co.).

Pokeweed antiviral protein: PAP was isolated from spring leaves using our modifications of the method of Irvin and Stirpe (8).

Immunotoxins: Immunotoxins were synthesized using a disulfide crosslinking reagent, N-succinimidyl 3(2-pyridyldithio)-propionate (SPDP), as previously described (3). The immunotoxins were freed from unconjugated PAP by gel filtration on Sephacryl 300 as before (3).   The conjugates were analyzed by electrophoresis on 10% polyacrylamide gels containing sodium dodecyl sulfate.   The amount of PAP linked to the antibody was determined in a homologous radioimmunoassay using radio-iodinated PAP as tracer (9).   The ratio of antibody to PAP was about 1:0.75 for 3A1-PAP and about 1:0.5 for 5E9-11.   For the purposes of calculating the efficiency of inhibition of protein synthesis, we have used an extinction coefficient of 1.2 absorbance units for a 1.0 mg of immunotoxin/ml solution and a molecular weight of 180,000 for the conjugate.

Inhibition of PHA-induced T-cell proliferation: Peripheral blood mononuclear cells were treated for 2 hr with immunotoxin and washed twice in medium containing 20% fetal calf serum. Cells (1×10^5 in 150 µl) were plated in 96-well dishes and 50 µl of a 1:80 dilution of phytohemagglutinin (PHA, Gibco) was added to each well.   After 3 days of additional incubation, DNA synthesis was measured by adding 1.0 µCi of tritiated deoxythymidine for 24 hr, then harvesting the trichloroacetic acid insoluble counts on a glass fiber filter, and counting the filter.

Protein synthesis assay: Protein synthesis was measured by the incorporation of tritiated leucine into trichloroacetic acid insoluble material (3).

Treatment of bone marrow cells with immunotoxin: Ten million cells/ml were incubated with immunotoxin for 16 hr at $37^{\circ}C$ in the above medium.   After incubation, the cells were washed twice in medium containing 5% fetal calf serum and assayed for CFU-GEMM (5).

RESULTS AND DISCUSSION

Fluorescence activated flow cytometric (FAFC) analysis of immunotoxin binding: To study the ability of the antibody portion of the immunotoxin to bind to the target cells, FAFC analysis was carried out by assaying for the PAP portion of the immunotoxin bound to the target cells by the antibody.   Under the assay conditions, unconjugated PAP did not bind to the cells.   The cells were briefly exposed for 15 min to 3A1-PAP immunotoxin (5.0 µg/ml) on ice and then incubated with affinity-purified rabbit

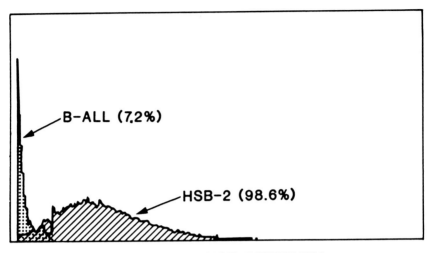

FLUORESCENCE INTENSITY

FIGURE 1.   FAFC analysis of immunotoxin binding to cells.
One million target T-lymphoblastic leukemia cells (▨ HSB-2)
and control Burkitt's lymphoma cells (▨ B-ALL) were
incubated with 3A1-PAP (5 µg/ml) on ice for 15 min.
Following washings, 5-10 µg/ml of affinity purified anti-PAP
antibodies were added and incubated for 15 min on ice.
Finally, the cells were developed with FITC-labelled anti-
rabbit IgG and analyzed for fluorescence intensity.

anti-PAP IgG.   The extent of immunotoxin bound to target cells
was measured by incubating the treated cells with FITC-labelled
anti-rabbit IgG and analyzing for the number of positive cells as
well as for the fluorescence intensity by FAFC.   Data in Figure 1
illustrate the strong binding of the immunotoxin to target cells.
Over 99.6% of the cells bound immunotoxin on their surface
compared to about 7% in a parallel control using B-ALL nontarget
cells.   These data further show that the presence of the toxin
polypeptide linked to the antibody did not interfere with the
ability of the antibody to bind target antigen.   5E9-11-PAP is a
potent immunotoxin as illustrated in Figure 2.   It inhibits protein
synthesis by 50% in HSB-2 cells at a concentration of about 80
pM.   3A1-PAP is an even more potent immunotoxin and inhibits

protein synthesis by 50% at a concentration of about 20 pM. Both immunotoxins were cytotoxic to CEM-CCL-119, another T-cell lymphoblastic line (data not shown). Because transferrin receptors are present on many cell types compared to the 3A1 antigen, 5E9-11-PAP is a less specific immunotoxin than 3A1-PAP.

Chloroquine is an agent that raises lysosomal pH. Data in Figure 2 also demonstrates that chloroquine potentiates the action of both 5E9-11-PAP and 3A1-PAP immunotoxins. By including 50 μM chloroquine, the concentration at which protein synthesis was inhibited by 50% was reduced from 80 pM to about

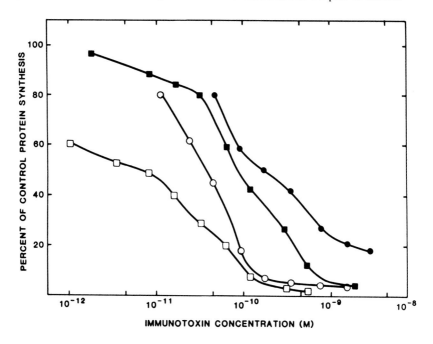

FIGURE 2. Immunotoxin mediated cytotoxicity of target cells: Potentiation by chloroquine. HSB-2 cells (1 x 10⁵) in a volume of 0.2 ml were incubated in the presence of different concentrations of PAP-immunotoxin for 18 hr at 37°C. The extent of cytotoxicity was determined by measuring ³H-leucine incorporated into proteins. ■——■ 3A1-PAP; ☐——☐ 3A1-PAP in the presence of chloroquine; ●——● 5E9-11-PAP; ○——○ 5E9-11-PAP in the presence of chloroquine.

7 pM for 5E9-11-PAP and from 20 pM to 3.5 pM for 3A1-PAP. If 5E9-11-PAP immunotoxin was incubated with nontarget cells (mouse leukemia AKR SL3) in the presence of chloroquine, no inhibition of protein synthesis was observed (2). In addition, the presence of an irrelevant PAP-containing immunotoxin directed against Thy 1.1 antigen present on mouse T-cells had no effect on protein synthesis by human HSB-2 cells (2). Therefore, the immunotoxin must be able to bind and internalize into the target cell before chloroquine can potentiate the activity of an antibody-toxin conjugate.

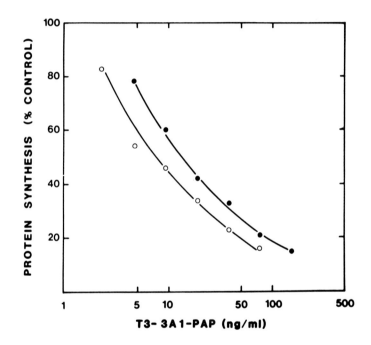

FIGURE 3. Effect of leucine methyl ester on immunotoxin activity. Target cells (HSB-2) were incubated with 3A1-PAP and leucine methyl ester (50 μM) for 18 hr at 37°C. The immunotoxin mediated inhibition of protein synthesis was determined by resuspending the treated cells in ^{3}H-leucine containing medium for 1 hr. Each value is a mean of triplicate cultures. ●——● 3A1-PAP; O——O 3A1-PAP in the presence of 50 μM leucine methyl ester.

The ability of chloroquine to enhance the activity of an immunotoxin is related to the kinetics of inhibition (2,10). The presence of 40 μM chloroquine reduced the lag period seen before the onset of protein synthesis inhibition induced by 5E9-11-PAP on HSB-2 cells. Chloroquine speeded the rate of protein synthesis inhibition by about 3- to 4-fold. At higher immunotoxin concentration, protein synthesis could be inhibited by 50% in 1 hr. The enhancement of immunotoxin activity by chloroquine was observed with all the PAP-conjugates we have tested. Similar effects on the kinetics of protein synthesis have also been observed with ammonium chloride (10). Leucine methyl ester, a compound known to induce osmotic changes resulting in the rupture of lysosomal structure (11), was not significantly effective in potentiating immunotoxin activity (Figure 3). Therefore, it may be possible that immunotoxin degradation by lysosomal enzymes (probable site for chloroquine action) is one of the major obstacles for the antibody-toxin conjugate before reaching the ribosomal target site in the cytosol.

In order to eliminate T-cells for allogenic bone marrow transplantation, we need to accumulate data about the efficiency with which human peripheral blood T-cells could be inhibited by T-cell-directed immunotoxins. Therefore, we studied the effect of immunotoxins on human peripheral blood T-cells by measuring the ability of peripheral blood T-cells to proliferate in the presence of a polyclonal mitogen. Figure 4 illustrates the sensitivity of the PHA-induced clonogenic growth of these cells to immunotoxin. The peripheral blood T-cells were incubated with PAP-immunotoxins, washed and then incubated with PHA, a potent mitogen. To quantitate the immunotoxin senstivity of PHA stimulated peripheral blood T-cells, cultures were pulsed with tritiated-deoxythymidine and the amount of DNA synthesized by cells was measured. The inability of treated cells (Figure 4a) to respond to PHA is clearly evident compared to the good mitogenic response of the control cells. As can been seen in Figure 4a, a concentration of 990 pM immunotoxin reduced DNA synthesis by 50% compared to PHA-stimulated cells not incubated with immunotoxin.

The 3A1-directed immunotoxin was more potent than the immunotoxin directed against transferrin receptor (Figure 4a). Similar observations were made in studies using lymphoblastic leukemic T-cells indicating that 3A1 antigen may be internalized faster or more efficiently than the transferrin receptor. The observed inhibition of mitogenic response by immunotoxins was specific since an irrelevant immunotoxin (31-E6-PAP) directed against mouse T-cells, as well as mixtures of free antibody

(20 μg/ml) and free PAP (3 μg/ml), did not inhibit PHA-induced mitogenic response (Figure 4b). PAP-immunotoxins are effective when incubated for only a short-time (10 min) with target cells (3). This is in contrast to observations made with ricin A-chain linked to T101 antibody where incubation with about 40 μg of immunotoxin/ml did not inhibit target cells. However, T101 linked to ricin was very cytotoxic to target cells (12).

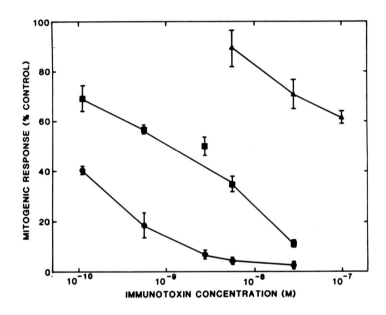

FIGURE 4. Inhibition of mitogen induced proliferation of human peripheral blood T-cells by immunotoxin. A. Peripheral blood mononuclear cells (PBMC) were incubated with 3A1-PAP (●——●), 5E9-11-PAP (■——■), and 31E6-PAP (▲——▲) for 2 hr at 37°C. The excess unbound conjugate was removed by washing and then cells were exposed to PHA (1:80 dilution) for 3 days. Following incubation, the cells were pulsed with ^{3}H-thymidine and the extent of DNA synthesis was measured.

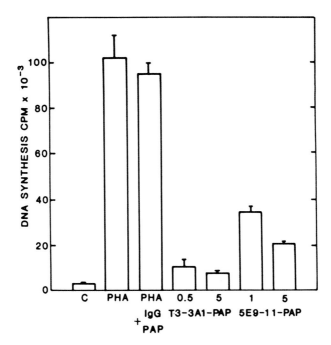

FIGURE 4B. PBMC were preincubated with a mixture of 3A1 IgG (20 μg/ml) and free PAP (3 μg/ml) for 2 hr at 37°C before the addition of PHA. As positive controls, 3A1-PAP (0.5; 5 μg/ml) and 5E9-11-PAP (1; 5 μg/ml) treated cells showed marked reduction in DNA synthesis.

Effect of immunotoxins on normal bone marrow cells (CFU-GEMM): To study the poossible use of the T-cell directed immunotoxin for eliminating leukemic T-cells in bone marrow preparations, experiments were carried out to investigate 1) the inhibition of clonogenic growth of target leukemia cells after immunotoxin treatment, and 2) the effect of immunotoxin treatment on the viability of stem cell populations. The latter parameter is critical in the successful re-engraftment/repopulation of the recipient after autologous/allogeneic bone marrow transplantation. Highly purified bone marrow cells treated with immunotoxin were grown in continuous culture on an irradiated allogenic stromal layer. Data in Table 1 indicate that

3A1-PAP did not interfere with the long-term functional capacity of multipotent hemopoietic stems cells at reasonably low concentrations of immunotoxin. The concentrations that did not inhibit CFU-GEMM measured at 4 weeks inhibited neoplastic T-cells by more than 3 logs (data not shown). 5E9-11-PAP at 1000 ng/ml inhibited completely the growth of CFU-GEMM, indicating the presence of transferrin receptors on the earliest human bone marrow stem cells detectable by currently available techniques. While human peripheral blood T-cells and human leukemic T-cells show the greater sensitivity to 3A1-PAP immunotoxin, normal bone marrow progenitors, as measured by CFU-GEMM assay, are relatively resistant to this immunotoxin in contrast to their sensitivity to the immunotoxin directed against transferrin receptor. Further, the extent of stem cell recovery was not affected by the addition of lysosomotropic agents to enhance immunotoxin activity (13).

TABLE 1
EFFECT OF IMMUNOTOXINS ON BONE MARROW
MULTIPOTENT STEM CELLS

Immunotoxin	CFU-GEMM/1 x 10^5 non-adherent cells[a] Concentration (nM)				
	0	1. 6	5.5	16	55
3A1-PAP	15	14	10	8	0
5E9-11-PAP	15	2	0	0	0

[a]CFU-GEMM was assayed after 4 weeks in culture (14).

In summary, this study indicates that both 3A1 antigen and transferrin receptor are potential determinants for immunotoxin targeting. PAP linked to 3A1 antibody eliminated effectively peripheral blood T-cells and leukemic T-cells and was not unacceptabley cytotoxic to normal bone marrow stem cells. Further, 3A1 antigen has been shown to be expressed in all T-ALL cells tested (14). Studies are in progress to evaluate the utility of this PAP-containing immunotoxins in the clinic.

REFERENCES

1. Vitetta ES, Krolick KA, Miyama-Inaba M, Cushly W, Uhr JW (1983). Immunotoxins: A new approach to cancer therapy. Science 209:641.
2. Ramakrishnan S, Houston LL (1984). Inhibition of human acute lymphoblastic leukemia cells by immunotoxins: Potentiation by chloroquine. Science 223:58.
3. Ramakrishnan S, Houston LL (1984). Comparison of the selective cytotoxic effects of immunotoxins containing ricin A chain or pokeweed antiviral protein and anti-Thy 1.1 monoclonal antibody. Cancer Res 44:201.
4. Ramakrishnan S, Houston LL (1984). Prevention of growth of leukemia cells in mice by monoclonal antibodies directed against Thy 1.1 antigen disulfide linked to two ribosomal inhibitors: Pokeweed antiviral protein or ricin A-chain. Cancer Res 44:1398.
5. Uckun FM, Ramakrishnan S, Houston LL (1985). Increased combination of a stable derivative of cyclophosphamide and a human B-cell specific immunotoxin containing pokeweed antiviral protein. Cancer Res 45:69.
6. Irvin JD (1983). Pokeweed antiviral protein. Pharmacol Ther 21:371.
7. Barbieri L, Stirpe R (1982). Ribosome-inactivating proteins from plants: Properties and possible uses. Cancer Surveys 1:489.
8. Houston LL, Ramakrishnan S, Hermodson MA (1983). Seasonal variations in different forms of pokeweed antiviral protein, a potent inactivator of ribosomes. J Biol Chem 25:9601.
9. Ramakrishnan S, Eagle MR, Houston LL (1982). Radio-immunoassay of ricin A-chain and B-chains applied to samples of ricin A-chain prepared by chromatofocusing and by DEAE Bio-Gel A chromatography. Biochim Biophys Acta 719:341.
10. Casellas P, Bourrie BJP, Gros P, Jansen FK (1984). ???? J Biol Chem 259:9359.
11. Thiele DL, Kurosaka M, Lipsky PE (1983). Phenotype of the accessory cell necessary for mitogen-stimulated T and B cell responses in human peripheral blood: Delineation by its sensitivity to the lysosomotropic agent, L-leucine methyl ester. J Immunol 131:2282.
12. Uckun, FM, Strong RC, Youle RJ, Vallera DA (1985). Combined ex vivo treatment with immunotoxins and mafosfamid: a novel immunochemotherapeutic approach for elimination of neoplastic T-cells from autologous marrow grafts. J Immunol (in press).

13. Uckun FM, Ramakrishnan S, Houston LL (1985). Immunotoxin mediated elimination of clonogenic tumor cells in the presence of human bone marrow. J Immunol (in press).
14. Bernard A, Boumsell L, Dauset J, Milstein C, Schlossman SF (1984). Leucocyte typing: Human leucocyte differentiation antigens detected by monoclonal antibodies. Springer-Verlag (Berlin), p.25.

VII. MONOCLONAL ANTIBODIES TO CELL SURFACE RECEPTORS

Monoclonal Antibodies and Cancer Therapy, pages 289–298
© 1985 Alan R. Liss, Inc.

PRODUCTION OF PROBES FOR THE STUDY
OF CELL RECEPTORS USING IDIOTYPE-ANTI-IDIOTYPE
MOLECULAR MIMICRY

D. Scott Linthicum and Michael B. Bolger

Department of Pathology, University of Texas Health
Science Center, Houston, Texas 77025
School of Pharmacy, University of Southern California
Health Science Campus
Los Angeles, Ca. 90033

CELL RECEPTORS AND ANTIBODIES

The concept of cell surface receptors which are
responsive to "outside chemical messages" was first put
forth by Ehrlich in 1900. His famous "side-chain" theory
(1) proposed that all cells possess many different receptor side chains (haptophores) which are capable of
reacting with foreign substances. After combining with
specific substances, the normal function of the involved
haptophore was "impaired" and a compensatory increase in
production of this specific haptophore resulted; excess
synthesis eventually resulted in secretion from the cell
and could be detected in serum. Although Ehrlich was specifically addressing the problem of immunity to toxins by
production of anti-toxin antibodies, his hypothesis set
the conceptual stage for a number of other cell surface
receptors yet to be discovered.
    Nearly fifteen years ago, Lennon and Carnegie (2) pro-
posed that functional impairment of certain endocrine and
neurological tissues was due to the presence of antibodies directed against specific cell surface membrane receptors for humoral agents such as polypeptide hormones or

Supported by grants from NIA/NIH P01 AG-03732, NIH
BRSG S07 RR05792 (MBB), American Parkinson Disease Foundation (DSL) National Multiple Sclerosis RG-1519-A-3 (DSL)

neurotransmitters. The interaction of autoantibody with receptors was expected to cause an "immunopharmacological block" through competition for the receptor with natural agents. They formulated this exciting hypothesis based on their observations of experimental allergic encephalomyelitis, an animal model for multiple sclerosis. This disease is induced by an autoantigen, myelin basic protein (MBP), specific to the central nervous system. A major disease-inducing determiniant of the molecule is located around the sole tryptophan residue. There is a striking resemblance between the structure of this region of MBP and that calculated by Smythies et al. (3) for a receptor for serotonin (5-hydroxytryptamine, 5-HT) and halucinogenic indoles (4). Close to the encephalitogenic region is a methylated arginine which Smythies et al. (5) have suggested would complete a hydrophobic pocket into which 5-HT could fit. Since the regions of the CNS that have the highest concentration of 5-HT nerve terminals (6) appear to be those affected in EAE, Carnegie (4)speculated that in EAE there was an immunopharmacological block of serotonergic receptors due to antigenic cross-reaction between the MBP and a receptor in synapses. Could it be that myelin basic protein was acting as a "molecular mimic" of the serotonin receptor? Unfortunately this hypothesis has remained largely untested to date, but it sparked a number of studies on the role of pathogenic antibodies to cell surface receptors and how antibodies to receptors can be used to further our understanding of them.

PATHOGENIC ANTI-RECEPTOR ANTIBODIES

In the past decade, research on experimental and clinical myasthenia gravis (MG) has served as the vanguard of our progress in understanding the pathogenic role of anti-receptor antibody (7). MG is a remitting and relapsing neuromuscular disease of autoimmune origin which is characterized by muscle fatigue ability that increases with exertion and improves with rest. Although the etiology is not known, it is clear that autoantibodies directed against the nicotinic acetylcholine receptor (AChR) causes impaired neuromuscular transmission, presumably through a immunopharmacologic block at the postsynaptic junction.

Autoantibodies directed against β2-receptors have been identified in patients with severe allergic rhinitis (hay fever) and asthma (8). These β2-receptor antibodies may be responsible for the clinically observed adrenergic hyporesponsiveness by preventing catecholamine binding and induced relaxation of airway smooth muscle, mucous glands, and mucosal blood vessels thereby leading to severe asthma.

Autoantibodies against polypeptide hormone surface receptors appear to be responsible for thyrotoxicosis (9) and insulin-dependent diabetes mellitus (10). Again as in the case of MG, autoantibodies reacting with the cell receptor causes a receptor block thereby making the cell refractory to normal humoral mediators. The etiology of such anti-receptor antibodies is unknown, but it may be that auto-anti-idiotype responses are responsible (see below).

A number of cell receptors, both surface and intra-cytoplasmic have been elusive, but advances in receptor biochemistry and immunochemical techniques are providing the new tools to make significant advances in this field. In most instances, the study of receptors is hampered by minute quantities of material available but in this regard monoclonal antibody technology is highly suited for these studies and when employed with the concept of "idiotypes and molecular mimcy" it becomes a powerful approach.

IDIOTYPES AND IDIOTOPES

Jerne (11) proposed that the immune system is composed of a network of idiotypes and anti-idiotypes which are intimately involved in immune response regulation. A given set of homogenous antibodies are immunogenic in their own right, in that their antigen combining sites (Fab regions) are comprised of amino acids unique to a particular variable region gene sequence. If these anti-bodies are used to immunize an animal, with the same gene-tic background, the reactive antibodies produced are referred to an anti-idiotypic, in that they react with antigenic determinants (idiotopes) on the first set of antibodies. It has been recently recognized that there are four types of anti-idiotypic antibodies.

The first type is directed against idiotopes associated with the Fab combining site of the heavy and light chains;

the second set are directed against idiotopes defined in
the "framework" of the variable region of the peptide
chains; the third type may react with L and H chain related
structures, and finally, the fourth type, react with
idiotopes which represent an internal image of the antigen
binding region and these complementary anti-idiotypes
apparently mimic the original ligand.

These antibodies which complement an "internal image"
have been referred to as "homobodies" by Lindemann (12);
Nisonoff and Lamoyi (13) have referred to these molecules
as having a "related-epitope" (RE) since it implies
"similarity", but not necessairly identity between structures in the anti-idiotype and antigen. As an example, in
developing a radioimmunoassay for thaumatin, a sweet
tasting protein, Hough and Edwardson (14) realized that
the antibodies cross-reacted with a wide variety of non-
protein sweet substances. The excellent correlation between the recognition of sweet substances by both
antibodies and the sweet-taste receptor is most likely
related to some fundamental relationship in structure of
the recognition site, and it was proposed that these antibodies may serve as a useful model for the sweet-taste
receptor in recognition of novel sweet substances. This
phenomena is most likely due to the "related epitopes"
between antibodies and the sweet-taste receptor.

Most studies concerned with immune responses and
idiotopes have utilized antigens which are devoid of known
biological function. Only recently have studies involving
biologically active substances such as hormones, anti-
hormone antibodies and anti-idiotypic antibodies brought to
light the importance of the phenomena of "related epitopes"
and "anti-receptor antibody" in the network regulation
diseases.

MOLECULAR MIMICRY AND RECEPTOR BINDING BY ANTI-
IDIOTYPIC ANTIBODIES

If antibodies (A) are raised against a given ligand
called B, some will form a particular complex (AB) which
may mimic the binding of B to its receptor protein C, (C
is the normal biological receptor). Hence, the anti-
idiotypic antibodies against idiotypic antibody A may have
common structures (related epitopes) with ligand B and
should bind receptor C (molecular mimicry). In support of

this assumption, Sege and Peterson (15) raised anti-idiotypic antisera directed against anti-retinol binding protein (RBP) antibodies and this antisera interact with pre-albumin, a normal receptor for RBP. Similar observations have been made for anti-insulin antibodies, viz., anti-idiotypic antibodies to anti-insulin react with the insulin receptor (16).

In a set of experiments by Schrieber et al (17), anti-alprenolol (a β_2 antagonist) antibodies (whole IgG) were use to generate rabbit anti-idiotypic antibodies; the resulting anti-idiotypic antisera reacted specifically with β-adrenergic receptors on turkey erythrocytes and could amplify epinephrine stimulated adenylate cyclase.

Similar findings were made by Homcy et al (18) using a similar approach with anti-alprenolol, but they used affinity purified anti-alprenolol antibodies to generate an anti-idiotypic response and found that their anti-receptor activity (anti-idiotype) was inhibitory for isoproterenol-mediated adenylate cyclase activity.

In the past several years three additional expermental models using polyclonal anti-idiotype antibodies (antisera) to cell surface receptors ahve been firmly established (See Table I and papers by Marasco, Farid and Greene in this volume.) A spectacular model involving anti-idiotypic antibodies to anti-BisQ (a potent agonist of the acetylcholine receptor) produced experimental and transient myasthenia gravis which correlated with the appearance of anti-idiotype antibodies in the serum is presented by Cleveland elsewhere in this volume.

The use of anti-idiotype antibodies in the study of receptors on lymphocytes has also been extensive. B cell malignancies offer a special opportunity since each B cell possess a unique cell surface immunoglobulin (idiotype) common to all members of the malignant clone. This receptor is practically tumor-specific, since it virtually absent on most other normal lymphocytes. Several approaches have been used to test the potential of anti-idiotype therapy in these cases. With this in mind, Lynch has presented his findings on immunoregulatory signals by anti-immunoglobulin antobodies elsewhere in this volume.

AUTO-ANTI-IDIOTYPE RESPONSES

As a natural part of the immune regulatory mechanism, the antibodies generated to a given immunogen are subsequently "down regulated" by an auto-antiidiotype response, and this response is also subjected to a "second wave" of "down regulation" by an anti-anti-idiotype response and so forth. With respect to the problem of related epitopes, internal images and anti-receptor antibodies there have been two systems examined with these aspects in mind. Shecter et al (19) discovered that mice immunized with insulin developed both antibodies to insulin (anti-ligand) and insulin receptor (anti-ligand anti-idiotype); the antibodies to insulin receptor displaced insulin from receptor and mimicked the actions of insulin in stimulating the oxidation of glucose and inhibiting lipolysis.

In a series of hybridoma experiments Cleveland et al (20) were able to isolate individual monoclonal antibodies, from mice immunized with BisQ-BSA, which reacted with the ligand BisQ, anti-BisQ antibodies (i.e. anti-ligand anti-idiotype) and AChR from Torpedo and rat muscle (anti-idiotypic had RE of the BisQ). This procedure enabled the investigators to "freeze in time", the various B lymphocyte clones which were activated during the "network" regulation of the response, thereby providing a series of anti-ligand and anti-idiotype clones.

An experimental model of reovirus infection in mice has demonstrated that the neurotrophic reovirus binds a neuronal receptor and anti-idiotype antibody to anti-reovirus hemagglutinin can bind the same neuronal receptor; therefore the role of "related epitopes" as a factor in the generation of anti-CNS receptor antibodies subsequent to a viral infection appears to be significant. Greene and Gaulton have reported these findings in this symposia.

TABLE I

GENERATION OF ANTI-RECEPTOR ANTIBODIES BY ANTI-IDIOTYPE MIMCRY

LIGAND	RECEPTOR	INVESTIGATORS
Retinol Binding Protein	Pre-Albumin Epithelial Cells	Seye and Peterson 1978
Insulin	Insulin	Sege and Peterson 1978
Alprenolol	β2 Adrenergic	Schrieber et. al. 1980
	β2 Adrenergic	Homcy et. al. 1982
Bis Q	Acetylcholine	Wasserman et. al. 1982
F-Met-Leu-Phe	Neutrophil Chemotaxis Peptide	Marasco and Becker 1982
Thyrotropin	TSH	Farid et. al 1982
Reovirus HA	Neuronal	Greene et. al. 1982

FUTURE GOALS

The two hypotheses 1) the binding site of an antibody to a potent structurally constrained ligand will resemble the receptor for the ligand with respect to specificility i.e., the anti-ligand-receptor for ligand, and 2) antibodies to the anti-ligand will bind to the receptor, i.e., anti-anti-ligand-anti-receptor have been substainitated in a number of studies presented in this symposia and elsewhere.

An important drawback of early studies, however, is that the precise nature of the anti-ligand and anti-idiotype antibodies is not really known because polyclonal antisera were used. The use of monoclonal antibodies in this experimental scheme provides a better understanding of the molecular characteristics of these antibodies and their interaction with each other and receptors. One needs to address the issues of ligand and receptor chemistry to determine if this approach is applicable to systems other than those described above. For example, can the molecular mimicry approach be used to study the cytoplasmic receptors for steroid hormones? Can an anti-idiotypic antibody mimic the molecular shape of a steroid hormone? What are the physical-chemical constraints which govern this working hypothesis? Are anti-receptor antibodies always capable of acting as agonists or antagonists? Do these characteristics predict if anti-receptor antibodies are going to be pathogenic? The use of monoclonal reagents should enable us to address these issues and define the molecular constitutions necessary to permit various interactions with types of receptors.

REFERENCES

1. Ehrlich P (1906). "Collected studies on immunity." New York: Wiley and Sons.
2. Lennon VA, Carneyie, PR (1971). Immunopharmacological Disease-Break in tolerance to receptor sites. Lancet 1:630.
3. Smythies JR, Beninyton F, Morin RD (1970). Specification of a possible serotonin receptor site in the brain. Neurosci Res Prog Bull 8:117.

4. Carnegie PR (1971). Properties, structure and possible neuroreceptor role of the encephalitogenic protein of human brain. Nature 229:25.

5. Smythies JR, Benington F, Morin RD (1972). Encephalitogenic protein: A beta-pleated sheet conformation (102-120) yields a possible molecular form of a serotonin receptor. Experientia 28:23.

6. Fuxe F, Hokfelt T, Ungerstedt U (1969). Distribution of monoamines in the mammalian central nervous system by histochemical studies. In Hooper G (ed) "Metabolism of Amines in The Brain," London: Macmillan, p10.

7. Patrick J, Linstrom J (1973). Autoimmune response to acetylcholine receptor. Science 180:871.

8. Venter JC, Fraser CM, Harrison LC (1980). Autoantibodies to B-adrenergic Receptors: A Possible Cause of Adrenergic Hyporesponsiveness in Allergic Rhinitis and Asthma. Science 207:1361.

9. Yavin E, Yavin Z, Schneider M, Kohn LD (1981). Monoclonal antibodies to the thyrotropin receptor: implications for receptor structure and the actions of autoantibodies in Graves' disease. Proc Nat Acad Sci 78:3180.

10. Flier JS, Kahn CR, Jarrett DB, Roth, J (1975). Antibodies that impair insulin receptor binding in an unusual diabetic syndrome with severe insulin resistance. Science 190:63.

11. Jerne NK (1974). Towards a network theory of the immune system. Ann Immunol (Paris) 125C:373.

12. Lindenmann G (1973). Speculations on idiotypes and homobodies. Ann Immunol (Paris) 124C:171.

13. Nisonoff A, Lamoyi E (1981). Implications of the presence of an internal image of the antigen in anti-idiotypic antibodies: Possible application to vaccine production. Clin Immunol Immunopath 21:397.

14. Hough CAM, Edwardson JA (1978). Antibodies to thaumatin as a model of the sweet taste receptor. Nature 271:381.

15. Sege K, Peterson PA (1978). Anti-idiotypic antibodies against anti-vitamin A transporting protein react with prealbumin. Nature 271:167.

16. Sege K, Peterson PA (1978). Use of anti-idiotypic antibodies as cell surface receptor probes. Proc Nat Acad Sci 75:2443.

17. Schreiber AB, Couraud PO, Andre C, Vray B, Strosberg, AD (1980). Anti-alprenolol anti-idiotypic antibodies bind to beta-adrenergic receptors and modulate catecho-

lamine sensitive adenylate cyclase. Proc Nat Acad Sci 77:7385.

18. Homcy CJ, Rockson SG, Haber E (1982). An anti-idiotypic antibody that recognizes the beta-adrenergic receptor. J Clin Invest 69:1147.

19. Shecter Y, Elias D, Maron R, Cohen IR (1983). Mice immunized to insulin develop antibody to the insulin receptor. J Cell Biochem 21:179.

20. Cleveland EL, Wasserman NH, Sarangar R, Penn AS, Erlanger BF (1983). Monoclonal antibodies to the acetylcholine receptor by a normally functioning auto-anti-idiotypic mechanism. Nature 305:56.

Monoclonal Antibodies and Cancer Therapy, pages 299–316
© 1985 Alan R. Liss, Inc.

ANTI-THYROTROPIN-ANTI-IDIOTYPES AS PROBES FOR
THYROTROPIN RECEPTOR STRUCTURE AND FUNCTION*

Nadir R. Farid

Thyroid Research Laboratory
Health Sciences Centre
St. John's, Newfoundland
Canada
A1B 3V6

ABSTRACT   A class of anti-idiotypes raised against
antibodies specific for hormones would be anticipated
to interact with the hormone receptors. We have
raised anti-TSH anti-idiotypes and found these to
interact with the high affinity binding site for TSH
on thyroid membranes, to induce adenylate cyclase
activation and iodide transport into dispersed thyroid
cells as well as to promote their organization into
follicular structures. The anti-TSH anti-idiotypic
antibody interacted with an $M_r \sim 200,000$ holoreceptor
on protein blots of thyroid membranes resolved on
SDS-PAGE in the absence of reductant. In another set
of experiments we raised anti-idiotypic antibodies
against monoclonal antibodies specific for the α and
β subunits of TSH respectively. Neither the α nor β
monoclonal antibody specific anti-idiotypic anti-
bodies interacted with the TSH holoreceptor. The
combination of the two anti-idiotypic antibodies,
however, did so and increased basal cyclase activity
compared to normal IgG and individual anti-idiotypes
as well as mediating TSH-specific cAMP dependent
physiologic changes. As a result of the second set
of experiments, we propose that the interaction of
TSH with its receptor involves two co-operative signals delivered by the two subunits rather than a
single signal requiring their combination.

* Supported by a grant from the Medical Research
Council of Canada.

Anti-idiotypic antibodies raised against highly purified hormones can be obtained in large amounts. They facilitate simple isolation of hormone receptors and are useful as probes for hormone-receptor interactions.

INTRODUCTION

The variable regions of the heavy and light chains of an antibody molecule contribute to the three dimensional attributes of the antigen binding site (1). In view of the unique structure of the antibody variable region, it is not surprising that it is immunogenic (2). The immunization of an appropriate experimental animal with a homogeneous antibody preparation results in an antiserum which combines specifically with structures within the variable region of immunizing antibody. These structures are called idiotypes and are defined by anti-idiotypic antibodies. Idiotypic determinants are known as idiotopes.

Anti-idiotypic antibodies arise not only by heterologous immunization but also autologously (auto-anti-idiotypes) in the course of a normal immune response (3). There is considerable evidence that idiotype/anti-idiotype interaction constitutes an important element in the communication between immuno-regulatory T cells, between these and B cells and in the regulation of B cells by circulating antibodies (for review see 3, 4).

Anti-idiotypic antibodies have been classified in a number of different ways (1, 3, 5). We classify them functionally into "internal image" and non-internal image anti-idiotypes (4). The former refers to those antibodies which combine with the antigen binding site, inhibit the binding of the antigen to the idiotype and simulate many biologic activities of the antigen and therefore represents an "internal image" of the immunizing antigen (6). This short review is concerned with the use of that class of anti-idiotypic antibodies as agents with which to probe hormone receptor as well as the interaction of receptors with hormone.

Sege and Peterson (7) first applied the "internal image" anti-idiotype concept to raising anti-insulin anti-idiotypic antibodies. The low bioactivity of the antiserum prepared, the fact that normal IgG mimicked some of the effects described and the lack of a mediator of insulin action (for review see 6) may have delayed the

wider adoption of this concept. Over the last five years,
anti-idiotypes have been raised to glycoprotein (8) and
peptide hormones (9, 10), β adrenergic antagonists (11, 12,
13), acetylcholine receptor agonists (14) and glucose (15,
16). In some instances, auto-anti-idiotypes were demonstrated following immunization with hormone (9, 17) or
neurotransmittor (18).

In view of the interest of my laboratory in autoimmune thyroid disease, the bias of our investigation toward anti-TSH anti-idiotypes is understandable.

DISCUSSION

Anti-TSH Anti-Idiotypic Antibodies

When this work was started in 1979, there was heated
debate as to whether the thyroid stimulating antibody of
Graves' disease was a true anti-TSH receptor antibody or
was raised to membrane sites close to the receptor (19,
20). Guided by the notion that anti-TSH anti-idiotypes
would recognize the domain in the receptor seen normally
by TSH, we proceeded to raise a series of anti-human (h)
TSH and anti-bovine (b) TSH anti-idiotypes to ask a number
of questions. We wanted to know whether it was feasible
to raise anti-TSH anti-idiotypes given the size and
structural difference between insulin (7) and TSH? whether
such antibodies would have biological activity? and whether
the anti-idiotypes would prove to be agonists i.e. simulate
TSH, at least in some respects?

The anti-TSH anti-idiotypes were found to be able to
displace ^{125}I-bTSH from thyroid plasma membranes dose
dependently (Fig. 1) and show an affinity of binding one
order of magnitude less than TSH itself. The binding of
the anti-idiotype was saturable and specific for the
receptor in that it was inhibited to 65% by 160 mU/ml bTSH.
Furthermore, the anti-idiotypes were found to stimulate
thyroid membrane adenylate cyclase (Fig. 2) as well as
biologic consequences dependent (at least in part) upon
cyclic AMP. These included the ability of dispersed
thyroid cells to become organized into follicular structures after seven days' culture (Fig. 3) and the ability
of these thyroid cells to take up ^{131}I (Fig. 4).

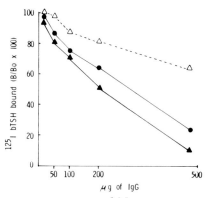

FIGURE 1.   Inhibition of ^{125}I-b-TSH binding to thyroid
membranes by anti-TSH anti-idiotype.
     Anti-TSH antibodies were raised by immunizing Sprague-
Dawley rats and the anti-TSH antibodies which were specifically isolated by TSH affinity column were used to immunize
rabbits. After appropriate absorption with rat IgG, the
biologic activity of the antibody preparations was tested
(21).
     The effects of NR (normal rabbit) IgG (△) and of
anti-idiotype IgG on ^{125}I-b-TSH binding to human (●) and
porcine (▲) thyroid membranes were studied. The curve
for NRIgG shown here was done on porcine membranes; the
influence of NRIgG on binding of radiolabeled ligand to
human membranes was similar. Since porcine tissue showed
greater sensitivity, it was used in all subsequent experiments. B denotes binding of ^{125}I-b-TSH to membranes in
presence of test material and Bo in their absence.
     (Reproduced with permission from the Eur. J. Immunol.).

     Interestingly, sera obtained from a rabbit 10 days
after the serum with which these biologic activities were
demonstrated caused a marked inhibition of TSH-induced
cyclic AMP accumulation in thyroid cells suggesting that
anti-anti-idiotypes (Ab3) had arisen in the interval (6).
This finding also emphasizes the cyclical nature of anti-
idiotype response with reciprocal fluctuation of the
complementary antibody (6, 9, 22).

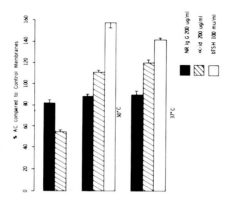

FIGURE 2. Stimulation of adenylate cyclase activity by anti-TSH anti-idiotype.

The upper panel shows relative AC activities at 30°C in the absence of Gpp(NH)p. Basal AC activity was 24 pM cAMP mg^{-1} protein/min^{-1}. bTSH stimulated activity is not different from basal and is not shown here. Anti-idiotype caused significant inhibition of AC activity compared to NRIgG (p < 0.05). When 10 μM Gpp (NH)p was added (middle panel) to the incubate at 30°C basal AC activity increased to 113 cAMP mg protein^{-1}/min^{-1}. At 37°C (lower panel) AC activity was further enhanced to 304 pM cAMP mg protein^{-1}/ min^{-1}. At 30°C and 37°C the anti-idiotype significantly activated enzymatic activity compared to baseline (p < 0.05). The bars represent means + SEM of six observations. (Reproduced with permission from Eur. J. Immunol.).

By that stage of the investigation, we had found out that the TSH receptor was a heterotetramatic glycoprotein of M_r ~ 200,000 with an immunoglobulin-like structure (23). The receptor comprises two light chains held by one or more disulphide bonds whose integrity is essential both for the TSH binding and the maintenance of the holo-receptor (23). We demonstrated directly that these anti-TSH anti-idiotypes did interact with a band of M_r ~ 200,000 in protein blots of thyroid plasma membranes resolved under non-reducing conditions. This interaction was blocked by preincubation of the blotted receptor with TSH but not with insulin or human chorionic gonadotropin (hCG) (24) (Fig. 5).

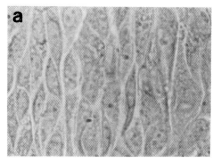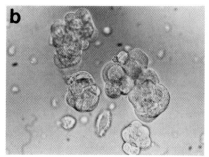

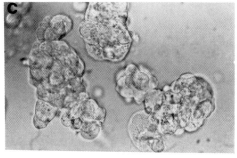

FIGURE 3. Influence of anti-idiotypes on follicular
organization of cultured thyrocytes.
(a) Cells cultured in absence of stimulator (in
presence of NRIgG). Note monolayer disposition and
fibroblast-like shape of cells.
(b) Cells cultured in presence of bTSH. Note the
three dimensional follicle-like structures.
(c) Cells cultured in presence of anti-idiotype.
Cells have adopted the three dimensional follicle-like
structure similar to the one obtained with bTSH. All
photographs were taken on the seventh day of culture under
the same magnification (x 520).
(Reproduced with permission from the Eur. J. Immunol.).

The interaction between the anti-idiotype with
receptor was completely abrogated when membranes were
resolved under reducing conditions (24).

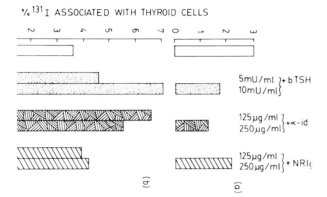

FIGURE 4. The influence of anti-idiotypic antibody on uptake of radioiodine by porcine thyrocytes.

(a) Radioiodine uptake was studied after incubation of thyroid cells with bTSH, NRIgG, or anti-id for 10 min (10^5 cpm). Na ^{131}I were then added and incubation continued for a further 10 min. Counts associated with pelleted cells were expressed as percentage of total counts added. Only the higher dosage of the experimental agents were used in these experiments. Both TSH and anti-id caused a decrease in the ^{131}I taken up by thyrocytes.

(b) The percentage of radio-iodine associated with thyrocytes 4 hr after incubation with bTSH, NRIgG, or anti-id. One hundred and twenty-five µg/ml of anti-id caused a significant stimulation of ^{131}I uptake ($p < 0.05$). The higher concentration (250 µg/ml) caused less stimulation, raising the possibility that the anti-id preparation contains in lesser relative concentration an antibody species which inhibits iodine concentration.

(Reproduced with permission from J. Cell. Biochem.).

These experiments demonstrated that an anti-TSH anti-idiotype had TSH-like effects which were exerted through the TSH receptor. As such this anti-idiotype which recognizes the receptor and no other thyroid membrane epitopes had all the attributes of the thyroid stimulating antibody of Graves' disease (19, 20). The hypothesis that the Graves' disease IgG may, at least in some instances, be due to anti-TSH auto-antibody was, therefore, enter-

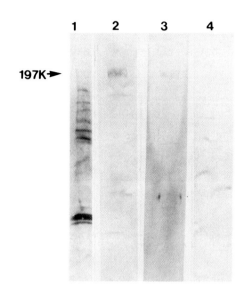

FIGURE 5. Binding of anti-TSH anti-idiotype to the
TSH holoreceptor band (M_r = 197K).
     Thyroid plasma membranes were resolved by SDS-PAGE
under non-reducing condition, transferred to nitrocellulose
paper and allowed to interact with IgG preparation. IgG
bound was detected with peroxidase-conjugated species
specific anti-IgG and developed with 4-chloro-napthol and
hydrogen peroxide. Lanes: 1) membrane polypeptides
stained with Commassie blue. 2) interaction of anti-
idiotype with holoreceptor. 3) virtual inhibition of this
interaction when paper strip was pre-incubated with native
TSH. 4) Pre-immune rabbit IgG.
     (Reproduced with permission from Endocrinology).

tained (21). This is unlikely to be a common occurrence
because anti-idiotypic responses are cyclical and short-
lived and would, therefore, not account for the sustained
presence of thyroid stimulating antibody (See 4, 19).
It is, however, conceivable that an anti-TSH anti-idiotype
initiates an immune response which, because of its anti-
receptor specificity, would then be maintained by the
presence of the TSH receptor. An anti-idiotype origin for
thyroid stimulating antibody cannot account for the con-
currence in most Graves' sera of antibodies directed

against thyroid "microsomal" antigens (25). Recent evidence suggests that a microsomal antigen may be an epitope on the TSH receptor (26) but far removed from that on which TSH and Graves' IgG interact (24, 26). It is thus most likely that Graves' IgG is a TSH-receptor auto-antibody (TRab) (19). We note here that other possible mechanisms for the appearance of anti-TSH receptor antibodies include an anti-idiotype against a TSH-like glycoprotein secreted by T lymphocytes induced by certain stimulants (27) and humoral reaction against a TSH receptor-like material on certain bacteria (28).

The anti-TSH anti-idiotype played an important role in our characterization of the isolated porcine TSH receptor.

Anti-TSH Subunit Anti-Idiotypic Antibodies

We next turned our attention to the mode of interaction of TSH with its receptor. TSH shares with FSH, LH and hCG a common α subunit which interacts non-covalently with a hormone-specific β subunit (29). The deduction that hormone specificity lies with β subunit has been adequately substantiated (29). The way in which the α and β subunits of TSH interact with the receptor to produce hormone specific signals was not, however, amenable to investigation because the free dissociated subunits are without biological effect. A number of models for the TSH receptor interaction may be envisaged. Thus, it is possible that the β subunits bind to a stereospecific site and the α subunit delivers the hormone signal or, conversely the α subunit may bind to a site common for glycoprotein hormone receptor and then β subunit deliver the TSH-specific signals. TSH interaction with receptor may be related to 2 signals delivered by the two subunits or to a one combinatorial signal.

In order to resolve this question, we have raised in rabbits, anti-idiotypic antibodies against rat monoclonals respectively specific for the α and β subunits of hTSH (30). The characteristics of these monoclonal antibodies are outlined in Table 1.

The binding of ^{125}I-hTSH to anti-β subunit monoclonal was inhibited by its complementary anti-idiotype in a dose-dependent manner; up to 48% at 500 ug IgG/ml. By contrast, ^{125}I-hTSH interaction with the anti-α subunit monoclonal was not influenced by anti-α anti-idiotype. Thus, whereas the anti-β subunit anti-idiotype is of the "internal image"

TABLE 1

CHARACTERISTICS OF ANTI-TSH SUBUNIT SPECIFIC MONOCLONALS

	Anti-α	Anti-β
Species	Rat	Rat
Ig isotype	IgM	IgG
Binding to ^{125}I-hTSH	+	+
Binding affinity (K_D)	5.9 M^{-9}	3.7 M^{-10}
Displacement of bound ^{125}I-hTSH by bTSH	< 5%	< 3%
Glycoprotein hormone causing displacement of bound ^{125}I-hTSH	hTSH, hFSH, hLH, hCG	hTSH
Inhibition of membrane bounding ^{125}I-bTSH	−	−
Inhibition of adenylate cyclase activation	+	++
Effect on bTSH-induced activation of cyclase		
a) added simultaneously	inhib.	inhib.
b) added 30 min after bTSH	stimul.	stimul.

variety, the anti-α anti-idiotype is not; it may be complementary to idiotopes in close proximity to the antigen binding site or may represent an epibody (5). Epibodies interact with a cross-reactive structure shared by antigenic epitopes and idiotopes expressed on complementary molecules.

The anti-idiotype preparations were without effect each alone or in combination when tested for their ability to inhibit ^{125}I-bTSH binding to thyroid plasma membranes, in spite of the ability of iodinated anti-idiotypes to show binding to thyroid plasma membranes. The binding of equimolar concentrations of the radiolabelled anti-idiotypes was additive. Some 40-65% of the bound anti-α, anti-β anti-idiotypes and their mixture was inhibited by 500 mU/ml of bTSH. The residual binding in the case of the anti-α anti-idiotype and particularly with the combination of anti-α and β anti-idiotypes was well above that for normal rabbit IgG and was attributed to the stabilization of the receptor by these antibodies (30).

Anti-α and anti-β anti-idiotypes each had some stimulatory activity on basal thyroid membrane adenylate cyclase compared to normal rabbit IgG. Equimolar mixture of the two anti-idiotypes resulted in a marked stimulation of adenylate cyclase comparable to that produced by 150 mU/ml of bTSH (Table 2). The more than additive influence of the two anti-idiotypes suggest co-operative interaction i.e. the binding of one antibody to the thyroid membranes increased the affinity of the other for the receptor (30). The combination of anti-α and anti-β anti-idiotypes was found to induce dispersed thyroid to organize into follicular structures and to promote the uptake of ^{131}I by these cells. The anti-β anti-idiotype alone showed some effect in both assays and anti-α was without influence on either.

TABLE 2

ADENYLATE CYCLASE ACTIVATION BY ANTI-α AND ANTI-β TSH
SUBUNIT ANTI-IDIOTYPES

| | ANTI-IDIOTYPES | | | | |
	Normal rabbit IgG	Anti-α^1	Anti-β^1	Anti-α^1+ anti-β^1	TSH[2]
Percent cyclase stimulation relative to buffer	−57±2	−7.3±3.1	−8.1±0.9	87.3±4.6	93±6.8

    1. IgG was tested at a concentration of 250 mgm/ml; in the anti-idiotype mixture, 125 mgm/ml of each was used. NRIgG and individual anti-idiotypes are inhibitory.

    2. 250 mU/ml crude bTSH (USV Laboratories, Mississauga, Ont.) was used.

    Lastly, the capacity of these antibodies to bind to protein blots of thyroid membranes resolved under non-reducing conditions was tested. Each of the two anti-idiotypes tested alone did not interact with the blotted peptides. Equimolar quantities of the two anti-idiotypes consistently yielded a clear band at $M_r \sim 200$ k. The seeming paradox between the binding of radiolabelled anti-idiotypes, the thyroid membranes (see above) and the inability to demonstrate binding to protein-blotted receptor can be resolved by noting that protein blots are extensively washed in 200 mM NaCl to minimize non-specific binding. This procedure removes antibodies of low binding affinity and again emphasizes the co-operative interaction of the two anti-idiotypes in binding to the TSH receptor.

Apparently, following binding to its receptor, TSH induces microaggregation of the receptor which is necessary for triggering adenylate cyclase activation (31). While it is conceivable that the combination of the two anti-idiotypes act through promoting receptor aggregation, we would need to invoke, in addition, specific interaction of each anti-idiotype with separate domains of the receptor and the bivalency of each of the two antibodies to account for the slight biologic influence of anti-β-anti-idiotype and the co-operative influence of the two anti-idiotypes particularly on protein blotted receptor. The lack of an "internal image" anti-anti-idiotype does not allow rigorous testing of the question of specificity.

We were able to reach a number of conclusions (30). The α and β subunits of TSH deliver two co-operative signals to the TSH receptor. The hormone specificity is indeed associated with the β subunit, the α subunit's contribution being through increasing the affinity of the receptor for subsequent β subunit interaction (although it has not been possible for us to find out the order in which the two subunits interact with the receptor). This co-operative interaction is apparently crucial for a receptor conformation requisite for the stimulation of the cyclase system. Studies comparing the interaction of free and receptor-bound bTSH with the monoclonal idiotypes also suggest that after binding to the receptor the bTSH molecule undergoes conformational change(s) such that new antigenic sites previously unrecognized by these mono-clonals are exposed (Table 1). The TSH receptor apparently comprises at least two functional domains; one of which is concerned with ^{125}I-bTSH binding and the second with stimulation of the cyclase system, a view consistent with work utilizing anti-TSH receptor monoclonal antibodies (32).

We further demonstrated the utility of the anti-TSH subunit anti-idiotypes by using their mixture to identify the TSH receptor and its subunits on protein blots of [^{3}H]-leucine labelled whole thyroid cell lysates (33). Fol-lowing identification, the bands were carefully cut and counted and the results used to monitor biosynthesis and turnover of the TSH receptor. TSH was found to accelerate the biosynthesis of its receptor with very efficient

incorporation of receptor subunits into the holoreceptor
($M_r \sim 200$ k). The effect of TSH upon new receptor
synthesis was bimodal both in terms of time and the TSH
dose: beyond optimal receptor labelling times, a progressive decrement in the labelling rate was observed
whether or not thyroid cells were grown in the presence of
TSH. Likewise, TSH dosage above an optimum of 100 mU/ml
caused decrement of the synthesis rate of the TSH receptor.
To measurably influence receptor biosynthesis, TSH had to
be in thyroid cell culture for several hours (greater
than 3 and less than 12) suggesting that TSH action is
mediated through transcription and/or mRNA stabilization.
TSH was also found to reduce the half life of the receptor.
The most dramatic effect of TSH on total thyroid cell
receptor half-life occurred between 12 and 15 hs of incubation. TSH receptor half-life decreased from 7.3 to 4 hs.
Interestingly, this coincided with the replacement of the
high affinity, low capacity TSH receptors on thyroid cell
plasma membranes and their replacement by low affinity
high capacity ^{125}I-bTSH binding sites. This last observation points to separate, longer range mechanism of TSH-
induced desensitization other than that through the
cyclase (33), which is well documented.

IMPLICATIONS

Anti-idiotypic antibodies have a number of potential
uses. They represent a reasonably economical approach
to raising anti-receptor antibodies (4, 6). The judicious
use of hormone analogue (where available) allows the use
of these antibodies to map the functional domains of the
receptors (34). From the point of view of preparing anti-
idiotypic reagents, it is worth noting that monoclonal
antibodies with such specificities have been selected in
the course of immunization with an antigen (18).

They have also been used as a basis of a new type of
immunoassay based on the inhibition of interaction between
idiotype and anti-idiotype by antigen (35). This type of
assay would be invaluable in screening large numbers of
sera for antibodies against newly recognized pathogens.

Furthermore, anti-idiotypic antibodies raised against
antibodies (or T cell receptors) specific for parasite
and microbal antigens were utilized to induce immunity
against trypanosomes (36), Sendai virus (37) and hepatitis
B antigen (38, 39). The observation (40) that synthetic

idiotypes can trigger specific anti-idiotype responses promises the advent of "vaccines" based on microbal specific synthetic anti-idiotype peptides.

Anti-idiotypes could also be used to modify immune response to major histocompatibility antigens in the course of allografting (41, 42), the induction of suppressor T cells that will modify IgE response to specific allergen (42) or autoimmune response to self antigen (see 4 for review).

Recent studies also hold promise for the use of anti-idiotypes (44, 45) to enhance immunological response to malignancy, although suppression of tumor rejection had previously been documented (46, 47).

Lastly, we would like to point out that the potential of auto-anti-idiotypic antibodies which arise in the course of an immune response may change previously held concepts of disease. We direct attention to the recent description in Type I diabetics who have never been treated with insulin of circulating anti-insulin antibodies (48) and also of anti-insulin receptor antibodies (49). The latter are probably anti-idiotypes to the insulin auto-antibody and may account for the relative insulin resistance seen in patients with Type I diabetes.

The scope of this article does not allow the discussion of the wider implications of the idiotype/anti-idiotype network within the immune system. We have attempted elsewhere (4) to pull together the evidence and theoretical consideration for the role of such a network in a "grand" scheme of the immune system.

ACKNOWLEDGEMENT

This work would not have been possible without the contribution of Dr. M. Nazrul Islam, Dr. Rosario Briones-Urbina, Miss Beverley S. Hawe and Mrs. Barbara Pepper. I thank Miss Gail O'Brien for secretarial assistance.

REFERENCES

1. Rajewsky K, Takemori T (1983). Genetics, expression and function of idiotypes. Ann Rev Immunol 1:569.
2. Jerne NK (1974). Towards a network theory of the immune system. Ann Immunol (Inst Pasteur) 125C:373.
3. Bona CA, Pernis B (1984). Idiotypic networks. In

Paul WE (ed): "Fundamental Immunology", Raven Press, New York, p 577.

4. Farid NR, Lo TCY (1985). Anti-idiotypic antibodies as probes for receptor structure and function. Endocrine Reviews (in press).

5. Bona CA, Finley S, Waters S, Kunkel HG (1982). Anti-immunoglobulin antibodies III: properties of sequential anti-idiotypic antibodies to heterologous anti-γ globulins. Detection of reactivity of anti-idiotype antibodies with epitopes of Fc fragments (homobodies) and with epitopes and idiotopes (epibodies). J Exp Med 156:986.

6. Farid NR, Briones-Urbina R, Islam MN (1984). Anti-idiotypic antibodies as probes for hormone-receptor interaction. Can J Biochem Cell Biol 62:

7. Sege K, Petersen PA (1978). Use of anti-idiotypic antibodies as cell-surface receptor probes. Proc Natl Acad Sci USA 75:2443.

8. Farid NR, Briones-Urbina R, Islam MN (1982). Biologic activity of anti-thyrotropin anti-idiotypic antibody. J Cell Biochem 19:305.

9. Shechter Y, Maron R, Elais D, Cohen IR (1982). Auto-antibodies to insulin receptor spontaneously develop as anti-idiotypes in mice immunized with insulin. Science (Wash DC) 216:542.

10. Amit T, Gavish M, Barkey RJ, Youdin MBH (1984). Anti-idiotypes to PRL antibody have PRL-like activity and bind to the PRL receptor. Program of the 7th International Congress of Endocrinology, July 1st-7th, Quebec City, PQ, Abst. #202.

11. Schreiber AB, Couraud PO, Andre C, Vray B, Strosberg AD (1980). Anti-alprenolol anti-idiotypic antibodies bind to β-adrenergic receptors and modulate catecholamine-sensitive adenylate cyclase. Proc Natl Acad Sci USA 77:7385.

12. Homcy CJ, Rockson SG, Haber G (1982). An anti-idiotypic antibody that recognizes the adrenergic receptor. J Clin Invest 69:1147.

13. Guillet JG, Kaveri SV, Durieu O, Delavier C, Hoebeeke J, Strosberg AD (1985). B-adrenergic agonist activity of a monoclonal antiidiotypic antibody. Proc Natl Acad Sci USA (in press).

14. Wassermann NH, Penn AS, Freimuth PI, Treptow N, Wentzel S, Cleveland WL, Erlanger BF (1982). Anti-idiotypic route to anti-acetylcholine receptor antibodies and experimental myasthenia gravis. Proc Natl

Acad Sci USA 79:4810.

15. Durino V, Lo TCY (1985). Identification of hexose transport components through the use of anti-idiotypic antibodies. (manuscript submitted).

16. Kay MMB (1985). Glucose transport protein is structurally and immunologically related to band 3 and senescent cell antigen. Proc Natl Acad Sci USA (in press).

17. Beall GN, Kruger SR (1983). Binding of ^{125}I-human TSH by gamma globulins of sera containing thyroid-stimulating immunoglobulin (TSI). Life Science 32:77.

18. Cleveland WL, Wassermann NH, Sarangarajan R, Penn AS, Erlanger BF (1983). Monoclonal antibodies to the acetylcholine receptor by a normally functioning auto-anti-idiotypic mechanism. Nature (Lond) 305:56.

19. Farid NR, Briones-Urbina R, Bear JC (1983). Graves' disease - the thyroid stimulating antibody and immunological networks. Mol Asp Med 6:355.

20. McKenzie JM, Zakarija M (1978). LATS in Graves' disease. Rec Prog Horm Res 33:29.

21. Islam MN, Pepper BM, Briones-Urbina R, Farid NR (1983). Biological activity of anti-thyrotropin anti-idiotypic antibody. Europ J Immunol 13:57.

22. Couraud PO, Lu BU, Strosberg DA (1983). Cyclic anti-idiotypic response to anti-hormone antibodies due to neutralization of autologous anti-antiidiotype anti-bodies that bind hormone. J Exp Med 157:1369.

23. Islam MN, Farid NR (1984). Structure of the porcine thyrotropin receptor: a 200 kilodalton heterocomplex. Experientia (in press).

24. Islam MN, Briones-Urbina R, Bakó G, Farid NR (1983). Both TSH and thyroid stimulating antibody of Graves' disease bind to an M_r 197,000 holoreceptor. Endocrinol. Endocrinol. 113:436.

25. Bakó G, Islam MN, Farid NR (1985). Photoaffinity labelling of the porcine thyrotropin receptor. Clin Invest Med (in press).

26. Islam MN, Tuppal R, Hawe BS, Briones-Urbina R, Farid NR (1985). In search of the antigens for thyroid "microsomal" auto-antibodies. Evidence for multiple epitopes on the thyrotropin receptor. (manuscript submitted).

27. Smith EM, Phan M, Kruger TE, Coppenhaver DH, Blalock JE (1983). Human lymphocyte production of immuno-reactive thyrotropin. Proc Natl Acad Sci USA 80:6010.

28. Weiss M, Ingbar SH, Winbald S, Kasper DL (1983). Demonstration of a saturable binding site for thyrotropin in yersinia entercolitica. Science (Wash) 219:1331.

29. Pierce JG, Parsons TF (1981). Glycoprotein hormones: structure and function. Ann Rev Biochem 50:465.

30. Briones-Urbina R, Islam MN, Ivanyi J, Farid NR (1985). Use of anti-idiotypic antibodies as probes for the interaction of TSH subunits with its receptor. EMBO J (manuscript submitted).

31. Avivi A, Tramontano D, Ambesi-Impiombato FS, Schlessinger J (1981). Adenosine 3',5'-monophosphate modulates thyrotropin receptor clustering and thyrotropin activity in culture. Science (Wash DC) 214:1237.

32. Valente WA, Vitti P, Yavin Z, Yavin E, Rotella CN, Grollman EF, Toccafondi RS, Kohn LD (1982). Monoclonal antibodies to the thyrotropin receptor: stimulating and blocking antibodies derived from the lymphocytes of patients with Graves' disease. Proc Natl Acad Sci USA 79:6680.

33. Briones-Urbina R, Farid NR (1985). Control of the biosynthesis and turnover of the thyrotropin receptor. (manuscript submitted).

34. Schecter Y, Elais D, Maron R, Cohen IR (1984). Mouse antibodies to the insulin receptor developing as anti-idiotypes. J Biol Chem 259:6411.

35. Potocnjack P, Znala F, Nussenzweig R, Nuzzenzweig N (1982). Inhibition of idiotype-anti-idiotype interaction for detection of a parasite antigen: a new immunoassay. Science (Wash DC) 215:1367.

36. Sacks DL, Esser KM, Sher A (1982). Immunization of mice against african trypanosomiasis using anti-idiotypic antibodies. J Exp Med 115:1108.

37. Ertl HC, Finberg RW (1984). Sendai virus-specific T cell clones: induction of cytolytic T cells by an anti-idiotypic antibody directed against a helper T-cell clone. Proc Natl Acad Sci USA 81:2850.

38. Kennedy RC, Alder-Storthz K, Henkel RD, Sanchez Y, Melnick JL, Dreeman GR (1983). Immune response to hepatitis B surface antigen: enhancement by prior injection of antibodies to the idiotype. Science (Wash DC) 221:853.

39. Kennedy RC, Dreeman GR (1984). Enhancement of the immune response to hepatitis B surface antigen. In

vivo administration of antiidiotype induces anti-HBS
that expresses a similar idiotype. J Exp Med 159:655.

40. McMillan S, Seiden MV, Houghten RA, Clevinger B,
Davie JM, Lerner RA (1983). Synthetic idiotypes:
the third hypervariable region of murine anti-dextran
antibodies. Cell 35:859.

41. Binz H, Wigzell H (1976). Successful induction of
specific tolerance to transplantation antigens using
autoimmunization against the recipients own natural
antibodies. Nature (Lond) 262:294.

42. Sachs DH, Auchincloss Jr H, Blueston JA (1983).
Modification of the immune response to H-2 antigens
by treatment with antiidiotypes. Transp Proc XV:
793.

43. Malley A (1983). Immunotherapeutic potential of
idiotype/anti-idiotype regulation of the IgE response.
Immunol Today 4:163.

44. Koprowski H, Herlyn D, Lubeck M, DeFreitas E, Sears
HF (1984). Human anti-idiotype antibodies in cancer
patients: Is the modulation of the immune response
beneficial for the patient. Proc Natl Acad Sci USA
81:216.

45. Nepom GT, Nelson KA, Holbeck SL, Hellstrom I,
Hellstrom KE (1984). Induction of immunity to a
human by in vivo administration of anti-idiotypic
antibodies in mice. Proc Natl Acad Sci USA 81:
2864.

46. Flood PM, Kripke ML, Rowley DA, Schreiber H (1980).
Suppression of tumor rejection by autologous anti-
idiotypic immunity. Proc Natl Acad Sci USA 77:2209.

47. Binz H, Meier B, Wigzell H (1982). Induction or
elimination of tumor specific immunity against a
chemically-induced rat tumor using auto-anti-idiotypic
immunity. Int J Cancer 29:417.

48. Palmer JP, Asplin CM, Clemons P, Lyen K, Tatpati O,
Raghu PK, Paquette TL (1983). Insulin antibodies
in insulin-dependent diabetes before insulin treatment. Science (Wash DC) 222:1337.

49. Maron R, Elias D, de Jongh BM, Bruining GJ, van Rood
JJ, Shechter Y, Cohen IR (1983). Autoantibodies to
the insulin receptor in juvenile onset insulin-
dependent diabetes. Nature (Lond) 303:817.

Monoclonal Antibodies and Cancer Therapy, pages 317–326
© **1985 Alan R. Liss, Inc.**

IMMUNE RESPONSES DIRECTED TO MONOCLONAL IMMUNOGLOBULINS ON MALIGNANT B CELLS[1]

Richard G. Lynch[2]

Departments of Pathology and Microbiology
University of Iowa College of Medicine
Iowa City, Iowa   52242

BACKGROUND

As is obvious from the contents of this book, a great deal of effort is currently directed to the production of monoclonal antibodies specific for antigens expressed on tumor cells and the development of therapeutic strategies in which the monoclonal antibodies can be used to eliminate tumor cells. The studies to be reviewed here take a somewhat different approach but to the same end. While most studies use monoclonal immunoglobulins to deliver an injurious agent to the surface of a tumor cell, the studies discussed below use the integral membrane monoclonal immunoglobulin of a malignant B cell as the molecular target of suppressive immunoregulatory signals; instead of functioning as an effector, the monoclonal immunoglobulin functions as a target.

The rationale for this approach derives from the knowledge that there exists in mammals an elaborate immunoregulatory apparatus that constantly orchestrates the expansion and contraction of normal B cell clones. The occurrence of immunoregulatory helper and suppressor cells raises the possibility that they might be directed to malignant B cells and influence their growth and differentiation.

[1]This work was supported by NIH Research Grants RO-CA32275.

[2]Present address: Department of Pathology, University of Iowa College of Medicine, Iowa City, Iowa 52242.

In a sequence of studies we have shown that murine plasmacytoma cells can be regulated by specific immunological signals (reviewed in 1). In 1972 we showed that idiotype-specific tumor immunity could readily be induced in a syngeneic system (2). Those studies, in effect, established that the idiotypes on myeloma proteins could function as tumor-specific transplantation antigens (TSTA). The finding that immunoglobulin idiotypes could function as TSTA has been confirmed in other studies with plasmacytomas, (3, 4, 5) and similar effects were subsequently observed with IgM-producing lymphomas (6, 7) and leukemias (8). Miller et al. (9) have employed an anti-idiotype strategy to treat humans with non-Hodgkin's lymphoma and Stevenson et al. (10) have used this approach in studies of human chronic lymphocytic leukemia. As more is learned about the mechanisms that are effective in the experimental animal studies this information may prove of use in developing clinical applications.

In addition to idiotype-specific suppression of murine plasmacytoma cells, we have shown that antigen-binding plasmacytoma cells can be suppressed by antigen-specific suppressor T cells (11). While an antigen-specific strategy would not be feasible in human B cell tumors because the antigen-binding property of the monoclonal immunoglobulin is not known, the observations in the mouse provide further evidence that malignant B cells can be regulated by normal immunoregulatory effectors. A major challenge to be met if immunoregulatory strategies are to be clinically useful is the development of systems that can specifically deliver suppressive signals to the tumor cell targets. In addition to anti-idiotypic and antigen-specific delivery systems, a recent report indicates that immunoglobulin isotype-specific delivery of suppressor signals may be feasible (12).

IDIOTYPE-SPECIFIC T CELL REGULATION
OF MURINE PLASMACYTOMA CELLS

That a myeloma protein could function as a TSTA was a surprising and paradoxical finding. It might have been expected that anti-idiotypic antibodies and/or idiotype-specific T cells would not influence plasmacytoma cells because: 1) the idiotype-specific effectors would be neutralized by the large amount of soluble, circulating idiotype secreted by the plasmacytoma cells, and

2) regulation of plasmacytoma cells by anti-idiotypes would require expression of the monoclonal immunoglobulin on the surface membrane of the plasmacytoma cells. While the expectation that anti-idiotypic effectors would be neutralized by circulating idiotype is a reasonable prediction, it is nonetheless clear that immunization with myeloma protein induces an idiotype-specific tumor immunity (2). In regards to the expression of membrane immunoglobulin by plasmacytoma cells, it is now clear that this is a regular occurrence. At the time of our initial experiments there was a general belief that plasmacytoma cells did not express surface membrane immunoglobulin. However, studies by Hannestad, et al. (13) showed that many plasmacytoma clones expressed surface membrane immunoglobulin. It was later shown that plasmacytoma cells expressed the messenger RNAs for both the secretory and membrane forms of immunoglobulin heavy chains. Differences in the biochemical nature of the membrane and secreted forms of IgA in murine plasmacytoma cells provide a means to distinguish the two forms (14).

The plasmacytoma tumor immunity and its idiotypic specificity stimulated efforts to identify the underlying mechanisms. It was recognized early that MOPC-315 cells were morphologically heterogeneous and that they appeared to undergo repetitive cycles of differentiation with each in vivo passage (15). MOPC-315 cells enclosed within peritoneal diffusion chambers exhibited a progressive change from small, stem cell-rich, non-secretory lymphocytoid cells to larger M315-secreting plasmacytoid cells.

In the original experiments that demonstrated tumor immunity against MOPC-315 some of the immunized mice developed tumors which were progressive, but which were not accompanied by the appearance of the IgA anti-TNP protein (M315) in the serum. However, when these tumors were transplanted to non-immunized mice, many of the tumors that developed were accompanied by the expected high levels of circulating M315. In subsequent studies it was demonstrated that M315-immunized mice developed idiotype-specific suppressor T cells that inhibited secretion of M315 but did not influence MOPC-315 proliferation or differentiation to plasmacytoma cells (16). Secretory inhibition could be adoptively transferred to normal mice with M315-immune T cells. There were several interesting aspects of these studies: 1) unlike the Id^{315}-specific suppressor T cells that

inhibited the clonal proliferation of MOPC-315 cells, the
T cell that inhibited secretion did not influence MOPC-315
proliferation; 2) The T cell that suppressed M315
secretion did not influence the cytologic differentiation
of MOPC-315 from lymphocytoid to plasmacytoid cells. This
latter observation suggested that inhibition of M315
secretion was effected at a late stage in plasmacytoma
cell differentiation. Other experiments demonstrated that
the inhibition of M315 secretion was reversible, further
suggesting that inhibition was mediated at the level of
the actual secretory cell. 3) Since the inhibition of
M315 secretion could be achieved across the 0.2 μ pores of
a diffusion chamber membrane, it indicated that a soluble
suppressor factor acted directly on the MOPC-315 secretory
cells.

   Subsequent studies conducted in vitro established
that the suppression of M315 secretion was dependent on
the dose of immune T cells and virtually total inhibition
could be achieved at high suppressor:target cell ratios
(17). The suppressor cells were shown to be $Lyt1^-2^+$ cells
that could recognize and bind to Id^{315}-sepharose columns.
Immune T cells co-cultured with MOPC-315 cells began to
inhibit secretion as soon as six hours after mixing.
Since the plasmacytoma cells were secreting M315 at the
time that the suppressor cells were added to the culture,
the suppressor T cells were shown to act directly on the
antibody secreting cell rather than on a secretory cell
precursor.

   Incorporation of ^{3}H-leucine into secreted and
intracellular M315 was inhibited by greater than 90% in
the presence of suppressor T cells (17). The suppression
of M315 synthesis was shown to be selective. Studies
performed in a diffusion apparatus in which the T cells
were separated from the MOPC-315 cells by a millipore
membrane provided a means to quantitate synthesis of total
proteins and M315 immunoglobulin by MOPC-315 cells. When
the cells were incubated in separate compartments of the
chambers for 48 hours and then pulsed with ^{3}H-leucine for
24 hours, a 50% decrease in total protein synthesis was
observed and the entire decrement could be accounted for
by the decrease in M315 synthesis. When suppressed
MOPC-315 cells were removed from the diffusion chambers
and cultured in the absence of T cells, secretion of M315
was re-established. In a recent study the suppressor T
cell has been shown to be specific for a V_H^{315} idiotope(s)
(18). In addition the induction of the specific

suppressor T cells was achieved by immunization by
purified V$_H$315. Thus, in this suppressor circuit, a
V$_H$315-recognition event occurs at the inductive and
effector stages.

The selective nature and the kinetics of inhibition
of M315 synthesis suggested a transcriptional or
translational mechanism of control. To address this
issue, polyadenylated RNA was isolated from control and
suppressed MOPC-315 cells (19). The RNA was
electrophoresed in 1.2% agarose gel under denaturing
conditions, transferred to nitrocellulose membranes, and
probed for RNA sequences complementary to cloned DNA
fragments specific for alpha-heavy-chain or lambda$_2$ light
chain gene segments. When polyadenylated RNA isolated
from non-suppressed and suppressed MOPC-315 cells was
hybridized to a radiolabelled probe specific for
alpha-constant region sequences, autoradiographs revealed
three major transcripts of 1.7, 2.1 and 3.0 kilobases (kb)
in length. It was found that the pattern of
alpha-transcript banding was comparable in suppressed and
non-suppressed MOPC-315 cells. Qualitative differences
were not detected whether MOPC-315 cells were co-cultured
directly or membrane-segregated from the suppressor T
cells.

Analysis of the RNA preparations with a hybridization
probe specific for the lambda$_2$ light chain constant region
revealed a single complementary transcript 1.2 kb in
length when the RNA was isolated from MOPC-315 cells that
had been co-cultured with normal T cells or membrane
segregated from normal T cells (19). Polyadenylated RNA
recovered from suppressed MOPC-315 cells had a marked
reduction in the amount of the lambda$_2$ transcript. When
the autoradiographs were analyzed by densitometric
techniques, the quantity of lambda$_2$ transcripts from
suppressed cells was less than 10% of the control. These
findings indicated that a diffusable product of the
suppressor cells produced a marked reduction in the
expression of lambda$_2$ mRNA in MOPC-315 cells.

When examined in a cell-free translation system, the
alpha-chain mRNA from suppressed MOPC-315 cells was shown
to be initiated and served as a template for a mature
sized alpha-polypeptide (20). The presence of a
functional alpha-heavy chain mRNA and the apparent absence
of heavy chain polypeptide synthesis in the suppressed
plasmacytoma cells presented a paradox. Furthermore,
while the suppressor T cells were specific for a V$_H$315

idiotope, the conspicuous alteration of mRNA expression was at the level of the light chain. In an effort to account for these findings, we proposed a model in which the light chain polypeptide functions as a regulatory subunit in the process of full expression of the immunoglobulin molecule. In normal immunoglobulin-secreting cells the expression of the light and heavy polypeptide chains occur as independent events, but the precise steps in the assembly and secretion of IgA molecules have not been completely defined. In the suppressed myeloma cell, the absence of a light chain polypeptide appears to prevent full expression of the heavy chain gene by a mechanism that operates distal to the occurrence of a functionally intact heavy chain mRNA. These findings are consistent with a model in which light chain polypeptides, once synthesized and released from their polysomes either: 1) facilitate the release of heavy chain polypeptides from their polysomes, or 2) protect heavy chains from degradation. The mechanism could also account for some of the patterns of heavy chain and light chain expression that have been observed in many neoplastic B cells (discussed in 20). Moreover, a regulatory role for light chain in the full expression of immunoglobulin is consistent with the changes that occur in the transition of a pre-B cell to an immunocompetent B cell (discussed in 20). The proposed model describes a mechanism in which regulation of expression of one chain of a two-chain protein in effect regulates expression of the other chain and therefore the whole molecule. Evidence for a similar mechanism in the expression of a family of adhesion molecules by leukocytes has recently been reviewed (21).

An interesting aspect of light chain mRNA regulation in MOPC-315 cells is the finding of coordinate regulation of the normal $lambda_2$ mRNA and the truncated $lambda_1$ light chain mRNA (19). In MOPC-315 cells an aberrantly rearranged $lambda_1$ gene produces a truncated mRNA that is translated into a rapidly degraded, short $lambda_1$ light chain polypeptide. When suppressed MOPC-315 cells were examined it was found that the concentration of the $lambda_1$ transcript precisely paralleled that observed for the $lambda_2$ mRNA. Since the concentration of the alpha-heavy chain mRNA in suppressed MOPC-315 cells is not significantly different from non-suppressed MOPC-315 cells, and there are no differences detected in the levels of J-chain mRNA in suppressed and non-suppressed MOPC-315 cells (Milburn, GL, Koshland M, Lynch RG; unpublished data), the inhibition of light chain mRNA expression is selective and is not merely a result of non-specific mRNA degradation. These findings establish that the Id^{315}-specific suppressor T cells selectively inhibit the expression of $lambda_2$ and $lambda_1$ light chain mRNAs in MOPC-315 cells. To produce such an effect, the suppressive factors must either decrease the rate of synthesis of light chain transcripts or enhance the rate of degradation of these transcripts in the nucleus or cytoplasm of the plasmacytoma cells. Since the aberrantly rearranged $lambda_1$ gene in MOPC-315 cells is located on the homologous chromosome from the productively rearranged $lambda_2$ chain (22), the coordinate regulation of $lambda_2$ and $lambda_1$ mRNAs appears to be mediated by a <u>trans</u> mechanism.

SUMMARY AND CONCLUDING REMARKS

The studies reviewed above show that lymphoid tumor cells can be useful model systems with which to investigate cellular and molecular immunoregulatory mechanisms. They also show that immunoregulatory strategies can be successfully employed to suppress the growth of malignant B cells. In addition to the advantages provided by their monoclonal nature and their availability in virtually unlimited number, tumor cells are useful for study because they frequently express aberrant features that may not occur in non-malignant lymphoid cells. For example, the co-expression of the productively rearranged $lambda_2$ light chain gene and the aberrantly rearranged $lambda_1$ chain gene in MOPC-315 cells provided the opportunity to detect the <u>trans</u>-acting, lambda-specific suppression of light chain gene expression. It is striking that while the Id^{315}-specific suppressor T cell recognizes a V_H^{315} idiotope, the conspicuous alteration in the target B cell is down-regulation of light chain mRNA expression. Since antigen-specific suppressor T cells can also inhibit immunoglobulin secretion by MOPC-315 cells (11) it will be of interest to see if that suppression also involves regulation of light chain expression.

A principle that has emerged from the study of MOPC-315 regulation is that, while a large number of different immunoregulatory effectors are targeted to the integral membrane M315 molecules on MOPC-315 cells

(reviewed in 1), the target cell consequences are
different in each case. Thus membrane M315 can be engaged
by TNP-antigen, antigen-specific helper and suppressor T
cell products, anti-idiotypic antibodies, anti-idiotypic T
cell products, and IgA-Fc receptors. Since engagement of
surface M315 molecules by different ligands can enhance or
suppress MOPC-315 proliferation and/or differentiation,
and promote or antagonize M315 expression, it appears that
surface M315 molecules function as molecular focusing
devices. The quality and intensity of the target cell
effect does not appear to be determined by engagement per
se, but is probably determined by a combination of the
captured regulatory effector and the existent
susceptibility of the target cell to that effector.

Studies of immunoregulatory events using tumor cells
as models may provide basic information about regulatory
mechanisms in normal lymphoid cells and may lead to new
strategies for clinical control of lymphoid neoplasms and
their paraneoplastic syndromes.

REFERENCES

1. Lynch RG, Rohrer JW, Odermatt B, Gebel HM, Autry Jr,
    Hoover RG (1979). Immunoregulation of murine myeloma
    cell growth and differentiation: A monoclonal model
    of B cell differentiation. Immunol Rev 48:45.
2. Lynch RG, Graff R, Sirinisinha S, Simms ES, Eisen HN
    (1972). Myeloma proteins as tumor-specific
    transplantation antigens. Proc Nat Acad Sci 69:1540.
3. Meinke GC, McConahey PJ, Spiegelberg HL (1974).
    Suppression of plasmacytoma growth in mice by
    immunization with myeloma proteins. Fed Proc 33:792.
4. Eisen HN, Sakato N, Hall SJ (1975). Myeloma proteins
    as tumor-specific antigens. Transplant Proc 7:209.
5. Freedman P, Autry Jr, Tokuda S, Williams RC (1976).
    Tumor immunity induced by pre-immunization with
    BALB/c mouse myeloma protein. J Nat Cancer Inst
    45:735.
6. Sugai S, Palmer DW, Talal N, Witz IP (1974).
    Protective and cellular immune responses to idiotypic
    determinants on cells from a spontaneous lymphoma of
    NZB/NZW$_{F1}$ mice. J Exp Med 140:1547.
7. Haugton C, Lanier LL, Babcock GF, Lynes MA (1978).
    Antigen-induced murine B cell lymphomas. II.
    Exploitation of the surface idiotype as tumor
    specific antigen. J Immunol 121:2358.

8. Krolick KA, Isakson PC, Uhr JW, Vitetta ES (1979). BCL$_1$, a murine model for chronic lymphocytic leukemia; use of the surface immunoglobulin idiotype for detection and treatment of a tumor. Immunol Rev 48:81.

9. Miller RA, Maloney DG, Warnke R, Levy R (1982). Treatment of B-cell lymphoma with monoclonal anti-idiotype antibody. N Engl J Med 306:517.

10. Stevenson KF, Hamblin TJ, Stevenson GT, Tutt AL (1980). Extracellular idiotypic immunoglobulin arising from leukemic B lymphocytes. J Exp Med 152:1484.

11. Rohrer JW, Lynch RG (1978). Antigen-specific regulation of myeloma cell differentiation in vivo by carrier-specific T cell factors and macrophages. J Immunol 120:1066.

12. Muller S, Hoover RG (1985). T cells with Fc receptors in myeloma; suppression of growth and secretion of MOPC-315 by Tα cells. J Immunol 134:644.

13. Hannestad K, Kao MS, Eisen HN (1972). Cell-bound myeloma proteins on the surface of myeloma cells: Potential targets for the immune system. Proc Nat Acad Sci 69:2295.

14. Hickman S, Wong-Yip YP (1979). Re-expression of non-glycosylated surface IgA in trypsin-treated MOPC-315 plasmacytoma cells. J Immunol 123:389.

15. Rohrer JW, Vasa K, Lynch RG (1977). Myeloma cell immunoglobulin expression during in vivo growth in diffusion chambers: Evidence for repetitive cycles of differentiation. J Immunol 119:861.

16. Rohrer JW, Odermatt B, Lynch RG (1979). Immunoregulation of murine myeloma: Isologous immunization with M315 induces idiotype-specific T cells that suppress IgA secretion by MOPC-315 cells in vivo. J Immunol 122:2011.

17. Milburn GL, Lynch RG (1982). Immunoregulation of murine myeloma in vitro: II. Suppression of MOPC-315 immunoglobulin secretion and synthesis by idiotype-specific T cells. J Exp Med 155:852.

18. Lynch RG, Milburn GL (1983). Id^{315}-specific T cells that suppress MOPC-315 IgA synthesis recognize a V$_H^{315}$ idiotope. Fed Proc 42:688.

19. Parslow TG, Milburn GL, Lynch RG, Granner D (1983). Suppressor T cell action inhibits the expression of an excluded immunoglobulin gene. Science 220:1389.

20. Milburn GL, Parslow TG, Goldenberg C, Granner DK, Lynch RG (1984). Idiotype-specific T cell suppression of light chain mRNA expression in MOPC-315 cells is accompanied by post-transcriptional inhibition of heavy chain expression. J Cell Molec Immunol 1:115.
21. Springer TA, Thompson WS, Miller LJ, Schmalsteiz FC, Anderson DC (1984). Inherited deficiency of the Mac-1, LFA-1, p150, 95 glycoprotein family and its molecular basis. J Exp Med 160:1901.
22. Hozumi N, Wu G, Murialdo H, Baumal R, Mosmann T, Winberry L, Marks A (1982). Arrangement of λ light chain genes in mutant clones of the MOPC-315 mouse myeloma cells. J Immunol 129:260.

Monoclonal Antibodies and Cancer Therapy, pages 327–344
© 1985 Alan R. Liss, Inc.

A SEARCH FOR "INTERNAL IMAGE" ANTI-IDIOTYPIC ANTIBODIES:
A SUBPOPULATION OF ANTI-f MET-LEU-PHE ANTI-IDIOTYPIC
ANTIBODIES BINDS TO THE FORMYL PEPTIDE CHEMOTAXIS
RECEPTOR OF THE NEUTROPHIL AND TO SEVERAL GENETICALLY
UNRELATED ANTI-f MET-LEU-PHE ANTIBODIES

Wayne A. Marasco, Jerome Charles and Peter A. Ward

Department of Pathology, University of Michigan
Medical School, Ann Arbor, MI 48109

ABSTRACT   Rabbit antibodies induced against formyl
Met-Leu-Phe, a potent neutrophil chemotactic factor
produced by Escherichia coli, bind numerous other
oligoformylpeptides with a rank order of reactivity
similar to the neutrophil formyl peptide chemotaxis
receptor.   Rabbit anti-idiotypic antibodies were
raised against the anti-f Met-Leu-Phe immunoglobulins
as demonstrated by the ability to block f Met-Leu-
[^{3}H] Phe binding to the anti-f Met-Leu-Phe immunogen.
To search for the presence of "internal image"
anti-idiotypic antibodies, we examined their ability
to bind to several genetically unrelated anti-f Met-
Leu-Phe antibodies and to the neutrophil formyl
peptide chemotaxis receptor. We found that some of
the rabbits produced anti-idiotypic antibodies that
were able to block f Met-Leu-[^{3}H]Phe binding to nearly
all rabbit, guinea pig and mouse anti-f Met-Leu-Phe
antibodies examined. Moreover, some of the anti-
idiotypic antibodies were able to bind to the formyl
peptide receptor on the neutrophil as evidence by 1)
the direct binding of anti-idiotypic IgG to the
neutrophil as detected by ^{125}I-Protein A, and 2) the
inhibition of fNle-Leu-Phe-Nle-[^{125}I]Tyr-Lys binding
to the membrane receptor. Thus, it appears that a
subpopulation of anti-idiotypic antibodies can bind to
any formyl peptide binding site, independent of their
idiotypic character.
Lastly we will show a rapid and cyclic appearance
and disappearance of the anti-idiotypic antibodies

which appears to be mediated by a auto-anti-anti-idiotypic antibody that shares binding characteristics with those of the anti-f Met-Leu-Phe immunogen.

INTRODUCTION

Anti-idiotypic antibodies have proven to be useful reagents for both functional and biochemical studies of cell surface receptors (1-11). It has recently been recognized that anti-idiotypic antibodies are a heterogenous population of molecules and that four types of antibodies may actually be induced (12-14). The first type is directed against idiotopes associated with the combining site of immunizing antibodies and is generally ligand inhibitable. The second type is composed of antibodies directed against idiotopes associated with the frame work of the V region and does not block ligand binding. A third type of anti-idiotypic antibody may interact with epitope- or idiotope-related structures of antibodies. The fourth type of antibody that may result from the immunization of antibodies apparently mimics the original antigen by presumably possessing an epitope in common with original antigen. These antibodies are said to constitute an "internal image" of the initial antigen and thus should bind to any receptor capable of binding the original antigen independent of its idiotypic character. Recently several reports have described systems in which these latter anti-idiotypic antibodies have been used to investigate the modulation and activation of specific membrane receptors. In some cases, the biological properties of antigens are indeed "mimicked" by these "internal image" like anti-idiotypic antibodies. In particular, antibodies raised against anti-hormone antibodies have been observed to bind hormone receptors and to trigger hormone-regulated physiological responses (3-8). In this report, we present experiments that are designed to identify "internal image" anti-idiotypic antibodies. Furthermore, we will show that the use of an idiotypic network is a feasible experimental approach for producing anti-cell receptor antibody without first purifying the receptor.

METHODS AND MATERIALS

Animal Immunization and Preparation of Antibodies.

Rabbit antibodies were raised against $fMLP_{10}$-BSA, $fMLP_{147}$-KLH and $fMLP_{12}$-Goat IgG and the IgG fractions were purified as previously described (1,2). For the production of ascites, mouse (B10.S) and guinea pig anti-$fMLP_{10}$-BSA antibodies were raised as previously described (2).

Anti-idiotypic antibodies were raised in rabbits by multiple intradermal injection of the IgG fraction containing the rabbit anti-f Met-Leu-Phe antibody (500 µg) in a 1:1 mixture with complete Freund's adjuvant. IgG fractions rather than specific antibodies were used as immunogen in order to avoid a purification step involving affinity chromatography with the possible leakage of the original antigen. Ten and thirty six days later, the rabbits were boosted with 1 mg and 500 µg of immunogen, respectively, in incomplete Freunds adjuvant.

Affinity Column Purification of Anti-Idiotypic Antibodies.

Rabbit anti-idiotypic antibody was purified by passage over a protein A-Sepharose CL-4B column using standard procedures. The purified IgG from the third bleeding of rabbit #2397 was filtered over a column of Sepharose 4B rabbit anti-f Met-Leu-Phe (2) previously equilibrated in Tris-HCL buffer (0.05 M Tris, 0.15 M NaCl, 0.02% NaN_3, pH 8.6). This removed over 95% of anti-idiotypic binding activity. The anti-idiotype was eluted with 0.05 M gly-cine-HCl, pH 2.3, immediately neutralized with 3 M Tris, and then dialyzed in phosphate-saline buffer. About 0.7% of the total IgG from the third bleeding represented specific anti-idiotypic antibodies.

Neutrophil Binding.

For the standard binding assay (15-16), 2.5 x 10^5 rabbit peritoneal neutrophils, obtained as previously described, and varying concentrations of f Nle-Leu-Phe-Nle-[^{125}I] Tyr-Lys (specific activity 1200 Ci/mmol) were incubated at 4°C in 100 µl Hanks' buffer plus 1.6 mM Ca^{++} and 0.1% α-lactalbumin. After 45 min, the suspension was rapidly filtered through a Whatman GF/C filter. The filters (in triplicate) were washed with five 2-ml aliquots of ice-cold Hanks' buffer containing 0.1% BSA and bound radioactivity was quantitated. Nonspecific binding, defined as the cpm bound in the presence of 1000-fold excess unlabeled peptide, was always less than 10% of the total binding.

Detection of Anti-Idiotype Binding to Rabbit Neutrophil by ^{125}I-Protein A.

^{125}I-Protein A was bound to neutrophils by a modification of the procedure previously described (2). In brief, 5.25×10^6 washed rabbit neutrophils in 825 μl of PBS buffer were incubated at 4°C for 1 hour with varying dilutions of purified preimmune or anti-idiotypic IgG. The cell suspension was centrifuged at 1500 rpm for 7 min at 4°C, washed twice, and resuspended in 100 μl of cold PBS buffer containing 65 ng of ^{125}I-protein A. The suspension was incubated for 30 min at 4°C, washed with 10 ml 4°C PBS, rapidly filtered through a Whatman GF/C filter and counted for cell bound ^{125}I-Protein A.

RESULTS

Preparation and Characterization of Anti-f Met-Leu-Phe Antibodies.

Antibodies against f Met-Leu-Phe, a potent leukocyte chemoattractant which is produced by Escherichia coli (17), were raised in rabbits, rats, guinea pigs and mice by immunization with synthetic f Met-Leu-Phe linked to bovine serum albumin (2). The antibody, further designated as Ab-1 and used as immunogen to produce anti-idiotypic antibodies, was the seventh bleeding from a single rabbit. The antibodies specifically bound f Met-Leu-(^{3}H)Phe with an equilibrium constant $K = 2.19 \times 10^6 M^{-1}$ and with an index of heterogeneity $a = 0.98$ (2). Specific antibody concentration of different bleeds varied from 100-300 μg/ml and represented 1-3% of the total IgG fraction. The specificity of the antibodies was studied by inhibition of f Met-Leu-(^{3}H)Phe binding by over 40 oligoformylpeptides with widely varying reactivity for the neutrophil formyl peptide chemotaxis receptor. Table 1 summarizes these results.

TABLE 1

CORRELATION BETWEEN NEUTROPHIL AND ANTIBODY
RECEPTOR ACTIVITY FOR 42 FORMYL PEPTIDES

Peptides Differing Only In	N^+	r^*
Formyl Group	5	0.94
Position 1	13	0.90
Position 2 - Non-Esterified	4	0.97
Position 2 - Benzyl Esters	5	0.36
Position 3	8	0.78
Beyond Position 3	7	0.29

+ N = Number of peptides compared
* r = Correlation coefficient

Comparison of the ability of the peptides to bind to the
antibody with their reactivity for the neutrophil formyl
peptide receptor demonstrated a strong correlation in the
rank order of reactivity of the numerous synthetic peptides. This strong correlation is seen across species
lines with both rabbit and rat antibodies (data not shown).
As with the neutrophil, the N-formyl group is manditory for
maximal antibody binding activity. In addition, bacterial
chemotactic factor-enriched butanol extracts from Escherichia coli filtrates can also bind to anti-f Met-Leu-Phe
(1,17). Significant differences, however, in the specificity of the antibody and neutrophil receptors are seen at
the carboxyl terminus of phenylalanine, and beyond the
phenylalanine ring (1). The antibody-containing IgG
fraction was injected into four allotypically matched
rabbits: MI, 3034, 3072, and 2397 to induce the synthesis
of anti-idiotypic antibodies (Ab2).

Inhibition of f Met-Leu-(^{3}H)Phe Binding to Rabbit Anti-f
Met-Leu-Phe by Various Rabbit Anti-Idiotypic Antibodies.

Anti-idiotypic activity was monitored in the serum of
the immunized rabbits by following its capacity to inhibit
the binding of f Met-Leu-(^{3}H)Phe to the rabbit anti-f Met-
Leu-Phe immunogen. As shown in Figure 1, all four rabbits

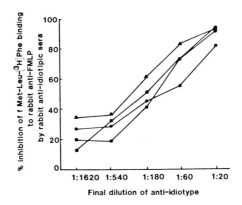

Figure 1.   Inhibition of binding of f Met–Leu–(^{3}H)Phe
to rabbit anti–f Met–Leu–Phe by various rabbit anti–idiotypic sera.   Various dilutions (50 µl) of anti–idiotypic
sera in PBS buffer were incubated for 1 hr at room temperature with a fixed dilution of rabbit anti–f Met–Leu–Phe
sera (25 µl) that was capable of binding 35 fmoles f Met–
Leu–(^{3}H)Phe at 7.75 nM f Met–Leu–(^{3}H)Phe.   Controls (not
shown) were pre–immune sera in all cases.   Radiolabeled
ligand (25 µl) was then added and the reaction was allowed
to proceed for an additional 30 minutes.   100 µl of 4°C
saturated ammonium sulfate was added, the tubes were
vortexed and incubated for an additional one hour at 4°C.
The precipitates were then washed with 10 ml 4°C saturated
ammonium sulfate and collected on glass fiber filters.   All
samples were run in triplicate and the values shown are the
means with S.E.M. (not shown) consistently < 10%.   (▲),
#2397; (■), #3034; (◆), #3072; (●), #MI.

produced anti–idiotypic antibodies with the capacity to
inhibit ligand binding.   However, their concentration in
serum and the time for the appearance and disappearance of
this activity varied (see below).   Pre–immune sera from
these same rabbits had no effect.   The results shown in
Figure 1 are from the third bleeding (21 days after the
primary immunization).

Transient Character of the Anti-Idiotypic Response to Ab-1.

Figure 2 demonstrates the transient character of the anti-idiotypic response to the anti-f Met-Leu-Phe antibodies in two of the rabbits (#2397 and #MI). As can be seen,

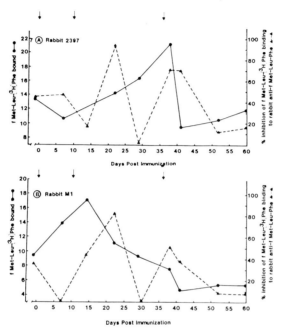

Figure 2. Time course of the transient appearance and disappearance of anti-idiotypic antibodies (Ab-2) (▲---▲) and "Ab-1 like" antibodies (●——●) in two rabbits (#2397 (upper) and #MI (lower)) immunized with rabbit anti-f Met-Leu-Phe. Anti-idiotypic antibodies (Ab-2) were analyzed by the ability of a 1:20 final dilution of sera to inhibit f Met-Leu-[^{3}H]Phe binding to a pre-determined amount of rabbit anti-f Met-Leu-Phe (see Fig. 1). "Ab-1 like" antibodies were quantitated by the number of fmoles of f Met-Leu-[^{3}H]Phe bound by a 1:20 final dilution of sera and at 7.75 nM f Met-Leu-[^{3}H]Phe. Non-specific binding was determined in the presence of 5 μM unlabeled f Met-Leu-Phe and did not exceed 5% of specific binding. Bound radioactivity was measured by means of an ammonium sulfate precipitation assay (Farr assay) (5). Arrows indicate times of injection of anti-f Met-Leu-Phe antibodies (Ab-1).

during the first 60 days after the primary immunization, two peaks of anti-idiotypic activity are found. The first peak, which is seen approximately 3 weeks after primary immunization, was transient in nature and in 3 of 4 rabbits was completely undetectable one week later. However, following a second boost with immunogen on day 36, a second peak of anti-idiotypic activity appeared which again was transient in nature and disappeared within two weeks. The transient character of the anti-idiotypic response to other anti-hormone antibodies has recently been described in other systems (5-8,14). We therefore investigated the presence of antibodies that might mask and/or neutralize the anti-idiotypic antibodies.

Formyl Peptide Binding Activity in Sera of Rabbits Immunized with Anti-f Met-Leu-Phe Antibodies.

In the sera of rabbits #2397 and #MI, we detected transient periods of "Ab-1 like" activity that varied markedly throughout the 60 day period examined (Figure 2). For rabbit #2397, a gradual increase in "Ab-1 like" activity is seen through day 38. However, a rapid loss of "Ab-1 like" activity is seen by day 41 which is 5 days after the second boost with immunogen. In contrast, for rabbit #MI an increase in "Ab-1 like" activity is seen following the primary immunization with the peak appearing 4 days after the first boost with immunogen. A gradual decline in "Ab-1 like" activity is seen throughout the remaining period that was examined.

To differentiate this "Ab-1 like" activity from that due to residual Ab-1 injected for immunization, the ligand-binding affinity of the "Ab-1 like" antibodies was examined. As seen in Table 2, the binding affinity of "Ab-1 like" antibodies from the peaks of formyl peptide binding activity from rabbits #2397 and #MI were different from that of the Ab-1 immunogen. We therefore suspect that the "Ab-1 like" response is due, in fact, to anti-idiotypic antibodies against Ab-2, which we will further designate as Ab-3 throughout this paper.

TABLE 2
BINDING AFFINITY OF THE "Ab-1 LIKE" ANTIBODIES[*]
(Ab-3) AND THE ANTI-f MET-LEU-PHE IMMUNOGEN
(Ab-1) FOR f MET-LEU-[^{3}H]PHE

ANTIBODY	EQUILIBRIUM BINDING CONSTANT (K_o) M^{-1}
IMMUNOGEN (Ab-1)	2.19×10^6
#MI (Ab-1 LIKE)	3.20×10^5
#2397 (Ab-1 LIKE)	4.22×10^5

[*]
The peaks of formyl peptide binding activity from rabbits
#2397 and #MI were analyzed at a 1:20 final dilution and
the anti-f Met-Leu-Phe immunogen at a 1:400 final dilution
for 1 hr at room temperature with increasing concentration
of f Met-Leu-[^{3}H]Phe. Non-specific binding was determined
in the presence of 100 μM unlabeled peptide.

Anti-Idiotypic Antibodies Inhibit f Met-Leu-(^{3}H)Phe Binding
to Various Genetically Unrelated Anti-f Met-Leu-Phe Antibodies.

To begin to differentiate among the four different
types of anti-idiotypic antibodies (Ab-2) that might be
induced by the anti-f Met-Leu-Phe antibodies (Ab-1), we
examined the ability of the anti-idiotypic antibodies
(Ab-2) to inhibit the binding of f Met-Leu-(^{3}H)Phe to
various genetically unrelated anti-f Met-Leu-Phe antibodies. Our rationale was that the binding of a subpopulation
of "internal image" anti-idiotypic antibodies occurs
independently of the idiotypic character of the anti-f
Met-Leu-Phe receptor and can thus bind to any receptor
capable of binding f Met-Leu-Phe. For all of the work that
follows in this paper, the third bleeding from rabbit #2397
was used.
    As seen in Figure 3, a portion of the anti-idiotypic
antibodies were able to bind, to a variable extent, all of

the anti-f Met-Leu-Phe antibodies examined. Thus, the anti-idiotypic antibodies inhibited the binding of f Met-Leu-(^{3}H)Phe to the anti-fMLP$_{147}$-KLH and anti-fMLP$_{12}$-Goat IgG antibodies produced in two different rabbits. In addition, this cross-reactivity occurred across species lines as evidenced by the inhibition of f Met-Leu-(^{3}H)Phe binding to mouse anti-fMLP$_{10}$-BSA and guinea pig anti-fMLP$_{10}$-BSA antibodies. All anti-idiotype producing rabbits except #MI generated antibodies that cross-reacted with anti-f Met-Leu-Phe antibodies that were genetically unrelated to the immunogen. The variable extent of cross-reactivity probably reflects several factors including the relative affinities and concentrations of the anti-f Met-Leu-Phe antibodies as well as steric considerations associated with anti-idiotype binding. In addition, the summation of all of the sub-populations of anti-idiotypic antibodies which may inhibit ligand binding are probably seen either by virtue of 1) being directed against one or more idiotopes within the combining site and/or 2) their being "internal image" anti-idiotypic antibodies.

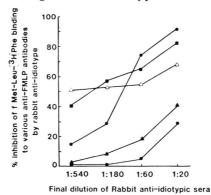

Figure 3. Ability of rabbit anti-idiotype (#2397) to inhibit the binding of f Met-Leu-(^{3}H)Phe to various genetically unrelated anti-f Met-Leu-Phe antibodies. The three sera listed: (●), rabbit anti-fMLP$_{10}$-BSA (immunogen); (■), rabbit anti-fMLP$_{147}$-KLH; (▲), rabbit anti-fMLP$_{12}$-Goat IgG; and the two ascites: (△), mouse anti-fMLP$_{10}$-BSA and (◆), guinea pig anti-fMLP$_{10}$-BSA were analyzed at a final dilution that would bind 35 fmoles f Met-Leu-(^{3}H)Phe at 7.75 nM f Met-Leu-(^{3}H)Phe. The assay was performed exactly as described in Figure 1.

Inhibition of f Nle-Leu-Phe-Nle-[^{125}I]Tyr-Lys Binding to Rabbit Neutrophils by Rabbit Anti-Idiotypic Sera.

We next investigated the possibility that the anti-idiotypic antibodies could also cross-react with the neutrophil formyl peptide receptor. Figure 4A shows that anti-f Met-Leu-Phe anti-idiotypic antibodies compete with f Nle-Leu-Phe-Nle-[^{125}I]Tyr-Lys for binding to the formyl peptide receptor on whole rabbit neutrophils.

Binding of f Nle-Leu-Phe-Nle-[^{125}I]Tyr-Lys has been shown to occur to a single class of non-cooperative binding sites (125,000-140,000 sites/cell) with an equilibrium dissociation constant (K_D) = 2.25 ± 0.50 nM (15). Preincubation of whole rabbit neutrophils at 4°C with pre-immune sera at a 1:10 dilution did not affect the K_D (2.84 nM) nor the total number of binding sites (135,000 sites/cell). Preincubation with anti-f Met-Leu-Phe anti-idiotypic sera resulted in a concentration dependent inhibition in the total number of binding sites per cell (30% reduction at 1:10 dilution (Figure 4B) and 45% reduction at 1:5 dilution (data not shown)). In Figure 4B, the Scatchard plots indicate that the inhibition is essentially due to a decrease in number of binding sites whereas no significant change in K_D occurs.

Direct Binding of Anti-f Met-Leu-Phe Anti-Idiotypic Antibodies to the Neutrophil, Detected by ^{125}I-Protein A.

Since the anti-idiotypic sera from bleeding 3 was shown to contain some Ab-1 like activity, it was necessary to demonstrate directly that the inhibition of fNle-Leu-Phe-Nle-[^{125}I]Tyr-Lys binding to the rabbit neutrophil formyl peptide receptor was due to direct binding of the anti-idiotypic antibody (Ab-2) to the cell and not due to fluid phase binding of the radiolabeled formyl peptide to "Ab-1 like" antibodies which could also result a decrease in formyl peptide binding to the cell.

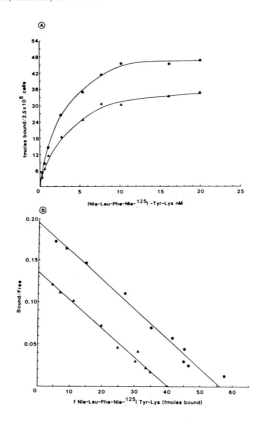

Figure 4. (A) Inhibition of binding of f Nle–Leu–Phe–Nle–[^125^I]Tyr–Lys to the formyl peptide receptor on whole rabbit neutrophils by anti-f Met–Leu–Phe anti-idiotypic sera. Whole rabbit neutrophils were preincubated for 1 hr at 4°C with a 1:10 final dilution of heat inactivated pre-immune (●) or anti-idiotypic sera (▲) and after extensive washing were assayed for f Nle–Leu–Phe–Nle–[^125^I]Tyr–Lys binding. Values shown are the means of two experiments. (B) Scatchard plots of the saturation binding data from A (16). The slope was determined by linear regression analysis. Preincubation of cells with pre-immune sera yielded a total number of binding sites of 134,100 sites/cell and an equilibrium dissociaton constant, K_D of 2.84 nM. For the whole rabbit neutrophils treated with anti-idiotypic sera, a reduction in the total number of binding sites to 96,300 sites/cell and K_D of 2.93 nM were obtained.

Table 3 demonstrates directly the ability of rabbit anti-f Met-Leu-Phe anti-idiotypic antibodies to bind to rabbit neutrophils. As can be seen, pre-immune rabbit IgG can also bind to the neutrophil in a dose-dependent fashion, but to a lesser extent than the anti-idiotypic IgG at each protein concentration tested.

Table 3
Direct Binding of Anti-Idiotypic Antibodies
to Rabbit Neutrophils

Cell Treatment	^{125}I-Protein A Binding[+] (cpm ± S.E.M.)	Fold Increase Over Control
Untreated	8,227 ± 1,621	---
210 µg anti-idiotypic IgG	33,225 ± 3,341	4.04
210 µg pre-immune IgG	24,051 ± 2,122	2.92
100 µg anti-idiotypic IgG	26,992 ± 3,813	3.28
100 µg pre-immune IgG	15,148 ± 619	1.84

[*] Purified IgG in PBS was incubated with 5.25×10^6 cells in 825 µl final volume for 1 hr at 4°C. The cells were then washed 2x with 4°C PBS before the addition of 65 ng ^{125}I-Protein A. After an additional 30 min incubation at 4°C, the cells were washed with 10 ml 4°C PBS, rapidly filtered through a Whatman GF/C filter and counted for cell bound ^{125}I-Protein A.

[+] All data points represent the mean of triplicate determinations.

An estimate of the number of binding sites per cell bound by anti-idiotype was made based on the differences in binding of pre-immune and anti-idiotype IgG to the PMN. These values (46,000 to 65,000 sites/cell) fall well within the range we and others have found for the number of formyl peptide receptors per cell and are in agreement with the reduction of the number of receptor sites seen by analysis of f Nle-Leu-Phe-Nle-[^{125}I]Tyr-Lys binding (Figure 4B).

DISCUSSION

In 1974, Jerne proposed that regulation of antibody production and expression was based on a network of inter-actions between immunoglobulins and anti-immunoglobulins, better defined as anti-idiotypic antibodies (12). These anti-idiotypic antibodies serve to establish a dynamic equilibrium of regulation which limit the extent of the immune response to a given antigen. Jerne further proposed that some of these anti-idiotypic antibodies may have antigenic similarities with the initial immunogen and may in fact constitute an "internal image" of the immunogen. In the case of anti-idiotypic antibodies directed against anti-hormone antibodies, these antibodies may bind to the hormone receptors and mimic some of the biological proper-ties of the hormone.

One approach used to study the type(s) of anti-idio-typic antibodies produced against an anti-hormone antibody is to examine the extent of the formers cross-reactivity. As shown in this study, a portion of the anti-f Met-Leu-Phe anti-idiotypic antibodies bind not only to the formyl peptide chemotaxis receptor of the neutrophil but also to several genetically unrelated anti-f Met-Leu-Phe antibod-ies. At least two explanations are possible for the apparent intra- and inter-species idiotypic cross-reactivi-ty of anti-f Met-Leu-Phe antibodies with the anti-idiotopic IgG and the further ability of the latter to react with the neutrophil formylpeptide receptor. First, it is possible that there are ligand recognition sites (idiotopes) in part of the neutrophil formylpeptide receptor and in the rabbit, mouse and guinea pig anti-f Met-Leu-Phe antibodies that are structurally or conformationally similar (2). Antibodies raised against these common idiotopes would allow cross-re-activity between the antibody and the receptor wherever found. Consistent with this hypothesis is our finding that the specificity of the anti-f Met-Leu-Phe binding site is very similar to that of the formyl-peptide neutrophil receptor. However, similarity of specificity among anti-bodies does not, in and of itself, suggest that the corre-sponding idiotypes will cross-react. An alternative explanation is one based on the "internal image" subpopu-lation of anti-idiotypic antibodies that can presumably possess an epitope in common with the foreign antigen and thus be viewed as containing a positive imprint of the foreign antigen (12). In this view, the extensive cross-reactivity we have described could be due to the presence in low concentrations of a unique subpopulation of anti-idiotypic "internal image" antibodies that possess an epitope in common with f Met-Leu-Phe, i.e., the putative "internal image" subset of anti-idiotype may contain in its variable region an antigenically similar epitope to f Met-Leu-Phe. This homology may enable the anti-idiotypic antibody to partially mimic the binding activities of f Met-Leu-Phe to the neutrophil and antibody receptors. However, these anti-receptor like anti-idiotypic antibodies would be expected to constitute only a small portion of the heterogenous anti-idiotypic response (2,12,14). Thus as shown in this study, only 0.7% of the anti-idiotypic IgG fraction is directed against the immunogen whereas only approximately 0.035% of the IgG fraction (or 5% of the anti-idiotypic IgG) will cross react with the neutrophil formyl peptide receptor.

Several studies have documented the ability of anti-idiotypic antibodies raised against anti-hormone antibodies to bind the corresponding hormone receptors (2-11). In addition, this anti-receptor anti-idiotypic response is usually transient, appears soon after immunization, but may be hardly detectable within days or a few weeks after its initial detection (5-8,14). Our study shows a cyclic appearance and disappearance of anti-idiotypic antibodies (Ab-2) in agreement with recent observations on the anti-idiotypic anti-receptor antibodies directed against the β-adrenergic receptor (14). The disappearance of these anti-idiotypic antibodies may be the result of an active removal/neutralization mechanism by a third kind of antibody "Ab-1 like" (Ab-3) auto-anti-idiotypic against (Ab-2). In addition, some of the Ab-3 antibodies appear to mimick the immunogen by maintaining some capacity to bind the f Met-Leu-Phe peptide. Thus, in agreement with predictions put forth by the network theory and with direct observations by several investigators on the β-adrenergic system (14) and the insulin system (18), the synthesis of anti-idiotypic antibodies that act as anti-receptor antibodies may constitute a potent stimulus for the synthesis of auto anti-anti-idiotypic antibodies (Ab-3) that could neutralize the potentially detrimental physiological effects of the hormone like anti-receptor "internal image" antibodies. Therefore if one is going to use anti-idiotypic sera as a probe against cell surface receptors, it is necessary to follow the time course of the immune response closely and to simultaneously monitor the presence of antibodies that may bind the hormone directly and/or neutralize the anti-receptor antibodies.

Despite the uncertainties as to the nature and origin of the cross-reactive anti-idiotypic antibodies, our findings together with those in the literature (reviewed in ref. #15) demonstrate that obtaining anti-idiotypic antibodies to antibodies directed to cellular ligands may be a general procedure for obtaining antibodies to the corresponding cellular receptors. Our data also suggest that due to the low concentration of these putative "internal image" anti-idiotypic antibodies in immune sera, use of hybridoma technology to produce monoclonal "internal image" anti-receptor antibodies will have practical advantages for obtaining antibodies to cellular receptors (19). This is especially true if one wishes to obtain antibodies to the binding sites of receptors since conventional anti-receptor antibodies (obtained by immunization with purified receptors) often result in most of the antibodies reacting with parts of the molecules other than the binding site (20-23).

ACKNOWLEDGEMENTS

This work was supported in part by NIH grants HL 28442 and HL/AI 33003.

REFERENCES

1. Marasco WA, Showell HJ, Becker EL (1982). Anti-f Met-Leu-Phe. Similarities in fine specificity with the formyl peptide chemotaxis receptor of the neutrophil. J Immunol 128:956.
2. Marasco WA, Becker EL (1982). Anti-Idiotype as antibody against the formyl peptide chemotaxis receptor of the neutrophil. J Immunol 128:963.
3. Sege K, Peterson PA (1978). Use of anti-idiotypic antibodies as cell-surface receptor probes. Proc Natl Acad Sci USA 75:2443.
4. Sege K, Peterson PA (1978). Anti-Idiotypic antibodies against anti-vitamin A transporting protein react with pre-albumin. Nature (Lond.) 271:167.

5. Schreiber AB, Couraud PO, Andre C, Vray B, Strosberg AD (1980). Anti-alprenolol anti-idiotypic antibodies bind to β-adrenergic receptors and modulate catecholamine-sensitive adenylate cyclase. Proc Natl Acad Sci USA 77:7385.

6. Homcy CJ, Rockson SG, Haber E (1982). An anti-idiotypic antibody which recognizes the β-adrenergic receptor. J Clin Invest 69:1147.

7. Wasserman NH, Penn AS, Freimuth PI, Treptow N, Wentzel S, Cleveland WL, Erlanger BF (1982). A new route to anti-acetylcholine receptor antibodies and experimental myasthenia gravis. Proc Natl Acad Sci USA 79:4810.

8. Farid NR, Briones-Urbina R, Nazrul-Islam M (1982). Biological activity of anti-thyrotropin anti-idiotypic antibody. J Cell Biochem 19:305.

9. Noseworthy JH, Fields BN, Dichter MA, Sobotoka C, Pizer E, Perry LL, Nepom JT, Greene MI (1983). Cell receptors for the mammalian reovirus. I. Syngeneic monoclonal anti-idiotypic antibody identifies a cell surface receptor for reovirus. J Immunol 131:2533.

10. Lambris JD, Ross GD (1982). Characterization of the lymphocyte membrane receptor for factor H (B1 H-globulin) with an antibody to anti-factor H idiotype. J Exp Med 155:1400.

11. Gaulton GN, Co MS, Royer H-D, Greene MI (1985). Anti-idiotypic antibodies as probes of cell surface receptors. Mol & Cell Biochem 65:5.

12. Jerne NK (1974). Towards a network theory of the immune system. Ann Immunol (Inst. Pasteur) 125C:373.

13. Lindenmann G (1973). Speculations on idiotypes and homobodies. Ann Immunol (Inst. Pasteur) 124C:171.

14. Couraud P-O, Lu B-Z, Strosberg AD (1983). Cyclical antiidiotypic response to anti-hormone antibodies due to neutralization by autologous anti-antiidiotype antibodies that bind hormone. J Exp Med 157:1369.

15. Walter RJ, Marasco WA (1984). Autoradiographic localization of formyl peptide chemotaxis receptors on rabbit peritoneal neutrophils. Exp Cell Res 154:613.

16. Marasco WA, Becker KM, Feltner DE, Brown CS, Ward PA, Nairn R (1985). Covalent affinity labeling, detergent solubilization, and fluid phase characterization of the rabbit neutrophil formyl peptide chemotaxis receptor. Biochemistry (in press).

17. Marasco WA, Phan SH, Krutzsch H, Showell HJ, Feltner DE, Nairn R, Becker EL, Ward PA (1984). Purification and identification of formyl-methionyl-leucyl-phenyl-alanine as the major peptide neutrophil chemotactic factor produced by escherichia coli. J Biol Chem 259:5430.

18. Shechter Y, Maron R, Elias D, Cohen IR (1982). Autoantibodies to insulin receptor spontaneously develop as anti-idiotypes in mice immunized with insulin. Science 216:542.

19. Cleveland WL, Wassermann NH, Sarangarajan R, Penn AS and Erlanger BF (1983). Monoclonal antibodies to the acetylcholine receptor by a normally functioning auto-anti-idiotypic mechanism. Nature 305:56.

20. Couraud P-O, Delavier-Klutchko C, Durieu-Trautmann O, Strosberg AD (1981). Antibodies raised against β-adrenergic receptors stimulate adenylate cyclase. Biochem Biophys Res Comm 99(4):1295.

21. Jacobs S, Chang KJ, Cuatrecasas P (1978). Antibodies to purified insulin receptor have insulin-like activity. Science 200:1283.

22. Lindstrom J (1977). Antibodies to Estrogen Receptor: Immunochemical Similarity of Estrophilin from Various Mammalian Species. In "Receptors and Recognition", Vol. A3, Cuatrecasas P and Greaves MF, eds. pp. 1-44, Chapman and Hall, London.

23. Greene GL, Closs LE, Fleming H, De Sombre ER, Jensen EV (1977). Antibodies to receptors for acetylcholine and other hormones. Proc Natl Acad Sci USA 74:3681.

Monoclonal Antibodies and Cancer Therapy, pages 345–357
© 1985 Alan R. Liss, Inc.

IDIOTYPIC ROUTES TO MONOCLONAL ANTI-RECEPTOR ANTIBODIES[1]

W.L. Cleveland, N.H. Wassermann, A.S. Penn, H.H. Ku,
B.L. Hill, R. Sarangarajan, and B.F. Erlanger

Departments of Microbiology (W.L.C., N.H.W., H.H.K.,
B.L.H., R.S., B.F.E.) and Neurology (A.S.P.), Columbia
University and the Cancer Center (W.L.C., N.H.W., H.H.K.,
B.L.H., R.S., B.F.E.) New York, New York 10032

ABSTRACT Idiotypic procedures have been developed for
the preparation of antibodies to receptors. These procedures do not require receptor for immunization and give
antibodies that are inherently combining site-specific.
In one of the procedures, which was applied to the
acetylcholine receptor (AChR), antibodies were first
raised to a structurally constrained agonist (BisQ) of
the AChR using a bovine albumin conjugate of BisQ
(BisQ-BSA). The specificity of these antibodies was
similar to the specificity of the AChR in its activated
state. In the second step of the procedure, rabbits were
immunized with anti-BisQ antibodies in order to raise
anti-idiotypic antibodies. The anti-idiotypic antibodies reacted with cross-reactive determinants found on
AChR preparations from Electrophorus electricus, Torpedo
californica, and rat muscle. In some of the rabbits,
signs of transient experimental myasthenia gravis were
seen. In a second, more direct form of the procedure,
mice were immunized with BisQ-BSA and splenocytes were
immortalized by fusion with myeloma cells. Screening of
the fusion revealed a substantial number of clones
secreting auto-anti-idiotypic antibodies, some of which
reacted with receptor. One clone, F8-D5, was selected
for further analysis. It bound to both anti-BisQ and

---

[1]This work was supported by the NIH (NS-15581,
NS-17904, and AI-17949) and the Muscular Dystrophy
Association.

AChR, and binding to one was inhibited by the other. Binding to both was also inhibited by BisQ, decamethonium, and α-bungarotoxin. In immunofluorescence with <u>Torpedo</u> tissue, staining patterns were identical to those obtained with anti-AChR antisera raised by direct immunization with AChR. Preliminary results suggest that immobilized F8-D5 can be used to isolate receptor. Experiments with a vesicle system containing reconstituted AChR indicate that F8-D5 inhibits ion flux. Mice bearing ascites tumors of F8-D5 developed muscle weakness that could be temporarily relieved by neostigmine. The auto-anti-idiotypic procedure has also been used successfully to prepare antibodies to the adenosine receptor. The specificities of the anti-receptor antibodies are discussed in terms of the classical concept of idiotypy as well as the internal image concept.

INTRODUCTION

In a previous study, we demonstrated that an idiotypic procedure could be used to prepare conventional antibodies to the combining site of the acetylcholine receptor (1). This procedure was inspired by the findings of Sege and Peterson (2), who demonstrated that anti-insulin antibodies could be used to raise anti-idiotypic antibodies that reacted with the insulin receptor, and by other studies which indicated that antibodies can mimic the active sites of nonimmunoglobulin molecules (3,4). In our study, a derivative of a synthetic agonist, BisQ (Fig. 1), of the AChR from <u>Electrophorous</u> <u>electricus</u> was coupled to bovine albumin (BSA) and used to raise anti-BisQ antibodies in a rabbit. Affinity-purified anti-BisQ antibodies were then used to raise anti-idiotypic antibodies in a second rabbit. This approach was basically successful and a number of interesting findings emerged.

A characterization of the anti-BisQ antibodies by radioimmunoassay using a panel of ligands known to bind the AChR revealed that the rank order of binding was similar for both AChR and anti-BisQ antibodies (1). Moreover, it was found that agonists were bound better than antago-antagonists. This suggested that the anti-BisQ antibodies possessed a specificity that was similar to the combining site of the AChR in its activated state. It should be

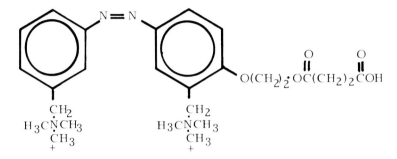

Figure 1. Derivative of BisQ for preparation of BisQ-BSA conjugate: 4-(succinoyloxyethyloxy)-3,3'-bis   (α-(tri-methylammonio)methyl)azobenzene.

noted that BisQ, which is an agonist in its trans-configu-ration, is a rigid structure. Given its   potency as an agonist and its rigidity, it is reasonable to expect that it is closely complementary to the AChR combining site when the latter is in its activated state. This property may be responsible for the similarity of the anti-BisQ antibodies to the activated state of the receptor combin-ing site.

Secondly, three out of three rabbits immunized with anti-BisQ antibodies developed titer to the acetylcholine receptor, as measured by complement fixation and ELISA with receptor preparations from rat, Electrophorus electricus, and Torpedo californica (1). Although titers were rather low and transitory, useful amounts of antisera could be obtained.

Two of the three rabbits also showed signs of experi-mental myasthenia gravis as revealed by tests for weakness and fatigability, and also by electromyography. Severity of symptoms correlated with anti-AChR titer as measured by ELISA (1). Signs of weakness, which appeared 7 days after the first boost, peaked 14 days later. At this point, a

second boost was given and both the titer and severity of
weakness declined. Two additional boosts led to further
declines.

Encouraged by our success in preparing conventional
antisera to the AChR combining site, we next attempted to
prepare monoclonal antibodies, as this would bypass the
problems of low and transitory titer. At this point, it
occurred to us that the two-step procedure of Sege and
Peterson might be replaced by a one-step procedure in
which cells secreting auto-anti-idiotypic antibodies
(i.e., anti-anti-BisQ) as a result of BisQ-BSA immunization are immortalized by fusion to myeloma cells (5). On
the basis of our rabbit experiments, we expected that a
portion of the anti-anti-BisQ antibodies would cross-react
with receptor. This strategy was inspired by the idiotype
network theory proposed by Jerne in 1974 (6). A basic
prediction of this theory is that immunization with
antigen stimulates not only the production of anti-antigen
antibodies, but also the production of auto-anti-idiotypic
antibodies which react with the anti-antigen antibodies.

A Balb/cCr mouse was immunized i.p. with BisQ-BSA in
complete Freund's adjuvant. After 23 days it was boosted.
After 5 additional days, splenocytes were harvested and
fused to non-Ig producing myeloma cells using standard
methods.   To avoid neutralization of anti-anti-BisQ by
anti-BisQ, which might occur in polyclonal cultures, the
fusion mixture was initially distributed into approximately 1000 microplate wells.   This insured that each well
would contain at most several clones.   After 14 days,
supernatants were harvested and tested by indirect ELISA
using three different antigens: BisQ-RSA, affinity-purified rabbit anti-BisQ antibodies, and purified Torpedo
AChR.   The second antibody in these assays was peroxidase-labeled goat anti-mouse Ig.   The use of rabbit
anti-BisQ facilitated the indirect ELISA, which would not
have been possible with mouse anti-BisQ antibodies. Moreover, it restricted detection to auto-anti-idiotypic antibodies that react with idiotopes shared across species.
The importance of thsi will become evident in the discussion of the internal image concept given below.

The ELISA screening revealed that 14% of the wells
were positive for BisQ-RSA, whereas 7.4% were positive for
rabbit anti-BisQ. Of the latter population, about 1/3
(i.e., 2.4% of the total) were positive for AChR. All of
the wells positive for AChR were contained in the set

positive for rabbit anti-BisQ. None of the wells positive
for BisQ-RSA were in the rabbit anti-BisQ set. One of the
cultures positive for receptor (F8-D5) was selected for
further study. After subcloning twice by limiting dilution, F8-D5 retained its ability to bind both AChR and
rabbit anti-BisQ (Fig. 2).

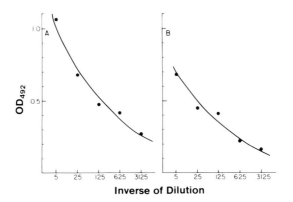

Figure 2. Binding of <u>Torpedo</u> AChR (a) and rabbit anti-
BisQ (b) by F8-D5 (5, reprinted with permission).

F8-D5 was further tested by ELISA in a series of
experiments aimed at defining its specificity more completely. Its binding to microplate wells coated with AChR
could be inhibited with rabbit anti-BisQ, 50% inhibition
occurring with 3 ug of affinity-purified antibody per well
(Fig. 3). In the reciprocal expeirment, 0.9 ug of AChR
gave 50% inhibition. Other ligands known to react with
the AChR combining site were also shown to inhibit the
binding of F8-D5 to AChR and to rabbit anti-BisQ, as shown
in Table 1. These results reinforce the conclusion that
F8-D5 is specific for determinants intimately associated
with the combining sites of AChR and rabbit anti-BisQ. It
should be noted that BisQ is a small ligand (molecular
weight = 486) and is therefore not likely to block reaction with non-idiotypic determinants near the combining
site as a result of steric hindrance.

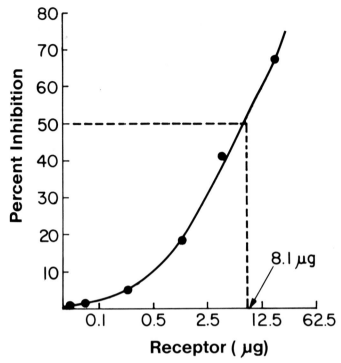

Figure 3. Inhibition of binding of F8-D5 to anti-BisQ by Torpedo AChR (5, reprinted with permission)

TABLE 1
INHIBITION OF BINDING OF F8-D5 TO ANTI-BisQ
AND TO TORPEDO AChR

Inhibitor	IC$_{50}$ (mM)*	
	Torpedo	anti-BisQ
BisQ	0.04	0.04
Decamethonium Br	0.06	0.07
Carbamylcholine Cl	0.05	0.1
Hexamethonium Br	0.37	0.29
α-Bungarotoxin	5.5 x 10-3	0.7 x 10-3

*IC$_{50}$ = concentration that caused 50% inhibition.

WORK IN PROGRESS

In collaborative studies with J. Lindstrom of the Salk Institute, F8-D5 has been shown to block influx in a vesicle system containing reconstituted <u>Torpedo</u> AChR. At an antibody to receptor ratio of 2:1, in the presence of 1mM carbamylcholine, ^{134}Cs influx was inhibited by about 80%. These results further confirm the specificity of F8-D5 for the combining site of AChR.

We have also begun experiments to test the utility of F8-D5 as a cytochemical reagent. Indirect immunofluorescence with <u>Torpedo</u> tissue revealed a staining pattern similar to that obtained with rabbit antisera raised by immunization with purified AChR (Fig. 4) (7).

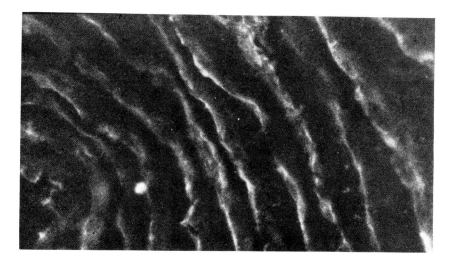

Figure 4. Immunofluorescence of sectioned <u>Torpedo</u> tissue after reaction with F8-D5 and fluorescein-labeled rabbit anti-mouse Ig.

The auto-anti-idiotypic strategy which was used to obtain F8-D5 has the compelling advantage of not requiring receptor for immunization. It therefore might be useful for studying the numerous ligand-receptor systems in which the receptor has not been isolated. Indeed, monoclonal antibodies prepared with the auto-anti-idiotypic strategy could in principle be used to isolate receptors. To test this possibility, we immobilized F8-D5 on diaminodipropyl-amine agarose beads (Pierce Chemical Co.) using gluta-raldehyde as the cross-linking reagent (8). The immobi-lized antibody was incubated with a crude preparation of AChR from <u>Torpedo californica</u>. Hexamethonium bromide was used to elute receptor after extensive washing. Receptor was quantitated using iodine-labeled -bungarotoxin. Es-sentially all of the receptor bound and could be eluted. However, entirely pure preparations were not obtained, as revealed by SDS-PAGE. Futher optimization of this proce-dure is in progress.

Recent preliminary results indicate that Balb/cCr mice bearing ascites tumors of F8-D5 show signs of muscle weakness. Two mice that were each injected with 10^7 F8-D5 cells showed detectable signs of ascites tumors on day 8. On day 12 they began showing signs of muscle weakness. By day 14, both were quadriplegic. One of these mice was injected with neostigmine. After 30 minutes, support by both hind and forelimbs was temporarily restored. The other mouse, injected with an equal volume of distilled water, showed no improvement. These results provide <u>in vivo</u> confirmation of the specificity of F8-D5 revealed by <u>in vitro</u> assays.

An important question is whether the auto-anti-idio-typic strategy will work with other ligand-receptor sys-tems. We have therefore begun to explore other systems. Recent, successful preliminary results (9) have been ob-tained with the adenosine receptor (for reviews see refs. 10,11). Our strategy was essentially identical to that used with the BisQ system. First rabbit antisera were raised against N-6-adenosine-caproyl-BSA. Adenosine-specific antibodies were isolated by affinity chroma-tography using a column prepared by coupling N-6-adeno-sinecaproic acid to aminohexyl-Sepharose 4B. After im-munization and boosting with adenosine conjugate, splen-cytes were immortalized using standard hybridoma technol-ogy. Supernatants were first screened by ELISA using microplates coated with affinity-purified rabbit anti-adenosine antibodies. Two positive cultures were recloned and studied further. By radioimmunoassay, both inhibited the binding of (^{3}H)-adenosine to affinity purified rabbit anti-adenosine antibodies. Essentially complete inhibi-tion could be obtained. Moreover, antibodies from both clones bound to a partially purified preparation of adeno-sine receptor (Fig. 5), and binding could be inhibited by

N-6-cyclohexyladenosine 2-chloroadenosine and theophyl-
line. In future studies, these monoconal antibodies will
be used to purify the receptor, which has not yet been
isolated in pure form. This second success with the auto-
anti-idiotypic strategy raises the possibility that it may
have wide utility.

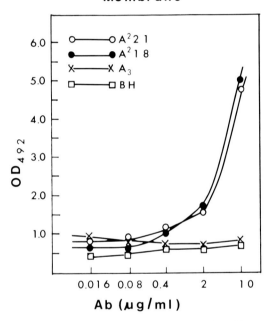

Figure 5. Binding of anti-idiotypic antibodies to bovine
bovine brain membrane preparation (0), monoclonal $A^2 21$;
(●) monoclonal $A^2 18$; (x) A3, a monoclonal anti-adenosine
antibody, (□) BH, an anti-thyrotropin stimulating hormone
antibody.

GENERAL DISCUSSION

An important question concerns the nature of the
idiotypic determinant recognized by F8-D5. Idiotypic
determinants, as defined by the classical studies of
Oudin (12) and Kunkel (13) and their respective coworkers,

are unique antigenic specificities that are presumably
associated with unique aspects of v-region sequences.
Antisera against classical idiotopes usually cannot be
absorbed with normal serum. Given the uniqueness of classical idiotopes, this is expected, since normal serum
contains a large diversity of v-region sequences.
Although not always the case, anti-idiotypic antisera are
often hapten- or antigen-inhibitable, which is consistent
with idiotypic determinants being associated with the combining site.

Conceivably, the antigenic determinant recognized by
F8-D5 is a classical idiotope. If so, our data indicate
that it is shared by both AChR and polyclonal anti-BisQ
antibodies. This assignment is challenged by the studies
of Oudin (12) and others (14), wh have shown that only 2-5%
of a large sample of rabbits immunized with the same
antigen produce antisera that show idiotypic cross-reac-
tions. If antibodies of similar specificity share idiotopes among themselves only rarely, then sharing idiotopes
with a nonimmunoglobulin receptor of similar specificity
is also likely to be infrequent. From this point of view,
one might expect infrequent sucess in using idiotypic procedures as a practical tool to prepare antibodies to
receptor combining sites. Since success does not seem to
be infrequent, it is relevant to consider alternative explanations.

F8-D5 can also be interpreted as an internal image of
BisQ. An internal image of an antigenic determinant is
defined as an idiotope which cross-reacts with the
antigenic determinant. The possible existence of internal
images was appreciated by Lindenmann (15) who called them
homobodies. Internal images were also included as an element of Jerne's idiotype network (6). Anti-idiotypic
antisera that have been interpreted in terms of the
internal image concept have the remarkable property of
reacting with essentially all antibodies that react with
the imaged determinant. This includes antibodies not only
from different individuals within the species, but also
antibodies from multiple species. They do not, however,
react with antibodies of different specificity (14,16).
Since the internal image idiotope is an approximate copy
of the antigenic determinant, it is entirely plausible
that the internal image react with nonimmunoglobulin
receptors having specificity for the imaged determinant.
It should be appreciated that although internal images are

conceptually quite different from classical anti-idiotypic antibodies, they satisfy similar operational criteria, i.e., they are inherently site-specific and will not usually be absorbed with normal serum.

On the basis of binding assays, it appears that F8-D5, as well as the auto-anti-idiotypic antibodies that react with adenosine receptor could be interpreted as internal images. While this interpretation is appealing in many ways, it should be noted that as yet there is no three-dimensional structural data that support the internal image concept. Our use of this term is therefore tentative.

Although the internal image concept is more than ten years old, it has not been thoroughly explored, either theoretically or experimentally. One question which immediately arises is whether auto-internal images exist. It should be appreciated that the ability to raise internal images by immunization with exogenous antibody does not provide direct evidence that internal images play a role in physiological idiotype regulation. Although a much larger data base is needed for a firm conclusion, our data, as well as that of Shechter et al. (17), would suggest that auto-internal images can be a rather prominent feature of the network response, at least when the immunogen is a ligand of a self receptor.

In conclusion, we wish to point out that ligand-receptor systems that are part of self are of special interest in connection with the self-nonself discrimination problem. When these systems are reflected into the idiotypic network, a blurring of the distinction between self and anti-self occurs. For example, an internal image of the ligand, i.e., an internal image of a self determinant, is also anti-self, since it reacts with receptor. Moreover, an anti-ligand antibody can be regarded as an internal image of the receptor combining site, but it is also anti-self, since it reacts with the ligand. A study of idiotype regulation in the context of ligand-receptor systems might lead to a penetrating understanding of this paradox, and identify a basis for the learning of self-nonself discrimination.

REFERENCES

1. Wasserman NH, Penn AH, Freimuth PI, Treptow N, Wentzel S, Cleveland WL, Erlanger BF (1982). Anti-idiotypic route to anti-acetylcholine receptor antibodies and experimental myasthenia gravis. Proc Natl Acad Sci USA 79:4810.
2. Sege K, Peterson PA (1978). Use of anti-idiotypic antibodies as cell-surface receptor probes. Proc Natl Acad Sci USA 75:2443.
3. Beiser SM, Tannenbaum SW (1963). Binding site topology of enzymes and antibodies induced by the same determinants. Ann NY Acad Sci 103:595.
4. Hough CAM, Edwardson JA (1978). Antibodies to Thaumatin as a model of the sweet taste receptor. Nature 271:381.
5. Cleveland WL, Wassermann NH, Sarangarajan R, Penn AS, Erlanger BF (1983). Monoclonal antibodies to the acetylcholine receptor by a normally functioning auto-anti-idiotypic mechanism. Nature 305:56.
6. Jerne NK (1974). Towards a network theory of the immune system. Ann Immunol (Inst Pasteur) 125C:373.
7. Erlanger BF, Cleveland WL, Wassermann NH, Hill BL, Penn AS, Ku HH, Sarangarajan R (1984). Anti-idiotypic antibody to the acetylcholine and adenosine receptors. In Changeux JP, Hucho F, Maelicke A, Neumann E (eds): "Molecular Basis of Nerve Activity," New York: Walter de Gruyter & Co., in press.
8. Reichlin M (1980). Use of glutaraldehyde as a coupling agent for proteins and peptides. Meth Enzymol 70A:159.
9. Erlanger BF, Cleveland WL, Wassermann NH, Hill BL, Penn AS, Ku HH, Sarangarajan R. Anti-receptor antibodies by the auto-anti-idiotypic route. 9th International Subcellular Methodology Forum, Surrey, England, Sept. 1-4, 1984, in press.
10. Daly JW, Bruns RF, Snyder S (1981). Adenosine receptors in the central nervous system: Relationship to the central actions of methylxanthines. Life Sci 28:2083.
11. Wolf J, Londos C, Cooper DMF (1981). Adenosine receptors and the regulation of adenylate cyclase. Adv Cyc Nuc Res 14:199.

12. Oudin J, Michel M (1963). Une nouvelle forme d'allo-typie des globulins du sérum de lapin apparement liée à la fouction et à la spécificité antecorps. CR Acad Sci 251:805.

13. Kunkel HC, Jannik M, Williams RC (1963). Individual antigenic specificites of isolated antibodies. Science 148:1218.

14. Urbain J, Slaoui M, Mariamé B, Leo O (1984). Idiotypy and internal images. In Köhler H, Urbain J, Casenave P-A (eds): "Idiotopy in Biology and Medicine," New York: Academic Press, Inc., p. 15.

15. Lindenmann J (1973). Speculations on idiotypes and homobodies. Ann Immunol (Inst Pasteur) 124C:171.

16. Bona CA (1984). Parallel sets and the internal image of antigen within the idiotypic network. Fed Proc 43:2558.

17. Shechter Y, Maron D, Elias D, Cohen IR (1982). Auto-antibodies to insulin receptor spontaneously develop as anti-idiotypes in mice immunized with insulin. Science 216:542.

Monoclonal Antibodies and Cancer Therapy, pages 359–365
© 1985 Alan R. Liss, Inc.

BIOCHEMICAL CHARACTERIZATION OF A PROSTATE TISSUE ANTIGEN

Ann M. Carroll and Mark I. Greene

Department of Pathology, Harvard Medical School
and Department of Medicine, Tufts New England
Medical Center, Boston, Massachusetts

ABSTRACT   The biochemical properties of human prostate
cell surface antigens recognized by two monoclonal
antibodies (F77-129 and F77-55) were studied.   RIA
blocking studies indicate steric proximity of F77-129
and F77-55 epitopes.   Both monoclonals bind human
prostate and breast tumor cell lines and modulate
surface antigen expression of these cells at 37^OC.
Both antibodies also precipitate a 32-35 kd protein
from surface lactoperoxidase iodinated and ^{35}S-
cysteine internally labeled prostate and breast cells.
Combined modulation, precipitation and enzyme
modification data suggest the epitope-bearing surface
component is a transmembrane protein.

INTRODUCTION

The development of antibodies to tumor specific
antigens has long been a goal of cancer immunologists, and
monoclonal antibody technology (1) eliminated many of the
practical problems of this approach.   A major obstacle,
however, persists: the failure to demonstrate the widespread existence of tumor-specific antigens in spontaneous
animal malignancies (2,3) and in human cancer patients (4).
We have therefore utilized an alternative approach to
the development of clinically useful anti-tumor monoclonals, namely the elicitation of antibodies to normal
tissue differentiation antigens.   Criteria for this
approach are uniform antigenic expression within

1.   This work was supported by Grant 3PO1 CA 14723-11 and
a grant from the Council for Tobacco Research

the target tissue and anatomical restriction of antigen
display to that tissue. Also, for antibody-mediated
cytotoxic anti-cancer therapy, it is essential that the
target tissue be non-essential for survival of the whole
organism. One tissue which meets these criteria and is
also subject to a high incidence of malignant transformation is prostate (5). Currently available reagents
for prostatic cancer imaging (6) and therapy (7) are
unsatisfactory, and anti-prostate monoclonal antibodies
would be well suited for adjunctive therapy and imaging of
disseminated cancer.

RESULTS

A panel of monoclonal antibodies reactive to surface
antigens of the PC-3 human prostate adenocarcinoma cell
line has been developed, as described elsewhere (8).
Hybridoma supernatants were screened by RIA and FACS
analysis on a panel of human tumor cell lines, and two
hybridomas were selected for further study. Both F77-129,
an IgG-3, and F77-55, also an IgG3 showed high reactivity
to the immunizing PC-3 cell line and the Du-145 human
prostate carcinoma cell line; they also bound significantly
to three of four human breast cell lines tested. Binding
of F77-129 was restricted to these tissue types and showed
selective binding to normal and malignant prostate and
breast glandular epithelium in immunoperoxidase analysis
of human tissue sections (8,9). F77-55 also showed
binding to one colon and one ovarian tumor cell line.
Synthetic media purified F77-129 has been shown to have
high specific localization and excellent imaging
properties in PC-3 tumor xenografted nude mice, supporting
a possible role of this antibody as a tissue-specific
diagnostic imaging agent (9,10). Preliminary studies also
indicate a significant functional anti-tumor effect of
unlabeled F77-129 in PC-3 tumor bearing nude mice
(unpublished).
    The present work attempts to biochemically define and
compare the surface determinants recognized by the F77-129
and F77-55 monoclonals. A blocking RIA assay with
iodinated F77-129 and unlabeled F77-129, F77-55 or anti-
HLA antibody (BRL, Gaithersburg, MD) was done to determine
whether the 55 and 129 epitopes were sterically related.
Results in Table 1 show that pre-incubation of PC-3 target
cells with unlabeled F77-129 or F77-55 blocked

subsequent binding of iodinated F77-129 in the same
quantitative range. Anti-HLA, previously determined to
bind PC-3 cells in indirect RIA and immunofluorescence
studies, did not block binding of F77-129. These results
indicate steric proximity (and possibly overlap or identity)
of the F77-55 and F77-129 epitopes. Iodinated F77-129 has
also been used for Scatchard analysis with PC-3 target
cells; it binds a mean of 165,000 sites per cell with a
binding affinity of 1.6×10^9 M^{-1} (10).

We have previously shown that F77-129 binding to PC-3
cells at $37^{\circ}C$ causes surface antigenic modulation,
indicating a transmembrane nature. F77-55 also modulates
surface antigen expression on both PC-3 and BT-20 human
breast carcinoma target cells. By FACS log scale analysis
of BT-20 cells incubated with F77-55 at $37^{\circ}C$ versus $4^{\circ}C$
for one hour, a shift in the percentage of antigen-positive
cells (relative to negative controls) from 80% to 37% was
seen.

We have further investigated the biochemical nature
of the target antigen by a variety of enzyme treatments
and modifications. When PC-3 cells were prefixed in cold
methanol, antibody binding was not decreased. Pretreatment of PC-3 cells with neuraminidase and the N-
linked glycosylation inhibitor tunicamycin **did not alter**
F77-129 binding in indirect FACS analysis. Together, the
modulation and enzyme modification data suggest the 129
epitope is present on a transmembrane protein or glycoprotein or is a non-N-asparagine linked carbohydrate
residue of a surface glycolipid.

To determine whether surface protein(s) could be
specifically isolated with these monoclonals, PC-3 and
other human cells were radiolabeled, detergent extracted
and immunoprecipitated with antibody bound to protein-A
sepharose. Fig. 1 is an autoradiograph of an SDS-PAGE
(10%) gel containing samples of F77-129 immunoprecipitates
of NP-40 (2%) lysates of surface lactoperoxidase iodinated
PC-3 (lane A) and G-361 melanoma (lane B) cells. A 34-35
kd band was precipitated from PC-3 but not G-361 cells
under reducing conditions; a similar band has also been
precipitated from lysates of iodinated BT-20 breast cells.
A similar band (32-34 kd) was also specifically
precipitated from lysates of BT-20 and PC-3 cells (but
not G-361 or T cells) metabolically labeled with ^{35}S-
cysteine using either F77-129 or F77-55. Protein A

TABLE 1

% ^{125}I-F77-129 BINDING TO PC-3 CELLS[a]

^{125}I-129 μg	Direct Binding	Inhibition with anti-HLA	Unlabeled 129	Unlabeled 55[b]
.035	22.0	26.3	14.1	9.4
.018	26.5	29.3	13.9	13.8
.009	29.0	26.6	12.0	14.9

a   % of total radioactivity added per well; 5 X 10[4] cells per well

b   for inhibition, cells were pre-incubated 45 min with unlabeled antibody
    and cells were washed prior to addition of ^{125}I-F77-129.

sepharose pre-incubated with normal mouse serum or purified mouse immunoglobulin did not bind this component. In an additional experiment in which ^{35}S cysteine labeled BT-20 lysate was precipitated with F77-129, use of non-reducing sample buffer resulted in a lowered molecular weight (29 kd) of the specifically precipitated component, suggesting the presence of intrachain disulfide bonds. Also, in initial attempts to selectively remove cytoplasmic components from ^{35}S-cysteine labeled cells prior to detergent extraction (by dounce homogenization and high speed centrifugation) the 32-35 kd component remained in the membrane-enriched pellet. Analysis of ^{35}S-cysteine labeled culture supernatants provided no evidence for secretion of this component.

DISCUSSION

The anti-PC-3 antibodies F77-129 and F77-55 could be clinically useful for prostate and breast cancer patients due to the following factors: restricted tissue-specific expression, cell surface antigen expression and modulation, high affinity binding to a large number of sites and good in vivo localization properties. Further clinical development of these antibodies requires better biochemical definition of the target antigen(s).

The similar modulating and precipitating properties and the RlA blocking studies suggest the two antibodies bind sterically related epitopes, probably on the same surface molecule. The direct antigenic modulation by antibody establishes the transmembrane nature of this component, and indicates the target bears repetitive surface epitopes or, alternatively, has physiologically relevant ligand binding and internalization properties. The immunoprecipitation data indicate a protein structure similar in size to the prostatic antigen described by Wang et al (11). However, the antigen described by Wang et al is cytoplasmic and secreted, is not present on membranes and does not occur in breast. The tunicamycin results rule out an N-asparagine linked carbohydrate residue as epitope but O-linked sugars have not been ruled out. Endoglycosidase modification and testing of antibody binding to a panel of defined carhohydrate residues are currently in progress.

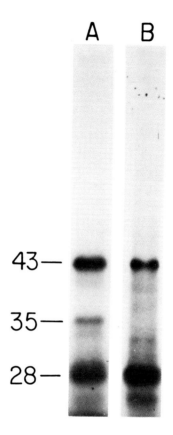

Fig. 1   F77-129-protein A sepharose immunoprecipitates of
lactoperoxidase iodinated PC3 (A) and G-361 (B) cells.

REFERENCES

1. Kohler, G and Milstein, C (1975). Continuous culture
   of fused cells secreting antibody of pre-defined
   specificity. Nature 25:495.
2. Hewitt, HB, Blake, ER and Waldern, AS (1976). A
   critique of the evidence for active host defense
   against cancer, based on personal studies of 27 murine
   tumors of spontaneous origin. Brit J Cancer 33:241.
3. Greene, MI (1980). The genetic and cellular basis of
   regulation of the immune response to tumor antigens
   Contemp Top Immunobiol 11:81.

4. Old, LJ (1981). Cancer Immunology: The search for specificity. G.H.A. Cloes Memorial lecture. Cancer Res 41:361.

5. Silverberg, E (1981). Cancer statistics. Cancer, N.Y. 31:13.

6. Counsell, RE, Klausmeier, WH, Weinhold, PA and Skinner, RW (1981). Radiolabeled androgens and their analogs. In Spencer (ed.): "Radiopharmaceuticals Structure-Activity Relationships", New York: Greene and Stratton pp 425-428.

7. Hechter, O (1984). Different physical, hormonal and chemical agents: present status and theoretical prospects for improved prostate cancer therapy. The Prostate 5: 159.

8. Carroll, AM, Zalutsky, M, Schatten, S, Bhan, A, Perry, LL, Sobotka, C, Benacerraf, B and Greene, MI (1984). Monoclonal antibodies to tissue-specific cell surface antigens. I. Characterization of an antibody to a prostate tissue antigen. Clin Immunol Immunopath 33:268.

9. Carroll, AM, Zalutsky, MR, Benacerraf, B, and Greene, MI (1984). Monoclonal antibodies to tissue-associated antigens as anti-tumor reagents. Surv Synth Path Res 3:189.

10. Zalutsky, M., Perry, LL, Schatter, S, Kaplan, W. Greene, MI and Benacerraf, B (1982). Imaging of human prostate tumors in nude mice using radio-iodinated antibodies. In Raynaud (ed): "Nuclear Medicine and Biology", vol 4, Paris: Pergamen Press, pp. 275-288.

11. Wang, MC, Valenzuela, LA, Murphy GP and Chu, TM (1979). Purification of a human prostate specific antigen. Invest Urol 17:159.

ACKNOWLEDGEMENT: We thank Ms. Ruth DeMattia for skillful secretarial assistance in typing of the manuscript.

Monoclonal Antibodies and Cancer Therapy, pages 367–379
© 1985 Alan R. Liss, Inc.

USE OF MONOCLONAL ANTI-IDIOTYPIC ANTIBODIES
AS SPECIFIC VACCINES AND AS PROBES
OF THE MAMMALIAN REOVIRUS TYPE 3 RECEPTOR[1]

Glen N. Gaulton, Man Sung Co, and Mark I. Greene

Department of Pathology Harvard Medical School
and Department of Medicine Tufts University
Medical School, Boston, MA 02111

ABSTRACT   Syngeneic monoclonal anti-idiotypic
antibodies which recognize the cellular receptor
of mammalian reovirus type 3 have been used to
isolate reovirus receptors by immunoprecipitation
from a panel of both normal and transformed cells.
Reovirus type 3 receptors appear identical on all
cells analyzed thus far, with a molecular weight
of 67,000 Da and a heterogenous pI of 5.8-6.0.
Structural homology of reovirus receptors to the
mammalian beta-adrenergic receptor was demonstrated by the indistinguishable immunoprecipitation and tryptic digest patterns of these
receptors. Anti-idiotypic antibodies were also
shown to precipitate beta-adrenergic ligands which
were bound to the cell surface. Lastly, syngeneic
monoclonal anti- idiotypic antibodies have been
utilized as vaccines for the induction of anti-
reovirus type 3 specific CTL and DTH T cell
responses and for the production of anti-reovirus
type 3 neutralizing antibodies.

[1] This work was supported by grant PO1-NS16998
-04 from the National Institutes of Health.

INTRODUCTION

Previous work from our laboratory has detailed the construction and characterization of anti-idiotypic antibodies which specifically recognize the cell surface receptor of reovirus type 3. These antibodies were produced following immunization with a monoclonal anti-reovirus type 3 antibody (9BG5) which binds to the viral hemagglutinin (HA) and displays potent neutralization capacity (1-5). Using genetic recombinant viruses Fields and colleagues (5,6) have shown that the viral outer capsid HA protein is the specific viral attachment molecule of reovirus. Both polyclonal and monoclonal anti-idiotypic (anti-id) antibodies to the reovirus type 3 receptor have now been purified. These antibodies display indistinguishable binding characteristics. The specificity of anti-id antibodies was confirmed by their capacity to: 1) Mirror the tropism of reovirus type 3 binding; 2) Inhibit the binding of type 3 virus to cellular targets; and 3) Mimic many of the physiological effects of virus which are related to cell attachment.

Reovirus anti-id antibodies serve as unique and highly specific probes of the reovirus type 3 receptor. Such reagents enable a more comprehensive biochemical approach to understanding the tropism of reovirus, its pathology, the use of anti-id antibodies as anti-viral vaccines, and finally the potential role(s) which anti-id antibodies may play in virally induced autoimmunity.

METHODS

Preparation of anti-id antibodies. The immunization, purification and characterization of polyclonal reovirus anti-id antibodies has been described by Nepom et al (1). Monoclonal anti-id antibodies were constructed by immunization with the reovirus neutralizaing antibody 9BG5 (5) followed by syngeneic fusion, as described by Noseworthy et al (3). The initial screening of

both polyclonal and monoclonal anti-ids was
accomplished by the ability of anti-id antibodies
to block the binding of the 9BG5 monoclonal to
purified reovirus type 3 HA using a solid phase
RIA (1,3). One monoclonal designated 87.92.6 was
selected as specific to the reovirus receptor
based on its ability to inhibit 9BG5 and virus
binding, and its similar pattern of cell and
tissue tropism as compared to reovirus type 3.

   Immunoprecipitation techniques. Cells to be
used were first surface radio-iodinated using the
enzyme lacto- peroxidase method ( ). Breifly, 2 x
10^7 cells were mixed with 1mCi Na ^{125}I (NEN,
Boston, MA) in 50ul of 0.2M phosphate buffer (pH
7.2) and 25ul of a 1% B-D-glucose solution. 50ul
of hydrated enzymobead reagent (Bio-Rad,
Richmond,CA) was then added and the reaction
incubated at room temperature for 30 minutes. The
cells were then washed extensively in ice cold PBS
and the membranes solubilized by the addition of
1% triton X-100, 0.5% NP-40 for 30 minutes on ice.
The debris were cleared by centrifugation at
35,000xg for 60 minutes and the solubilized
membrane proteins used immediately or frozen at
-20°C. Lysates of iodinated cells ($2-5\times10^5$ cpm)
were then incubated with 50ug of purified anti-id
antibody or control immunoglobulin at room
temperature for 45 minutes. 25ul of sepharose
protein A (Pharmacia, Piscataway, NJ) was then
added and the incubation continued for 30 more
minutes at room temperature with gentle agitation.
Pellets were harvested in a Beckman microfuge,
washed three times in detergent solubilization
buffer, twice in PBS and resuspended in SDS-gel
sample buffer. SDS-PAGE was conducted on
discontinuous 5/10% gels under reducing conditions
as described (8).

   Precipitation of membrane bound beta-ligands.
For the analysis of beta-adrenergic ligand binding
to reovirus receptors 1x10^7 R1.1 cells were
incubated with ^{125}I- iodohydroxybenzylpindolol
(IHYP, 20,000 cpm), with or without 25mM
isoproterenol (ISO), for 30 minutes at 37°C. Cells
were then washed in PBS and the membranes
solubilized in 0.5% digitonin. The debris were

cleared by centrifugation and reovirus receptors
immunoprecipitated by the addition of anti-id
antibodies and protein A sepharose as described
above. After washing the pellets were counted in a
Packard gamma counter.

Immunization protocols. Syngeneic Balb/C mice
were immunized with highly purified reovirus
antibodies by subcutaneous injections in the
dorsal flanks. In some instances anti-id
antibodies were coupled using glutaraldehyde to
the carrier protein keyhole limpet hemocyanin
(KLH) prior to immunization. Mice were injected on
day0 with anti-id in the presence of Freunds
complete adjuvant, on day14 with anti-id in
incomplete Freunds adjuvant, and boosted at weekly
intervals thereafter with anti-id in saline.

RESULTS

Isolation of the Reovirus Type 3 Receptor.

        Preliminary biochemical characterization of
the type 3 reovirus receptor was accomplished by
immunoprecipitation of receptors from reovirus
binding cells using anti-id antibodies. A panel of
reovirus binding cells, both from tissue culture
and fresh isolates, were surface radio-iodinated
with ^{125}I and then immunoprecipitated with anti-
id. Immunoprecipitations were extensively washed
and then run on SDS-PAGE under reduced conditions.
In each instance a single band of Mr = 67,000 was
detected in anti-id precipitates which was absent
in control precipitates. Figure 1 shows the
results of a representative experiment of
immunoprecipitations conducted on (A) murine B and
T cells and (B) the BW5147 (murine thymoma), B3C8
(murine T cell hybridoma) and CEM (human lymphoid)
cell lines. The additional bands seen in B cell
immunoprecipitates correspond to surface labeled
immunoglobulin which is co-precipitated along with
the reovirus receptor by sepharose protein A.
Immunoprecipitations have since been conducted on
monkey, rabbit and rat lymphoid and neuronal cells
all with similar results (7,9). Thus, the basic

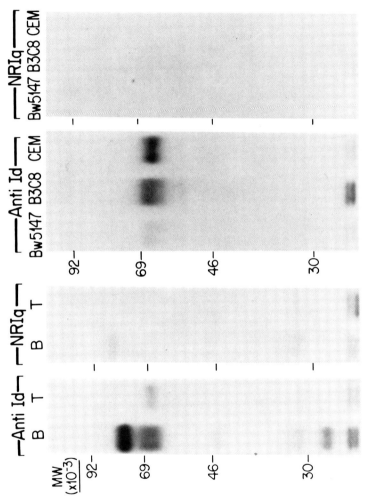

FIGURE 1. SDS-PAGE ANALYSIS OF ANTI-ID IMMUNOPRECIPITATES

structure of reovirus receptors appears to be highly conserved.

2-D gel analysis of isolated receptors has demonstrated that the reovirus receptor has a slight microheterogeneity of charge (PI 5.8-6.0) possibly corresponding to multiple glycosylation patterns (7). Receptors have also been shown to be sensitive to neuraminidase and tunicamycin (3,7) and to be monomeric (7).

Confirmation that the 67,000Da band seen in these gels represents the reovirus receptor was achieved by western blot analysis. Purified membranes of reovirus binding cells were run on gels then electroblotted onto nitrocellulose paper and incubated with radiolabeled anti-id, reovirus type 3 or control antibody. Incubations conducted with anti-id and type 3 virus contained a prominant band at 67,000Da which was absent in controls (7,9).

Homology of Reovirus and Beta-Adrenergic Receptors.

Recent reports in the literature have documented that a number of viruses utilize essential cell proteins as viral binding sites. For example, LDH virus binds to Ia proteins on the surface of macrophages (10), EBV binds to the C3d receptor CR2 on B cells (11) and HTLV-3 binds to the OKT4 protein on human T cells (12). Our initial search, based on surface proteins which have a common size and tissue distribution pattern, led us to examine the mammalian beta-adrenergic receptor as a likely candidate for reovirus attachment.

Our analysis of the homology of reovirus and beta-adrenergic receptors was initially conducted by comparing these receptors at the structural level. The reported molecular weight of both beta-1 and beta-2 mammalian adrenergic receptors is 53-67,000Da (13,14), similar to that of reovirus receptors. More detailed comparisons were conducted using purified beta-2 receptor obtained from Dr. Charles Homcy (Massachusetts General Hospital, Boston, MA). Purified beta-2 receptor was first immunoprecipitated using anti-id antibody. Purified beta-adrenergic receptor was specifically immunoprecipitated by anti-id but not by control antibody (15), thus demonstrating that reovirus and beta-adrenergic receptors share the idiotope recognized by anti-id; and more importantly since anti-id mimics the binding pattern of reovirus type 3, that both receptors bind reovirus type 3.

2-D gel analysis was next conducted on immuno-precipitated beta and reovirus receptors. The expected homology of molecular weight (67,000Da) was accompanied by an indistinguishable isoelectric pattern (PI 5.8-6.0), even to the extent of subtle microheterogeneity (15). Partial tryptic digests of these receptors were also identical; major degradation fragments of 57, 50 and 45Kd were seen (15).

More direct proof of the functional identity of reovirus receptors as beta-adrenergic binding proteins was achieved by examining whether anti-id antibodies would co-precipitate beta ligands bound to the cell surface. The radiolabeled beta-antagonist IHYP was first bound to intact cells, then after washing, cells were solubilized in detergent and immunoprecipitated with anti-id. The results of this experiment are shown in Table 1. Anti-id immunoprecipitates contained approximately 18-times the level of labeled beta-ligand compared to control immuno-precipitates. The specificity of this interaction was further verified by the competition of IHYP binding in the presence of the unlabeled beta-agonist isoproterenol (ISO). Taken together these results demonstrate that reovirus and beta-adrenergic receptors share considerable structural homology, and that both receptors contain binding sites for reovirus type 3, anti-id and beta ligands.

Jerne's network theory predicts that the presence of anti-id antibodies will elicit an anti-anti-id anitbody response (16). In the case of internal image anti-id antibodies, a subset of these anti-anti-id (internal image anti-anti-id) will resemble the primary antibody in the specificity of its epitope binding. Thus, syngeneic immunization with reovirus anti-id should induce anti-reovirus immunity.

Table 1

Precipitation of Membrane bound
^{125}I-Iodohydroxybenzylpindolol by Anti-Id

Precipitation Condition	CPM in Precipitate
IHYP + Anti-Id	$1,897 \pm 42$
IHYP + Normal Rabbit Ig	86 ± 12
IHYP + ISO + Anti-Id	105 ± 19

Induction of Specific Anti-Reovirus Immunity Using Anti-Id.

Despite the fact that antigen receptors on B and T cells are encoded by distinct genetic loci (17,18), common idiotopic domains have been repeatedly observed on B and T cell receptors (19,20). While it is not known if this shared idiotypy originates by conformational mimicry or domains shared by T and B receptor genes, stimulation of both B and T cell receptors by anti-receptor antibodies has been shown to induce cellular activation (21,22).

Our attempts to induce T cell mediated anti-reovirus immunity using syngeneic anti-id antibody have recently been pulished (23,24). Immunization with purified anti-id stimulated a potent and type specific delayed type hypersensivity (DTH) response as determined by footpad swelling assay. These responses showed a classical DTH time course and morphologic response; maximal responses were detected at 28-32 hours with extensive invasion of mononuclear cells. DTH responses were dose dependent on the amount of anti-id, with as little as 100ng being effective (23).

In contrast to these observations the induction of a type specific anti-viral cytolytic activity was only detected when anti-id was administered in a cell bound form. Immunization with 3×10^5 irradiated anti-id bearing 87.92.6 hybridoma cells stimulated a CTL response which was indistinguishable in magnitude and specificity from reovirus type 3 induced cytolytic activity (23).

To elicit anti-viral antibody responses syngeneic mice were immunized with either KLH coupled or self agglutinated anti-id. Immunization with nonlinked anti-id failed to induce immunity presumably reflecting requirements for antigen bridging of T helper with B cells in the antibody forming response. As seen in Table 2 anti-id immunization was effective in a dose dependent fashion analogous to that seen previously for the induction of T cell mediated DTH responses. Similar immunizations have also been conducted on a variety of genetically unrelated mouse strains and in rabbits. In each instance responses were indistinguishable from those seen in the syngeneic Balb/C system, thus confirming that the reovirus anti-id hybridoma 87.92.6 represents a true internal image of the viral HA neutralization domain.

Table 2

Dose Dependence of Anti-Id Immunization

Dose	50% Neutralization Titer	
	Type 3	Type 1
10^7 Reovirus Type 3	3200	100
25ug anti-id	200	10
50ug anti-id	200	10
100ug anti-id	800	10
150ug anti-id	1000	10
200ug anti-id	800	10
200ug control anti-id1	10	10

1 anti-sendai virus anti-id

DISCUSSION

The studies presented here, which utilize the reovirus type 3 anti-id system, demonstrate the wide range of experimental applications of anti-id antibodies. Anti-id antibody can be used to construct specific probes of receptors for ligands, to isolate and quantitate the numbers of receptor sites, to compare receptors of diverse function and to induce immunity to ligand. Reovirus anti-id antibodies have been productively utilized for each of these applications.

The most striking observation of these studies is the demonstration that beta-adrenergic receptors can serve as reovirus binding proteins on the cell surface. Our results thus far suggest that beta-adrenergic receptors comprise the primary cellular targets of reovirus, What remains unknown is 1) whether reovirus utilizes these receptors in unique ways to gain entry into cells and to initiate the replicative cycle and 2) whether reovirus binding acts in an agonist or antagonist fashion on beta-receptors.

These observations also have important implications to the possible mechanisms of virally induced autoimmunity. As exemplified by reovirus, anti-id antibodies which react with cellular components could be induced following viral exposure. Along these lines, potent autoimmune reactivity is associated with both type 1 and 3 reovirus infections. Notkins, Weiner and colleagues (25-27) have shown that reovirus infection triggers the generation of autoantibodies which react at multiple sites with endocrine glands, and which result in an often fatal polyendocrine disease. Whether anti-id antibodies are responsible for specific disease pathology is not known, however, model systems might be constructed based on the observation of anti-receptor mediated diseases such as myasthenia gravis and some forms of insulin-independent diabetis mellitus (28,29).

REFERENCES

1. Nepom JT, Weiner HL, Dichter MA, Tardieu M, Spriggs DR, Gramm C, Powers ML, Fields BN, Greene MI (1982). Identification of a hemagglutinin specific idiotype associated with reovirus recognition shared by lymphoia and neuronal cells. J. Exp. Med. 155:155.

2. Nepom JT, Tardieu M, Epstein RL, Noseworthy JH, Weiner HL, Gentsch J, Fields BN, Greene MI (1982). Virus binding receptors:Similarities to immune receptors as determined by anti-idiotypic antibodies. Surv. Immunol.Res.1:255.

3. Noseworthy JH, Fields BN, Dichter MA, Sobotka C, Pizer E, Perry LL, Nepom JT, Greene MI (1983). Cell receptors for the mammalian reovirus. 1. Syngeneic monoclonal anti-idiotypic antibody identifies a cell surface receptor for reovirus. J. Immunol. 133:2533.

4. Kauffman RS, Noseworthy JH, Nepom JT, Finberg R, Fields BN, Greene MI (1983). Cell receptors for the mammalian reovirus. 11. Monoclonal anti-idiotypic antibodies block viral binding to cells. J. Immunol. 133:2539.

5. Burstin SJ, Spriggs DR, Fields BN (1982). Evidence for functional domains on the reovirus type 3 hemagglutinin. Virol. 117:146.

6. Lee PWK, Hayes EL, Joklik WK (1981). Protein s1 is the reovirus cell attachment protein Virol. 108:156.

7. Co MS, Gaulton GN, Fields BN, Greene MI (1985). Isolation and biochemical characterization of the mammalian reovirus type 3 cell surface receptor. Proc. Natl. Acad. Sci. USA in press.

8. Samuel CE, Joklik WK (1974). A protein synthesis system for interferon-treated cells that discriminates between cellular and viral mRNAs. Virol.58:476.

9. Gaulton GN, Co MS, Greene MI (1985). Anti-idiotypic antibody identifies the cellular receptor of reovirus type 3. J. Cell. Biochem. in press.

10. Inada T, Mims C (1984). Mouse Ia antigens are receptors for lactate dehydrogenase virus.

Nature (London) 309:59.

11. Fingerorth JD, Weis JJ, Tedder TF, Strominger JL, Biro PA, Fearon DT (1984). Epstein-Barr virus receptors of human B cells is the C3d receptor CR2. Proc. Natl. Acad.Sci. USA 81:4510.

12. Dalgleish AG, Beverley PCL, Clapham PR, Crawford DH, Greaves MF, Weiss RA (1985). The CD4 (T4) antigen is an essential component of the receptor for the aids retrovirus. Nature (London) 312:763.

13. Cubero A, Malbon CC (1984). The fat cell B-adrenergic receptor.J. Biol. Chem. 259:1344.

14. Homcy CJ, Rockson SG, Countaway J, Egan D (1983). Purification and characterization of the mammalian B2-adrenergic receptor.Biochem. 22:660.

15. Co MS, Gaulton GN, Tominaga A, Homcy CJ, Fields BN, Greene MI (1985). Structural similarities between the mammalian beta-adrenergic and reovirus type 3 receptors. Proc. Natl. Acad. Sci. USA in press.

16. Jerne NK (1974). Towards a network theory of the immune system. Ann. deImmunol. 125C:373.

17. Yanagi Y, Yoshikai Y, Leggett K, Clark SP, Aleksander I, Mak TW (1984). A human T cell-specific cDNA clone encodes a protein having extensive homology to immunoglobulin chain. Nature (London) 308:148.

18. Hedrick SM, Nielsen EA, Kavaler J, Cohen DI, Davis MM (1984). Sequence relationship between putative T-cell receptor polypeptide and immunoglobulins. Nature (London) 308:153.

19. Krawinkel U, Cramer M, Berek C, Hammerling G, Black SJ, Rajewski K, Eichmann K (1976). On the structure of the T-cell receptor for antigen. Cold Spring Harbor Symposia on Quantitative Biology. 41:285.

20. Binz H, Frischknecht H, Shen FW, Wigzell H (1979). Idiotypic determinants on T-cell subpopulations. J. Exp. Med. 149:910.

21. Fothergill JJ, Wistar RJr, Woody JN, Parker DC (1982). A mitogen for human B cells: anti-Ig coupled to polyacrylamide beads activates blood mononuclear cells independently of T

cells. J. Immunol. 128:1945.

22. Imboden JB, Weiss A, Stobo JD (1985). The antigen receptor on a human T cell line initiates activation by increasing cytoplasmic free calcium. J. Immunol. 134:663.

23. Sharpe AH, Gaulton GN, Ertl HJC, Finberg R, McDade KK, Fields BN, Greene MI (1985). Cell receptors for the mammalian reovirus IV Reovirus specific cytolytic T cell lines which have idiotype receptors recognize anti-idiotype B cell hybridomas. J. Immunol. 134:1.

24. Sharpe AH, Gaulton GN, McDade KK, Fields BN, Greene MI (1984).Syngeneic monoclonal anti-idiotype can induce cellular immunity to reovirus. J. Exp. Med. 160:1195.

25. Onodera T, Jenson AB, Yoon JW, Notkins AL (1978). Virus-induced diabetes mellitus: reovirus infection of pancreatic B cells in mice. Sci. 201:529.

26. Haspel MV, Onodera T, Prabhakar BS, Horita M, Suzuki H, Notkins AL (1983). Virus-induced autoimmunity: monoclonal antibodies that react with endocrine tissues. Sci. 220:304

27. Tardieu M, Powers ML, Hafler DA, Hauser SL, Weiner HL (1984). Autoimmunity following virus infection: demonstration of monoclonal antibodies against normal tissue following infection of mice with reovirus and demonstration of shared antigenicity between virus and lymphocytes.Eur. J. Immunol. 14:561.

28. Dwyer DS, Bradley RJ, Urquhart CK, Kearney JF (1983). Naturally occuring antiidiotypic antibodies in myasthenia gravis patients. Nature (London) 301:64

29. Cohen IR, Elias D, Maron R, Shechter Y (1984). Immunization to insulin generates anti-idiotypes that behave as antibodies to the insulin hormone receptor and cause diabetes mellitus. In Kohler H, Urbain J, Cazenave P-A (eds): "Idiotypy in Biology and Medicine" New York: Academic Press Inc., p365.

VIII. MONOCLONAL ANTIBODIES TO LYMPHOKINES

Monoclonal Antibodies and Cancer Therapy, pages 383–395
© 1985 Alan R. Liss, Inc.

MONOCLONAL ANTIBODIES TO HUMAN IL-2 AND THE IL-2 RECEPTOR

Christopher S. Henney, Steven Gillis, Steven K. Dower and David L. Urdal

Immunex Corporation
51 University St., Seattle, WA 98101

INTRODUCTION

Lymphokines, a group of immunoregulatory glycoproteins produced by lymphocytes, have attracted enormous attention of late, largely because of the perceived usefulness of these hormones as clinical therapeutics. Additionally, monoclonal antibodies against lymphokines are seen by many as a route to development of a new class of diagnostic assays for the quantitative assessment of cell-mediated immunity.

To date, attempts to produce monoclonal antibodies to lymphokines have been troubled by the difficulties associated with purification of sufficient antigen. The incidence of lymphokine producing cells in normal lymphoid tissue is quite low and the proteins themselves are largely undetectable in serological fluids. Lack of adequate quantities of protein not only limits the amounts of immunogen available, but also precludes many conventional routes for screening antibodies produced following immunization. Thus, solid-phase immunoassays, such as enzyme-linked immunoadsorption, which require access to antigen in quite large amounts, are usually not feasible for anti-lymphokine antibody detection. Neutralization of the biological activity of lymphokines is thus the only path available for antibody screening and is a far from trivial technology.

To overcome the difficulties of antigen availability, we have developed two broad strategies (i) identification of lymphokine producing cell lines which can be use as a source of protein and also of genetic material and thus provide avenues to cloning and expressing lymhokine genes and (ii) identification of immunodominant amino acid stretches (which can be duplicated by solid-phase peptide synthesis) from partial protein sequence data and which can be used to develop anti-peptide antibodies which also recognize the intact lymphokine molecule.

In our quest to develop monoclonal antibodies to interleukin-2 (IL-2) and its membrane receptor, we have used adaptations on the first of these approaches (1, 2). With another lymphokine, CSF 2α (IL-3) we have used the second approach (see accompanying paper by Conlon et al. (3)).

This paper briefly reviews our strategies for the development of monoclonal antibodies to IL-2 and its homologous receptor and indicates some of the uses to which these reagents are currently being put.

MATERIALS AND METHODS

Anti-IL-2 Monoclonal Antibodies.

Spleen cells harvested from BALB/c mice previously immunized with partially purified rat IL-2 (4) were fused with the drug-marked myeloma SP-2. Several of the resultant hypoxanthine-aminopterin-thymidine-(HAT)-resistant hybrid cell clones secreted a soluble product that significantly inhibited (>50%) IL-2 dependent T cell proliferation when tested in conventional T cell growth factor microassays (5). Of the potential anti-IL-2 secreting hybridomas, a clone designated 4E12B2H5 was selected for further characterization, based on the capacity of this cell line's supernate to totally inhibit IL-2 dependent T cell proliferation. In fact, when tested at a dilution of 1:20 in the presence of the co-precipitating matrix Igsorb (The Enzyme Center, Boston, MA), 4E12B2H5 culture supernate completely abrogated tritiated thymidine ((^{3}H)TdR) incorporation of T cell lines as monitored after 24-h culture in the presence of IL-2 (1).

Peritoneal ascites containing large concentrations of anti-IL-2 antibody were produced by intraperitoneal challenge of BALB/c female mice (6-8 wk of age) with 2 X 10^6 4E12B1H5 hybridoma cells. Mice were challenged with cells 1 week after intraperitoneal injection with 0.5 ml of pristane. Ten to fourteen days after the administration of 4E12B2H5 hybridoma cells, intraperitoneal ascites were harvested, clarified by centrifugation, and frozen (-20°C) until used for purification of anti-IL-2 IgG.

IgG purification was achieved by successive binding/elution from protein A-coupled Sepharose (Pharmacia). A small volume (2-5 ml) of hybridoma ascites was passed over a 10-ml protein A-Sepharose column equilibrated in 0.9% NaCl. Anti-IL-2 IgG was removed from the column by elution with 200 mM glycine HCl buffer, pH3. Purified antibody was then dialyzed overnight against NaCl-Hepes, pH 7.2, and frozen (-20°C) until use. The capacity of the antibody to inhibit IL-2 dependent T cell line proliferation was assayed in 200 µl cultures containing 4×10^4 IL-2-dependent T cell line cells (CTLL-2) (5), 3 U/ml IL-2, and various concentrations of anti-IL-2 IgG. Replicate cultures also contained Igsorb at a final dilution of 1:200. Inhibition of proliferation was assessed by a 4-h pulse of (^{3}H)TdR (20 Ci/mM, New England Nuclear).

The effect of anti-IL-2 on T cell mitogen-induced proliferation was tested in replicate 200 µl cultures (RPMI 1640, 2% fetal calf serum (FCS), 50 U/ml penicillin, 50 µg/ml streptomycin, and 300 µg/ml fresh L-glutamine) of C57BL/6 splenocytes (10^6 cells/ml) containing 2 µg/ml Con A and various concentrations of anti-IL-2 IgG in the presence and absence of Igsorb (final dilution of 1:400). As a further control, separate Con A stimulation cultures were initiated that contained an identical concentration of a monoclonal anti-gp70 antibody of the same isotype as the anti-IL-2 antibody.

Antibodies to the Human IL-2 Receptor.

Female BALB/c mice 8 to 12 weeks of age were injected with 10^7 PHA activated human peripheral blood leukocytes (PHA/PBL) in 0.4 ml of complete Freunds adjuvant intradermally in the hind legs. A series of four weekly injections of 10^7 PHA/PBL was subsequently given. Sera were collected and tested individually for binding to PHA/PBL cells by an enzyme linked immunoabsorbant assay (ELISA). The animal found to have the highest response received an additional 10^7 PHA/PBL in phosphate buffered saline, intraveneously. Four days later, the spleen of this animal was removed and used for fusion, as described elsewhere (1, 6). Subsequently, hybrid cells were selected in Click's medium containing 15% fetal calf serum, and HAT. Finally the cells were transferred to 96 well microtiter plates for growth and testing.

After 10 days in culture > 80% of the microcultures exhibited hybrid cell growth. A 100 µl aliquot of supernate was removed from each viable culture and tested in an ELISA assay for binding to PHA/PBL (IL-2 receptor positive) or PBL (IL-2 receptor negative). Of the approximately 320 supernatants screened, 35 demonstrated significant binding to PHA/PBL and little or no binding to PBL (2). These hybrids were then transferred to 1 ml cultures and gradually weaned to HAT-free medium. Of these hybrids, only one, designated 2A3, was able significantly to inhibit both mitogen and antigen induced proliferation of human PBL (IL-2 dependent functions). This hybrid was subcloned by limiting dilution cultures. Hybrid cells were reseeded (0.2-0.3 cells/well) in 200 μl cultures Clicks medium, containing 12% FCS and freshly prepared BALB/c thymocytes (3 X 10^5 cells/well), as feeder cells.

2A3 (γ_1, κ) monoclonal antibody was then purified from ascites fluid as described above (see also 2, 7).

RESULTS

Monoclonal Antibody to IL-2.

Figure 1 demonstrates the ability of 4E12B2H5 hybridoma supernate, or purified IgG derived from ascites, to inhibit the IL-2-driven (^{3}H)TdR incorporation of CTLL-2 cells. In the absence of anti-IL-2, or in the presence of parent myeloma SP-2 cell-conditioned medium, CTLL-2 cells cultured in the presence of IL-2 incorporated maximal amounts of (^{3}H)TdR during a 4-h pulse added 20 h after culture initiation. However, in the presence of a 1:20 dilution of crude 4E12B2H5 hybridoma culture supernate, IL-2-induced (^{3}H)TdR incorporation was markedly inhibited. Similar levels of inhibition were observed in CTLL-2 cell cultures containing IL-2 and 4E12B2H5 hybridoma-derived IgG (purified by protein-A Sepharose affinity chromatography). Greater than 90% inhibition of proliferation was observed in cultures containing either 10 or 1μg/ml of 4E12B2H5 IgG, whereas 10μg/ml of an irrelevant antibody of the same isotype (anti-gp70 IgG) in identical cultures had no effect on IL-2-driven CTLL-2 cell replication.

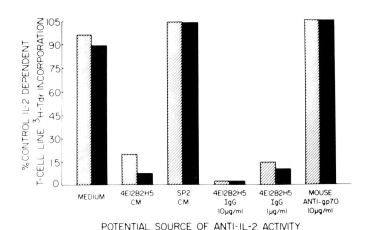

POTENTIAL SOURCE OF ANTI-IL-2 ACTIVITY

Fig. 1. (^{3}H)TdR incorporaton mediated by 4,000 CTLL-2 cells during hours 20-24 of culture in 200 µl volumes, containing 3 U/ml IL-2. Various hybridoma or control supernates and purified IgG were tested for the ability to inhibit IL-2 dependent T cell proliferation in the presence (■) or absence (▨) of Igsorb (1:200 final dilution). Control-conditioned media (CM) and hybridoma supernates were tested at a final dilution of 1:20 by volume. Purified IgG was assayed at the concentrations indicated.

Inhibition of T Cell Mitogenesis by Anti-IL-2.

Given (a) the capacity of monoclonal 4E12B2H5 antibody to inhibit IL-2-dependent T cell proliferation in both neutralizing and precipitating (in concert with Igsorb) cultures and (b) the hypothesis that IL-2 is the initiator of normal mitogen-induced T cell proliferation (8, 9), we were curious to determine what effect anti-IL-2 IgG would have on Con A-induced T cell mitogenesis. As shown in Table 1, inclusion of anti-IL-2 in cultures of Con A-stimulated normal murine spleen cells, severely inhibited resultant T cell proliferation, as assessed by (^{3}H)TdR incorporation during hours 72-76 of culture. Significant inhibition was observed with <1 μg/ml of 4E12B2H5 IgG. However, Con A stimulation conducted either in the absence of anti-IL-2 or in the presence of 20 μg/ml of anti-gp70 IgG resulted in splenocyte stimulation indices >25 times the background (^{3}H)TdR incorporation observed.

As was repeatedly seen in assays testing the effect of anti-IL-2 on T cell line proliferation, the ability of anti-IL-2 IgG to inhibit mitogenesis was dose-dependent and enhanced in Igsorb-containing cultures in which presumably IL-2 was removed from solution.

In further studies, anti-IL-2 antibody was used to inhibit the alloantigen-induced generation of cytotoxic T lymphocytes (CTL), another IL-2 dependent phenomenon. It was found that not only did anti-IL-2 serve to depress the lytic activity developing in mixed lymphocyte cultures (1), but also significantly curtailed proliferation and recovery of responsive T cells. Thus, the number of viable cells harvested from 5 day mixed lymphocyte cultures in the presence of 5μg anti-IL-2 was approximately one-third that seen in the absence of such antibody.

These results, using an IgG monoclonal antibody to IL-2, provide convincing serological evidence for the integral role that IL-2 plays in controlling antigen/mitogen induced T cell proliferation. These studies further suggest that such antibodies will prove immunosuppressive in vivo, a hypothesis currently being tested.

Monoclonal Antibodies to the IL-2 Receptor.

The likelihood that the 2A3 antibody, described in the materials above, was directed against the IL-2 receptor was strongly suggested by the studies reported in Figure 2. The right hand side of this figure demonstrates that purified 2A3 antibody is capable of inhibiting the absorption of IL-2 by PHA activated human lymphocytes at 0°C. In control experiments we found that 4F2, a monoclonal antibody directed against an activation antigen (10) not part of the IL-2 receptor, did not block absorption. In later studies, not shown here, 2A3 was also found to inhibit the binding of radiolabelled recombinant IL-2 to PHA-activated T cell and to a T cell leukemia.

Furthermore, Figure 2 shows the binding of ^{125}I labelled 2A3 IgG to resting and PHA activated human peripheral blood leukocytes. The data show that while resting T cells express less than 10^3 2A3 binding sites/cell on average, mitogen activation produced a population with about 20,000 2A3 binding sites/cell. While the activated population used in this experiment was 72 hrs in culture, we have found that IL-2 receptor (2A3 binding) sites appear on mitogen activated lymphocytes within 12 hours of exposure to lectin.

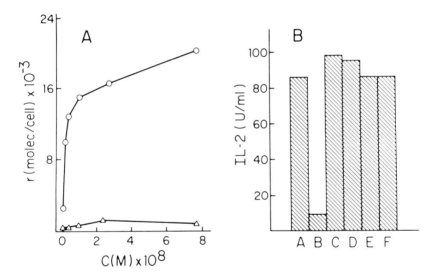

Fig. 2. Specificity of 2A3 Antibody. (A) Binding of [125]I-2A3 IgG to resting (△) and PHA activated (○) human PBL. ^{125}I-Antibody and cells were incubated together in binding medium for 1.5 hr on ice. Data are corrected for nonspecific binding of labelled antibody, which was measured in the presence of 5.7×10^{-6}M 2A3 IgG. Cell concentrations were: resting cells 3×10^7 cells/ml; activated cells 1.2×10^7 cells/ml. Resting and activated cells were 96% and 87% viable respectively, by trypan blue exclusion, at the end of the experiment.
(B) Inhibition of IL-2 absorption by 2A3 antibody. All incubations were performed on ice for two hours. A,

conditioned medium alone; B, conditioned medium with 1.9 x 10^7 PHA/PBL added; C medium, cells, and 210 µg/ml 2A3 IgG; D, medium, cells, and 64 µg/ml 2A3 IgG; E, medium, cells, and 19 µg/ml 2A3 IgG; F, medium, cells, and 9 µg/ml 2A3 IgG. All incubations were performed in a total volume of 300 µl, containing 100 µl of conditioned medium.

In further studies, we examined the ability of the antibody to bind to a variety of cells, including mouse CTLL-2, the indicator line we have used for human IL-2 biological activity (5), MLA-144, a gibbon ape T-lymphoma, concanavalin-A activated bovine T cells and human B-cells. 2A3 did not bind to any of these cell types. This indicates, that for the cells tested so far, the target antigen for 2A3 is present only on activated human T-cells, suggesting that the epitope recognized by the antibody is both cell type and species specific.

Further studies confirmed the specificity of 2A3, in showing that 2A3 and B1-49-9, a recently described antibody specific for the human IL-2 receptor, completely cross-complete for binding to activated human T-cells. Each antibody, when unlabelled, inhibited the binding of homologous ^{125}I-antibody and ^{125}I-cross reactive antibody with the same inhibition constant. Such findings suggest that 2A3 and B1-49-9 bind to the same epitope on human T cells. Furthermore, the antigen precipitated from detergent lysed T cell membranes by 2A3 was found to have a molecular weight between 55,000 and 60,000 and to be precleared from ^{125}I-labelled activated T cell lysates by B1-49-9. The reverse was also true. These data indicate that the two monoclonal antibodies recognize the same antigen, and that the antigen has the same molecular weight as that previously reported for the IL-2 receptor using other serological probes.

2A3 has an extremely high affinity constant, in excess of $10^{10} M^{-1}$. Furthermore, it can be radioiodinated to high specific activity with retention of its capacity to bind to the IL-2 receptor. These properties have allowed the construction of convenient and sensitive 2A3 based assays for the presence of receptor in its soluble form. One, the nitrocellulose dot assay, is illustrated in Figure 3b. Receptor containing fractions bound to nitrocellulose can be readily detected by radiolabelled 2A3 antibody; the limit of sensitivity being of the order of 0.03 µg of receptor protein.

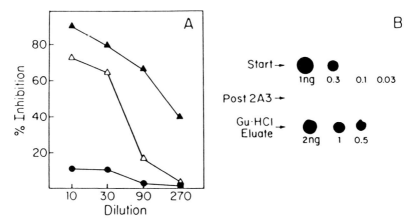

Fig. 3. Assays for soluble IL-2 receptor. (A) 50 μl of 0.25nM ^{125}I-2A3 IgG was mixed with 50 μl of dilutions of detergent lysates of HuT-102 cells prior to passage of the lysate through a 2A3 affinity column (▲), after passage (●), and after elution of bound receptor with 6M Gdn-HCl (△). Uncomplexed ^{125}I-2A3 was detected by the addition of 2 × 10^6 glutaraldehyde-fixed PHA-PBL, and specific inhibition of binding of the antibody to the cells was calculated. (B) Nitrocellulose dot assay. Five microliters of dilutions of detergent lysates of PHA-PBL was applied to dry nitrocellulose prior to the passage of the lysate through a 2A3 affinity column (Start), after passage (Post 2A3), and after elution of bound receptor with 6 M Gdn-HCl (Gdn-HCl eluate). The numbers below the dots refer to the amount of receptor that was detected in the original solution by the soluble receptor assay outlined in A.

We have recently used the 2A3 monoclonal antibody as an affinity reagent to purify sufficient IL-2 receptor for protein sequencing studies (7). As alluded to above,

2A3 was able to precipitate a 60,000 mw glycoprotein from the surface of metabolically (^{35}S methionine) labelled PHA activated human T cells. The purification of IL-2 receptor protein using 2A3 immunoaffinity adsorbtion, coupled with the 2A3 based assay for the detection of soluble receptor, has allowed a straightforward strategy for the cloning and expression of the IL-2 receptor gene, which has recently been successfully completed (7, 11). Purified IL-2 receptor was partially sequenced from the NH$_2$-terminus (7), unambiguous oligonucleotide probes were prepared from this sequence information and used directly to probe a complementary DNA library prepared from HuT-102 cell messenger RNA (11).

DISCUSSION

The results presented in this communication have detailed the capacity of a monoclonal IgG antibody directed against a determinant present on IL-2 to severely inhibit several proliferation-dependent in vitro T cell immune responses. In addition to curtailing IL-2 dependent T cell line proliferation, the addition of the antibody reagent to spleen cell cultures markedly inhibited both Con A-induced T cell mitogenesis and alloantigen-induced generation of cytotoxic T cells. The ability of anti-IL-2 monoclonal antibody to inhibit these responses provides strong serological evidence that the production and use of IL-2 is essential for mitogen and antigen induced T cell proliferation.

Taken together with previous studies, which showed that ligand-activated T cells could both absorb IL-2 and proliferate in response to in vitro stimulation with purified IL-2 (8, 9), the ability of antibody against IL-2 to inhibit both T cell mitogenesis and the in vitro generation of alloreactive cytotoxic T cells argues forcibly in favor of the pivotal role that IL-2 plays in controlling T cell proliferation.

In order to study interactions between IL-2 and its homologous receptor it became necessary to isolate and characterize the receptor in soluble form. Pivotal to this aim was the development of a monoclonal antibody to the receptor.

Three monoclonal antibodies have been described that are specific for the human IL-2 receptor (2, 7, 12, 13, 14, 15). The first, anti-Tac, resulted from the immunization of mice with longterm cultures of human T cells (12, 13). Among normal cells, anti-Tac was shown to react only with activated T cells and more recently to bind to the same molecule that binds to Interleukin 2 (15). The second, B1-49-9, also resulted from the immunization of mice with long term cultures of activated T cells (14). This antibody competitively inhibits the binding of anti-Tac to cells (unpublished work), and immunoprecipitates the same molecule from detergent lysates of radiolabelled cells (14); thus it can be argued that B1-49-9 recognizes the same antigenic epitope on the receptor molecule that is detected with anti-Tac. The third monoclonal antibody, 2A3, is the subject of this report. This monoclonal antibody was generated by sensitization of mice with activated peripheral blood T cells and presumably reacted with the same epitope that is recognized by B1-49-9 and thus, by inference, with anti-Tac. The very high affinity constant of 2A3 (see ref 2), far higher than that reported for other antibodies of this specificity, is of considerable practical importance. 2A3 provided an essential role in the recent successful cloning and expression of the IL-2 receptor gene, being used both in the purification of receptor from activated T cells and in the detection of gene products (7, 11).

The development of monoclonal antibodies to IL-2 and its receptor have been central to our current appreciation of the structure of these molecules and their interaction. The techniques developed and adapted for the production of these antibodies should prove of general usefulness in the detection, isolation and ultimately the characterization of other members of the lymphokine group of glycoproteins.

REFERENCES

1.   Gillis, S, Gillis, A, Henney CS (1981). Monoclonal Antibody Directed Against Interleukin 2. I. Inhibition of T Lymphocyte Mitogenesis and the In Vitro Differentiation of Alloreactive Cytolytic T Cells. J. Exp. Med. 154:983.
2.   Dower, SK, Hefeneider, SH, Alpert, AR, Urdal, DL (in press, 1985). Quantitative Measurement of Human IL-2 Receptor Levels with Intact and Detergent Solubilized Human T-cells. Mol. Immunol.
3.   Conlon, PJ, Luk, H, Park, L, Hopp, T, Urdal, D (in press, 1985). Characterization of a Monoclonal Antibody to CSF-2α (IL-3). In Monoclonal

Antibodies in Cancer Therapy. UCLA Symposia and Molelular and Cellular Biology New Series, vol. 27. Reisfeld, RA, Sell, S (eds): Alan R. Liss. (Accompanying manuscript).

4.   Watson, JD, Gillis, S, Marbrook, J, Mochizuki, D, Smith, KA (1979). Biochemical and biological characterization of lymphocyte regulatory molecules. I. Purification of a class of murine lymphokines. J. Exp. Med. 150:849.

5.   Gillis, S, Ferm, MM, Ou, W, Smith, KA (1978). T cell growth factor: parameters of production and a quantitative microassay for activity. J. Immunol. 120:2027.

6.   Gillis, S, Henney, CS (1981). The biochemical and biological characterization of lymphocyte regulatory molecules: VI generation of a B-cell hybridoma whose antibody product inhibits Interleukin 2 activity. J. Immunol. 126:1978.

7.   Urdal, DL, March, CJ, Gillis, S, Larsen, A, Dower SK (1984). Purification and chemical characterization of the receptor for interleukin 2 from activated human T lymphocytes and from a human T-cell lymphoma cell line. Proc. Natl. Acad. Sci. USA. 81:6481.

8.   Smith, KA, Gillis, S, Baker, PE, McKenzie, D, Ruscetti, FW (1979). T-cell growth factor-mediated T-cell proliferation. Proc. N.Y. Acad. Sci. 332:423.

9.   Ruscetti, FW, Gallo, RC (1981). Human T lymphocyte growth factor: regulation of growth and function of T lymphocytes. Blood 57:379.

10.   Cotner, T, Williams, JM, Christenson, L, Shapiro, HM, Strom, TB, Strominger, J (1983). Simultaneous flow cytometric analysis of human T cell activation antigen expression and DNA content. J. Exp. Med. 157:461.

11.   Cosman, D, Cerretti, DP, Larsen, A, Park, L, March C, Dower, S, Gillis, S, Urdal, D (1984). Cloning, sequence and expression of human interleukin-2 receptor. Nature 312:768.

12.   Leonard, WJ, Deppler, JM, Robb, RJ, Waldmann, TA, Greene, WC (1983). Characterization of the human receptor for T-cell growth factor. Proc. Natl. Acad. Sci. U.S.A. 80:6957.

13.   Robb, RJ, Greene, WC (1983). Direct demonstration of the identity of T cell growth factor binding protein and the tac antigen. J. Exp. Med. 158:1332.

14.   Hemler, ME, Malissen, B, Rebai, N, Liabeuf, A, Mawas, C, Kourilsky, FM, Strominger, JL (1983). A

55,000 Mr surface antigen on activated human T
lymphocytes defined by a monoclonal antibody.
Hum. Immun. 8:153 (1983).

15.   Wano, Y, Uchiyama, T, Fukui, K, Maeda, M,
Haruto, U, Yodoi, J (1984). Characterization of
human interleukin 2 receptor (Tac antigen) in normal
and leukemic T cells: co-expression of normal and
aberrant receptors on HuT-102 cells. J. Immunol.
132:3005.

Monoclonal Antibodies and Cancer Therapy, pages 397–411
© 1985 Alan R. Liss, Inc.

APPLICATIONS OF MONOCLONAL ANTIBODIES TO INVESTIGATIONS
OF GROWTH FACTORS, THEIR RECEPTORS AND TUMOR ANTIGENS,
AND AN ADJUVANT FORMULATION POTENTIALLY USEFUL FOR
IMMUNIZATION AGAINST MALIGNANT DISEASES

Anthony C. Allison and Alain B. Schreiber

Institute of Biological Sciences, Syntex Research
Palo Alto, CA 94304

ABSTRACT Methods for generating antibodies against
receptors for growth factors are discussed. These
antibodies have been useful for characterizing
receptors and analysing the mechanisms by which they
exert their biological effects. Cross linking and
internalization of the EGF receptor is required for
mitogenesis. Studies with monoclonal antibodies have
defined two families of protein angiogenic factors,
one basic and the other acidic. These may have
synergistic effects with other angiogenic factors,
including TGFα, prostaglandins and heparin, to
promote the neovascularization required for growth of
solid tumors. A monoclonal antibody has been used to
define a 120 kilodalton membrane protein antigen
associated with squamous carcinoma cells. This is
being developed for the detection of cancer of the
cervix by immunocytology. Tumor-associated antigens
identified by monoclonal antibodies and other methods
might be used for specific immunization. A non-toxic
adjuvant formulation which elicits cell-mediated and
humoral immune responses against a variety of
antigens has been developed. This has been used with
killed virus antigens to protect cats against feline
leukemia. It may be useful for prophylaxis against
or therapy of other neoplasias.

INTRODUCTION

The central theme of this meeting is tumor antigens. Although the main emphasis is on the potential uses of monoclonal antibodies for cancer therapy, other aspects of tumor immunity are being considered, including the definition of tumor antigens (for which purpose monoclonal antibodies are useful) and their possible application to immunization against malignant diseases. The affiliations of persons attending this meeting show that they have a wide range of interests, and presumably the interests of readers of the published proceedings will be even wider. Hence we are making a broad presentation covering different aspects of the work of our institute relevant to the general themes being discussed at the meeting, rather than a presentation focused on one particular topic. Because of time and space limitations the coverage of each subject cannot be deep, but the references cited should provide documentation sufficient for most purposes. Readers requiring access to more detailed information can refer to us.

MONOCLONAL ANTIBODIES TO RECEPTORS FOR GROWTH FACTORS

One of the main interests of our institute is the definition of factors affecting cell growth and differentiation, how these events are mediated within different cell types by activating several protein kinases and other mechanisms, and how they can be controlled by small molecules and analogs of naturally occurring mediators. Examples of enhanced growth factor effects that would be useful in practice are increasing the growth and milk yield of farm animals and facilitation of wound healing. Opposing the effects of growth factors might limit the growth of malignant cells or the vascularization of solid tumors and of the retina in diabetes mellitus.

Apart from possible practical applications, this subject is of fundamental importance in molecular and cell biology. The excitement generated during the past three years by the demonstration of homology between oncogene products and growth factors and their receptors underlines the point. Monoclonal antibodies and gene cloning have played a major part in defining the structure and activities of growth factors and their receptors.

Purified hormone receptor has been available in sufficient amounts as starting immunogen only in the case of the nicotinic acetylcholine receptor isolated from the electric eel (1). For most hormone or growth factor receptors one of the following experimental strategies was chosen for the definition of the immunogen:

1) selection of cells or cell membranes bearing a large number of molecules of a particular receptor. This approach to generate antibodies has the advantage that the receptor need not be purified. However the selection of monoclonal antibodies requires a panel of screening assays and immunoprecipitation of the receptor to ensure specificity of the antibody. Another drawback of this approach is that the antibodies only recognize surface-expressed epitopes of the receptor and are often directed to carbohydrate determinants.

2) The receptor may be partially purified by cell solubilization and combinations of gel filtration, affinity chromatography and electrophoretic separation techniques. Small amounts of protein, often denatured by solubilization procedures involving detergents, are used to generate antibodies. These antibodies may prove to become good tools for alternative receptor purification and metabolic studies. Because they recognize denatured receptor they are likely to be of less value in functional studies.

3) Antibodies to ligands may be used as immunogens for the induction of anti-idiotypic antibodies. Some of these anti-idiotypic antibodies interact with the anti-receptor ligand antibodies in a fashion similar to the ligand, thus behaving as an "internal image" of the ligand (see for review 2). Such anti-idiotypic antibodies will by virtue of this molecular mimicry bind to the receptor through the ligand-binding domain. This strategy, which has been demonstrated for the insulin (3), β-adrenergic (4), acetylcholine (5), TSH (6) and chemotactic peptide (7) receptor systems, circumvents the requirement for purified

receptor. However, the low frequency of relevant
anti-idiotypic antibodies has limited its
usefulness.

Monoclonal antibodies have been generated to
different epitopes and domains of the EGF receptor and
provide a good illustration of the various approaches
described above. EGF is a polypeptide of 53 residues that
binds to a 1200 residue transmembrane glycoprotein
receptor, as a result of which the cytoplasmic domain of
the receptor becomes phosphorylated, shows increased
tyrosine kinase activity and eventually stimulates cell
growth. At the time when studies were initiated, purified
EGF receptor was not available in amounts sufficient for a
full immunization schedule. Schreiber et al. (8, 9)
therefore used as immunogen intact A-431 cells, which bear
an unusually high number of EGF receptors. Igs secreted
by the hybridomas were screened for specific binding to
A-431 cells and to several cell lines bearing EGF
receptors and for lack of reactivity with cell types
devoid of EGF receptors. Further selection was made
according to either competition of binding with
radiolabeled EGF, immunoprecipitation of complexes of EGF
cross-linked to receptor or immunoprecipitation of a
functional receptor-tyrosyl protein kinase.

One IgM antibody competed for growth factor binding
and behaved as a full agonist for all early and delayed
EGF-mediated biologic effects on cultured cells (8).
Other monoclonal antibodies (9) did not possess intrinsic
bioactivity but were used in the isolation and
microsequencing of the EGF receptor (10). On the basis of
sequence and homology data, antibodies were generated to
synthetic peptides corresponding to predicted
intracellular portions of the EGF receptor (11). Such
antibodies did not bind to intact cells but interfered
with the protein kinase activity of isolated
EGF-receptor. Studies with these intact antibodies, their
monovalent Fab fragments and cross-linking with a second
layer of antibodies, have led to important conclusions
concerning transmembrane signaling via the EGF receptor.
Indeed it is now evident that:

1)   the EGF-receptor, when properly triggered,
     contains all the biochemical attributes necessary
     for the initiation of biological effects. The
     growth factor molecule is not _per se_
     indispensable; rather it represents one of many

"allosteric regulators" of the receptor,
appropriate antibody representing another.
2) Receptor cross-linking and subsequent
internalization are apparently necessary and
sufficient for productive signal transduction.

TUMOR GROWTH FACTORS

Two other growth factors show sequence homology with
EGF. One is transforming growth factor type I (TGFα),
which is secreted in small amounts by several different
kinds of tumor cells and has the capacity to stimulate the
growth of the same tumor cells (12). It has been
suggested that this type of autocrine secretion increases
the growth rate of tumors (13). In collaborative studies
we have found that TGFα produced by recombinant DNA
technology introduced into the hamster cheek pouch
efficiently induces neovascularization, so it must be
considered as a potential tumor angiogenic factor (14).
Recently it has been found that vaccinia virus
encodes a polypeptide homologus to EGF and TGFα (15,
16). The viral gene has presumably evolved from a gene
picked up from a host cell. If the virally encoded
product is on the surface of the virus, it could allow
attachment to the membrane of target cells through the EGF
receptor. Production of EGF-like growth factors could
explain the proliferative responses of host cells to
infection by poxviruses such as fibroma virus of rabbits,
Yaba virus of monkeys (both classified as tumor-inducing
viruses) and molluscum contagiosum virus of humans.

GROWTH FACTORS FOR ENDOTHELIAL CELLS

One of the requirements for growth of solid tumors is
neovascularization, and attempts have been made to define
a "tumor-angiogenesis factor" (17). Because tumor
products are not proteins peculiar to tumors but are
products of normal cell types inappropriately expressed,
our approach has been to analyse the effects of known
mitogens for endothelial cells and to prepare panels of
monoclonal antibodies which allow rapid definition of the
relatedness of angiogenic factors, including those derived
from tumors.

Several growth factors for endothelial cells have been isolated from bovine neural tissue. Cationic polypeptides include Fibroblast Growth Factor (FGF) and Brain-Derived Growth Factor type I (BDGF I). Acidic polypeptides include Endothelial-Cell Growth Factor (ECGF), acidic FGF, Eye-Derived Growth Factor (EDGF) and BDGF type II. All these growth factors have been shown to interact with heparin, which promotes angiogenesis in vivo. We have recently generated a large number of monoclonal antibodies to purified pituitary FGF and purified brain ECGF. Some of the antibodies inhibited binding of the ligands to their respective cellular receptors. These antibodies also neutralized the bioactivity of the growth factors, showing their mediation through the receptor-binding step. Several of the anti-pituitary FGF antibodies cross-reacted with purified cationic mitogens isolated from placenta, corpus luteum (corpus luteum angiogenic factor?), adrenal cortex, liver, macrophages (macrophage-derived growth factor?), and brain FGF (18). This immunological cross-reactivity indicates that cationic FGF is not a specific neuropeptide, but rather belongs to a family of molecules stored and/or synthesized in a variety of organs (which, interestingly, are all well vascularized). The anti-ECGF monoclonal antibodies neutralized up to 80% of the mitogenic activity of crude bovine brain extract for human endothelial cells, indicating that ECGF is the principal neurally derived endothelial mitogen (19). Recognition of epitopes on ECGF by the antibodies was altered in the presence of heparin, showing that interaction of heparin with ECGF produces a change in the tertiary structure of the protein (20). Several anti-ECGF antibodies cross-reacted with both acidic FGF and EDGF, but not cationic FGF (21) and also bound to endothelial mitogens derived from liver, melanoma and retinoblastoma cells. Hence there appear to be two major families of protein endothelial cell mitogens based on immunological criteria. These various findings, now being extended by amino-acid sequencing and DNA cloning, illustrate the value of monoclonal antibodies for the analysis of growth factors.

Already TGFα has been found to be angiogenic and some angiogenic factors derived from tumors have been shown to belong to the family of acidic protein angiogenic factors. It seems likely that other tumor cells will produce proteins belonging to the family of cationic angiogenic factors. In addition tumor cells produce prostaglandins such as PGE_2, which is angiogenic (22). They may also produce heparin or related molecules, which act synergistically with protein mitogens. Thus there is no such entity as a "tumor angiogenesis factor"; instead, several angiogenic factors secreted by tumor cells (and even by cells invading tumors such as macrophages) can act synergistically in different combinations to produce the neovascularization required for growth of solid tumors. Hence attempts at therapy by counteracting the effects of any one angiogenic factor are not likely to be generally successful.

A MONOCLONAL ANTIBODY DEFINING A SURFACE ANTIGEN OF BASAL EPIDERMAL CELLS AND SQUAMOUS CARCINOMA CELLS

This investigation has been carried out jointly with Dr. Vera Morhenn of Stanford University (23). Several monoclonal antibodies were raised by immunizing mice with skin cells recovered from psoriatic plaques and fusing their splenocytes with SP2/08A2 cells. Many antibodies were found to bind to all human epidermal cells, but one IgG_1 monoclonal antibody, designated VM-2, recognized an antigen expressed in skin only on cells in the basal and suprabasal layer of the epidermis and the external root sheath of hair follicles. Further studies showed that VM-2 also binds to squamous carcinoma cells from the skin, lung, esophagus and cervix. The binding was demonstrable by immunoperoxidase or gold-silver staining of sections of tissues containing these tumors and by solid-phase enzyme-linked immunoassays in cultured tumor cells. VM-2 binds to an antigen expressed to different degrees on human squamous carcinoma cells from skin (SCL-1), cervix (HeLa), vulva (A-431) and lung (A-459). VM-2 does not show detectable binding to normal fibroblasts, endothelial cells or hemopoietic cells.

The antigen to which VM-2 binds is on the cell surface, as shown by reactions using living cells and surface labeling with lactoperoxidase- catalysed iodination. The antigen is stable to fixation with acetone, ethanol, paraformaldehyde and glutaraldehyde. Antigen labeled biosynthetically with $[^{35}S]$-methionine in culture or by surface iodination, solubilized with detergent and immunoprecipitated with VM-2, showed on

SDS-polyacrylamide gel electrophoresis a major doublet band at 120 kilodaltons and a minor band at 100 kilodaltons. Bands of similar molecular weight were observed from several different positive cell types, including normal epidermal cells.

The observations suggest that VM-2 recognizes a 120 kilodalton antigen expressed on the surface membrane of basal epithelial cells which is normally lost as the cells differentiate. However, in malignant squamous cells the antigen continues to be expressed, so that it can be considered a tumor-associated antigen. If the antigen is found in superficial epithelial cells in sections of tissues or recovered by exfoliative cytology, such as cervical smears, it can be useful for the diagnosis of carcinoma or dysplasia preceding carcinoma. Because 95% of all cervical carcinomas are of squamous origin, we are assessing the usefulness of the VM-2 antibody for the diagnosis of this condition by immunocytology.

The value of the Papanicolau cytological screen for early diagnosis of cancer of the cervix is well established, but the procedure is labor-intensive and can give ambiguous results, particularly in dysplasias and when infection increases the number of leukocytes in smears. We have already established that VM-2 immunostaining is easily read, even by inexperienced personnel, and should be suitable for automation. Preliminary comparisons suggest a success rate for diagnosis of squamous carcinoma of the cervix at least equal to conventional cytology. Careful comparative follow-ups are required to establish whether immunocytology has any advantage over Papanicolau cytology, for instance in defining dysplasias that are more likely to be pre-malignant or in detecting recurrences after local excision. At the very least, our studies with the VM-2 antibody provide a fresh look at an important approach to cancer prevention that has remained essentially unchanged for forty years.

AN ADJUVANT FORMULATION INCREASING CELL-MEDIATED AND HUMORAL IMMUNE RESPONSES TO A WIDE RANGE OF SPECIFIC ANTIGENS

The antigen of cervical carcinoma cells just described is one of several human tumor-associated

antigens recently defined. The structures of some
glycolipid tumor-associated antigens have been established
and partial amino-acid sequences of some glycoprotein
tumor-associated antigens have been determined. Since the
immunogenicity seems to lie in the protein moeities of
these antigens, synthetic peptide and recombinant
DNA-produced homologs should soon be available. These can
in principle be used for diagnosis, for antibody-based
therapy (with or without coupled toxins) or for
immunization. The last point raises general questions:
whether prior immunization can prevent neoplasia and
whether specific immunization can be used for therapy of
established malignant disease.

The answer to both questions is clearly yes.
Immunization of mice against polyoma virus-induced tumors
established the general importance of cell-mediated
immunity in surveillance against virus-induced tumors
(24). Immunization of chickens with live virus to prevent
Marek's disease is a well-established procedure (25). A
striking example of immunogenicity of a non-virus-induced
tumor is that of ultraviolet-induced tumors of the skin
(26).

A great deal of work on experimental animals shows
that immunization even when tumors are already present can
prevent their recurrence. Elsewhere in this volume Hanna
and his colleagues describe how they are attempting to
extend these results to human patients with carcinoma of
the colon. However, a word of caution must be
interjected. The Prehns (27) summarize compelling
evidence that immune responses can in some circumstances
actually increase tumor growth, so the wrong kind of
intervention may do more harm than good. It is therefore
essential to elicit protective rather than inappropriate
immune responses.

A variety of synthetic peptide and recombinant
DNA-produced viral, bacterial and parasitic antigens have
become available during the past few years. To elicit
effective immune responses these antigens must be
administered with an adjuvant. Adjuvants accepted for
human use, such as aluminum salts, elicit antibody
formation but not the cell-mediated immunity which is
required for protection against some viruses and tumors.
Freund's complete adjuvant, which does elicit
cell-mediated immunity, is unacceptable for human use
because large granulomas are formed at injection sites.

To overcome this problem we have developed an adjuvant formulation that has activity comparable to Freund's complete adjuvant but lacks the undesirable effects of the latter (28). The adjuvant is N-acetylmuramyl-L-threonyl-D-isoglutamine (threonyl-MDP), a synthetic analog of the adjuvant-active component of mycobacterial cell walls. Instead of the mineral oil component of Freund's adjuvant we use a formulation based on pluronic polymer L121, which forms two phases with antigen localized at the interface in a two-dimensional array that seems favorable for eliciting immune responses. Antigen so presented presumably cross links receptors on the surface of T-lymphocytes, providing the first signal for activation; the second signal is provided by interleukin 1 produced by macrophages and interdigitating cells stimulated by threonyl-MDP. The latter is not pyrogenic and does not produce arthritis or anterior uveitis, which are the main undesirable complications of the use of MDP, lipopolysaccaride and other bacterial products. We have also found that interleukin-1ß is a growth factor for human B-lymphocytes, which contributes to the generation of B-lymphocyte memory. A second property of pluronic polymer L121, capacity to activate complement by the alternative pathway, may also be relevant. Complement activation allows localization of antigens on the surface of follicular dendritic cells which is required for the generation of B-lymphocyte memory.

Using killed feline leukemia virus antigens produced in cell culture, in the adjuvant formulation just described, we have protected the great majority of cats against virus challenge (29). This immunization procedure may well be applicable to other retroviruses, including HTLV-1 and HTLV-3, to hepatitis-B virus (with consequent protection against hepatoma in Taiwan and other areas of high susceptibility) and to tumor-associated antigens. Experiments to test some of these possibilities are in progress.

Peptide antigens are traditionally considered as haptens which have to be coupled to carrier proteins (T-lymphocyte immunogens) to elicit immune responses. Selection of a traditional macromolecular carrier is not straightforward. Some carriers such as thyroglobulin are contraindicated because of potential elicitation of thyroid autoimmunity. Other carriers which are ethically acceptable, such as bacterial toxins, present problems.

Most humans are already immunized, so re-exposure may
elicit allergic reactions or epitope-specific
suppression. The latter is the phenomenon demonstrated
experimentally when prior immunization with a carrier and
exposure to a hapten-carrier complex induces suppression
of immune responses to the hapten (30).

Audibert and her colleagues have covalently coupled
MDP to peptides to elicit immune responses (31). In our
hands that procedure has given erratic results, so we have
attempted to understand what carriers are really doing and
to identify a universal non-immunogenic carrier (32). A
traditional, macromolecular, immunogcnic carrier has two
roles. The first is to anchor the peptide or other hapten
to the surface of antigen-presenting cells, while the
second is to elicit T-cell-dependent immune responses.
Since the latter can be overcome by administration of
allogeneic cells (the so-called allogeneic effect), it
seems likely that elicited formation of lymphocyte growth
factors is required. If that is so, adjuvants should
by-pass the second requirement, and anchoring peptide
haptens to the interface of the two phases of the vehicle,
and subsequently to the plasma membrane of the
antigen-presenting cell, should substitute for the first
requirement. The attachment of a lipophilic tail to a
peptide should therefore suffice as a carrier in the
presence of a suitable vehicle and adjuvant. In support
of this interpretation, coupling a peptide to fatty acids
has been found to make it immunogenic (33). Carbohydrates
coupled to fatty acids are also more immunogenic than free
carbohydrates (34), as might be expected from the
well-known immunogenicity of glycolipids. Coupling of
haptens and proteins to phosphatidylethanolamine, which
achieves the same end, can be used for antigen
presentation in liposomes (35, 36).

CONCLUSION

Those who seek common themes running through this
presentation can find them in the application of
immunological methods, in particular monoclonal
antibodies, to define the properties of tumor-associated
antigens, growth factors and their receptors. Growth
factors may affect the growth of tumor cells themselves,
and also contribute to neovascularization of solid

tumors. The antigen which we have found associated with carcinoma of the cervix could have important diagnostic applications. Coupling of toxins to VM-2 antibody, or other antibodies against the same antigen, can be considered for therapy of squamous carcinomas not amenable to local treatment. It would of course be necessary to establish that their use would not have serious side effects in skin and other stratified epithelia where basal cells contain the antigen. Definition of tumor-associated antigens raises the possibility of immunization, and that requires an adjuvant formulation. Our knowledge of lymphocyte growth factors and the requirements for generation of T- and B-lymphocyte memory were useful in the development of an adjuvant formulation that has already proven successful to prevent feline leukemia virus infections. It could have other applications for prevention and therapy of malignant diseases.

ACKNOWLEDGEMENTS

The following participated in various projects described in this paper, and we are glad to acknowledge their collaboration: N. Byars, R. Derynk (Genentech), D. Gospodarowicz (University of California, San Francisco), J. Kenney, J. Kowalski, T. Maciag (Revlon) and V. Morhenn (Stanford University).

REFERENCES

1. Fuchs S, Sourajon MC, Mochly-Rosen D (1984). Antibodies to the acetylcholine receptor. In Greaves M (ed): "Receptors and Recognition Series B," Chapman and Hall, Vol. 17, pp 163-200.
2. Strosberg AD, Schreiber AB (1984). Antibodies to receptors and idiotypes as probes for hormone and neurotransmitter receptor structure and function. In Greaves M (ed): "Receptors and Recognition Series B," Chapman and Hall, Vol. 17, pp 15-42.
3. Sege K, Peterson PA (1978). Anti-idiotypic antibodies against anti-vitamin A transporting protein react with prealbumin. Nature 271:167-168.

4. Schreiber AB, Couraud P-O, Andre C, Vray B, Strosberg AD (1980). Anti-alprenolol anti-idiotypic antibodies bind to β-adrenergic receptors and modulate catecholamine sensitive adenylate cyclase. Proc Natl Acad Sci USA 77:7385-738_.

5. Wasserman NH, Penn HS, Freimuth PI, Treptow N, Wentzel S, Clevel WL, Erlanger BF (1982). Anti-idiotypic route to anti-acetylcholine receptor antibodies and experimental myasthenia gravis. Proc Natl Acad Sci USA 79:4810-4814.

6. Farid NR, Pepper B, Urbina-Briones R, Islam NR (1982). Anti-idiotypic antibodies against anti-thyrotropin interact with the TSH receptor. J Cell Biochem 19:305-309.

7. Marasco WA, Becker EL (1982). Anti-idiotype as antibody against the formyl peptide chemotaxis receptor of the neutrophil. J Immunol 128:963-968.

8. Schreiber AB, Lax I, Yarden Y, Eshbar Z, Schlessinger J (1981). Monoclonal antibodies against the receptor for EGF induce the early and delayed effects of EGF. Proc Natl Acad Sci USA 78:7535-7539.

9. Schreiber AB, Libermann TA, Lax I, Yarden Y, Schlessinger J (1983). Biological role of epidermal growth factor-receptor clustering. J Biol Chem 258:846-853.

10. Downward J, Yarden Y, Mayer E, Serace G, Tolty N, Stockwell P, Ullrich A, Schlessinger J, Waterfield M (1984). Close similarity of EGF receptor and V-erb-B oncogene protein sequences. Nature 307:521-527.

11. Lax I, Bar-Eli M, Yarden Y, Libermann TA, Schlessinger J (1984). Antibodies to two defined regions of the transforming protein pp 60[src] interact specifically with the EGF receptor kinase system. Proc Natl Acad Sci USA 81:5911-5915.

12. Todaro GJ, De Larco JE (1978). Growth factors produced by sarcoma virus-transformed cells. Cancer Res 38:4147-4154.

13. Sporn MB, Roberts AB (1985). Autocrine growth factors and cancer. Nature 313:745-747.

14. Schreiber AB, Derynck R, submitted.

15. Blomquist MC, Hunt LT, Barker C (1984). Vaccinia virus 19-kilodalton protein relationship to several mammalian proteins, including two growth factors. Proc Natl Acad Sci USA 81:7363-7367.

16. Brown JP, Twardzik DR, Marquardt H, Todaro GJ (1985). Vaccinia virus encodes a polypeptide homologous to epidermal growth factor and transforming growth factor. Nature 313:491-492.
17. Folkman J (1983). Angiogenesis: initiation and control. Ann NY Acad Sci 401:212-227.
18. Massoglia S, Kenney J, Schreiber AB, Allison AC, Gospodarowicz D., in preparation.
19. Maciag T, Friesel R, Mehlman T, and Schreiber AB (1984). Heparin binds endothelial cell growth factor, the principal endothelial cell mitogen in bovine brain. Science 225:932-935.
20. Schreiber AB, Kenney J, Kowalski J, Friesel R, Mehlman T, Maciag T (1985). The interaction of endothelial cell growth factor with heparin: characterization by receptor and antibody recognition. Proc Natl Acad Sci USA (in press).
21. Schreiber AB, Thomas K, Barritault D, Maciag T (1985). J Cell Biol, submitted.
22. Form D, Auerbach R (1983). PGE_2 and angiogenesis. Proc Soc Exp Biol Med 172:214-218.
23. Morhenn V, Schreiber AB, McMillan B, Soriero O, Allison AC. A monoclonal antibody specific for proliferating skin squamous cells: use in the diagnosis of cervical neoplasia. J Clin Invest, in the press.
24. Allison AC (1980). Immune responses to polyoma virus and polyoma virus-induced tumors. In Klein G (ed) "Viral Oncology," New York: Raven Press, pp 481-487.
25. Nazerian K (1980). Marek's disease: a herpesvirus-induced malignant lymphoma of the chicken. In Klein G (ed) "Viral Oncology" New York: Raven Press, pp 665-682.
26. Fisher MS, Kripke ML (1982). Suppressor T-lymphocytes control the development of primary skin cancer in ultraviolet-irradiated mice. Science 216:1133-1134.
27. Prehn RT, Prehn LM (1985). On the autoimmune nature of cancer. Cancer Research, in press.
28. Allison AC (1985). Immunological adjuvants and their mode of action. In Bell R, Torrigiani G (eds) Schwabe, Basel: "New Approaches to Vaccine Development," pp 133-156.

29. Braemer AC, Peterson M, Rennike G, Bass E, Allison AC, Byars N (1984). Effect of inactivated FeLV vaccines on the development of persistent viremia. Proceedings of the Conference of Research Workers on Animal Diseases (in press).

30. Herzenberg LA, Tokuhisa T, Hayakawa K (1983). Epitope-specific regulation. Ann Rev Immunol 1:609-620.

31. Audibert F, Jobinet M, Chedid L, Arnon R, Sela M (1982). Successful immunization with a totally synthetic diphtheria vaccine. Proc Natl Acad Sci USA 79:5042.

32. Allison AC, Byars N, Waters RV (1985 in press). Immunological adjuvants: efficacy and safety considerations. Rev Infect Dis.

33. Hopp TP (1984). Immunogenicity of a synthetic HbsAg peptide: enhancement by conjugation to a fatty acid carrier. Molecular Immunol. 21:13-16.

34. Wood C, Kabat EA (1981). Immunochemical studies of conjugates of isomaltosyl oligosaccharides to lipid. I. Antigenicity of glycolipids and the production of specific antibodies in rabbits. J Exp Med 154:432-449.

35. Okada N, Yasuda T, Tsumita T, Okada H (1982). Activation of the alternative pathway of guinea pig by liposomes incorporated with trinitrophenylated phosphatidyl-ethanolamine. Immunology 45:115-120.

36. Shek PN, Heath TD (1983). Immune response mediated by liposome-associated antigens. III. Immunogenicity of bovine serum albumin covalently coupled to vesicle surface. Immunology 50:101-106.

Monoclonal Antibodies and Cancer Therapy, pages 413–429
© 1985 Alan R. Liss, Inc.

CHARACTERIZATION OF A MONOCLONAL ANTIBODY
TO CSF-2α (IL-3)

P.J. Conlon, H. Luk, L. Park, T. Hopp and D. Urdal

Immunex Corporation
51 University Street
Seattle, WA 98101

ABSTRACT The colony stimulating factor CSF-2α (IL-3)
has been purified to homogeneity, the protein
sequenced, and the gene encoding this lymphokine
cloned. Knowledge of the protein sequence permitted
the synthesis of peptides corresponding to the
amino terminus of the molecule. These peptides,
after conjugation to palmitic acid, were used to
immunize mice. Spleen cells from mice immunized
with one of these peptides (CSF-2α$_{1-14}$) were fused
with the myeloma cell line NS-1. The fusion resulted
in the isolation of two hybridoma cell lines,
designated 6A5 and 4D4, that secreted antibodies
that were specific for the immunizing peptide.
The antibodies did not react with a closely related
peptide CSF-2α$_{7-16}$. The antibodies were capable,
however, of recognizing CSF-2α protein as judged
by the ability of the antibodies to remove CSF-2α
activity from culture medium of PHA-stimulated
LBRM-33-5A4 cells and to immunoprecipitate
radiolabeled CSF-2α protein.

INTRODUCTION

The differentiation of hematopoietic progenitor
cells is influenced by glycoprotein molecules termed
colony stimulating factors (CSF) (1,2,3). These
factors stimulate the proliferation of progenitor
cells in vitro to lineage-specific cell types, including
eosinophils (4), megakaryocytes, neutrophils (5),

macrophages (6), mast cells (7,8) and possibly lymphocytes (9).

Previously, we reported that the murine T cell lymphoma LBRM-33-5A4 produced several biochemically distinct CSFs in addition to IL-2 (10). These CSF's, termed 2α, 2β and 2γ, also differed in their biological properties. CSF-2α and CSF-2β appeared to be glycosylated forms of the same protein and identical to the multi-lineage factor, interleukin 3 (11,12,13) (also known as hematopoietic cell growth factor (14,15), mast cell growth factor (16), and persisting cell growth factor (7,8)).

CSF-2α was purified to homogeneity and the protein sequenced (17,18). Based on this sequence, peptides were chemically synthesized, conjugated to palmitic acid and used as immunogens in mice. We report here the isolation and characterization of two anti-peptide monoclonal antibodies, 6A5 and 4D4 which recognize the mature CSF-2α protein. These monoclonal antibodies, when covalently coupled to agarose, could remove CSF-2α biological activity from LBRM-33-5A4 conditioned medium. Further experiments are underway to determine the in vivo role of CSF-2α using these monoclonal antibodies.

MATERIALS AND METHODS

Mice.

Female Balb/c mice (6-8 wks of age) were obtained from the Jackson Laboratories, Bar Harbor, ME.

Cell Lines.

The murine lymphoma cell line LBRM-33-5A4 (19) was used as a source of CSF-2α and IL-2 and was maintained as previously reported (10,17). The myeloma cell line NS-1 was maintained in culture in RPMI-1640, supplemented with 10% fetal bovine serum, penicillin (50 µg/ml), streptomycin (50 µg/ml) and fresh L-glutamine (300 µg/ml). The factor dependent cell lines FDC-P2 and CTLL-2 were maintained in culture as previously described (10). The hybridoma W6/32 (20) was obtained from the

American Type Culture Collection (Rockville, MD) and
was used as a control for the experiments detailed herein.

Synthesis of Peptide Immunogens.

Two peptides were synthesized. The first
incorporated amino acid sequences found in the
amino-terminal region of colony stimulating factor
amino acids 1-14 (CSF-$2\alpha_{1-14}$). The second peptide
corresponds to the N-terminal sequence for IL-3 reported
by Ihle (13) and contains amino acids 7-15 (CSF-$2\alpha_{7-16}$).
Each was comprised of the appropriate amino acids, and
a carboxy-terminal hydrophobic segment, Gly-Lys-Lys-Gly,
in which both lysines were derivatized by coupling
palmitic acid to their epsilon amino groups (referred
to as carboxy terminal dipalmityl, or CDP) (Figure
1). The entire synthesis was carried out using the
Merrifield synthesis procedure (21) with
N-alpha-tert-butyloxycarbonyl (BOC) protected amino
acids and standard side chain protection, except in
the case of the lysines that were derivatized with
palmitic acid. For these, the lysines were coupled as
the alpha BOC, epsilon α-fluorenylmethyloxycarbonyl
(FMOC) derivatives. Subsequently, the FMOC group was
removed with piperidine and the palmitic acid was
coupled using the same carbodimide procedure as for
normal BOC amino acids. The resulting alpha BOC,
epsilon palmityl lysyl residue could then be deprotected
with trifluoroacetic acid, and the synthesis was
continued as usual. After cleavage from the resin
with hydrofluoric acid, the peptides were partially
purified by gel filtration on Bio-Gel P10 in 95%
acetic acid 5% water. Trinitrobenzene sulfonic acid
(TNBS) reactive peptide material eluting from the
column was pooled and lyophilized. The resulting
white powder was suspended in saline for immunizations
and for coating plates in the Elisa assays. Such
suspensions were usually opalescent or milky appearing,
suggesting that a micellar or liposomal aggregate had
been formed.

Immunization and Fusion.

A group of 10 Balb/c mice were injected

subcutaneously every 14 days with 25 µg of CDP-peptide (either CSF-2α_{1-14} or CSF-2α_{7-16}) emulsified in Freund's adjuvant. After two injections, serum was collected and the presence of antibodies to the peptide measured by an enzyme-linked immunosorbent assay (Elisa). Animals with high titer antibodies to CSF-2α_{1-14} (> 1:2500) were then sacrificed, their spleens removed and fused to the NS-1 myeloma cells (22).

Anti-CSF-2α Peptide Antibody Detection.

Seven to ten days following fusion, antibodies to the CSF-2α_{1-14} and CSF-2α_{7-16} peptides were measured by Elisa. Fifty µl of CDP-peptide (5 µg/ml in PBS, pH 7.2) was added to individual wells of a 96 well polyvinyl microtiter plates (Linbro/Titertek, Flow Laboratory, McLean, VA) and incubated overnight at 37°C. After incubation, the plates were blocked with 1% BSA in PBS, pH 7.2 for 90 min. Culture supernatant was then added to the wells and incubated for 90 min at room temperature. Following extensive washing, 50 µl of a 1:500 dilution of alkaline phosphatase conjugated goat anti-mouse Ig (Sigma) was added for 1 hour at room temperature. After 10 washes with PBS, 50 µl of substrate solution (pH 9.0, 1 mg/ml phosphatase substrate in .02M Na_2CO_3, .03M $NaHCO_3$ and 10^{-3}M $MgCl_2$) were added. The amount of antibody bound was then quantified by measuring the absorbance at 405 nm (A405) on a multiskan Elisa plate reader (Titertek, Flow Laboratories). Samples were assayed in triplicate and the average of the absorption at 405 nm recorded.

Ascites Production of Antibody.

Pristane primed Balb/c mice were injected intraperitoneally with 3 x 10^6 hybridoma cells. Ascitic fluid was collected 14-17 days later, centrifuged and the ascites stored at -20°C until needed.

Antibody Purification and Coupling to Gels.

Anti-CSF-2α_{1-14}, and a control monoclonal W6/32 of the same isotope, were purified by affinity chromatography using Protein A-sepharose according to the procedure of Ey, et al. (23). Briefly, ascites fluid containing the monoclonal antibodies was applied to a Protein A-sepharose column (2 ml) equilibrated in 0.1M Hepes pH 7.4. The column was washed extensively with 0.1M Hepes until no detectable protein was observed in the eluant. Protein A bound antibody was then eluted with 0.1M citrate buffer pH 3.5. Purified antibody in 0.1M Hepes pH 7.5, was coupled to Affigel-10 (Biorad Laboratories, Richmond, CA) according to the manufacturer's instructions. Supports containing 6-12 mg of antibody per ml gel were routinely obtained by this procedure.

Radioimmuneprecipitation of ^{125}I-labeled CSF-2α was performed by incubating 25 μl of Affigel-10 beads containing 8 mg/ml gel of W6/32, 6A5 or 4D4, with 30 μl of 0.05M Tris pH 7.5 buffered saline containing 3% BSA and 500,000 cpm of ^{125}I labeled CSF-2α. PBS-1% Triton X-100 (100 μl) was added to the mixture and the incubation continued overnight at 4°C. The Affigel-10 beads were then washed five times with PBS-1% Triton X-100 and suspended in 40 μl of sample buffer (0.06M Tris-HCl, pH 6.8, 2% SDS, 10% glycol, 5% 2-mercaptoethanol). This suspension was boiled for 3 minutes and then 30 μl of the supernatant analyzed by SDS polyacrylamide gel electrophoresis according to the stacking gel procedure of Laemmli (24). Gels were dried and exposed to Kodak X-mat AR film at -70°C.

Affinity Chromatography of CSF-2α.

    1 ml columns (Biorad) of Affigel-10 containing anti-CSF-2α_{1-14} antibodies, 6A5 and 4D4, or the control antibody W6/32, were equilibrated in PBS. Media (5 ml) conditioned by the growth of phytohaemagglutinin-stimulated LBRM-33-5A4 cells was passed through the column at a flow rate of approximately 0.5 ml/min, one ml fractions were collected. The column was washed with PBS and bound activity was eluted by 0.1 M glycine pH 3.0. Assays for IL-2 and CSF-2α were then performed on the fractions as previously described (10).

H$_2$N-Ala-Ser-Ile-Ser-Gly-Arg-Asp-Thr-His-Arg-Leu-Thr-Arg-Thr-Leu-Asn   CSF-2α sequence

H$_2$H-Ala-Ser-Ile-Ser-Gly-Arg-Asp-Thr-His-Arg-Lys-Thr-Gly-Lys-Lys-Gly-COOH CSF-2α_{1-14}

      Pa   Pa

H$_2$N-Asp-Thr-His-Arg-Leu-Thr-Arg-Thr-Leu-Abu-Gly-Lys-Lys-Lys-Gly-COOH CSF-2α_{7-16}

FIGURE 1. Synthesis of peptide immunogens. The upper sequence is the N terminal 16 amino acids of CSF-2α, as determined in our laboratory by combined protein and nucleic acid sequencing. Below it are the structures of the two chemically synthesized peptides. The first 14 residues of CSF-2α_{1-14} correspond to our protein sequence information for CSF-2α, which disagrees with the nucleic acid-derived sequence at positions 11 and 13. The CSF-2α_{7-16} sequence corresponds to the N terminal sequence for IL-3 reported by Ihle (13) with the Asn substituted by aminobutyric acid (Abu) to avoid forming the unstable Asn-Gly peptide bond. Palmitic acid moieties attached to the epsilon amino groups of lysines are indicated by Pa.

CSF-2α Purification and Radiolabeling.

CSF-2α was purified to homogeneity from media conditioned by PHA stimulated LBRM cells as previously described (10,17) and summarized below. Protein was first sequentially precipitated from conditioned medium by the step-wise addition of ammonium sulfate to 30%, 50%, and finally to 80% saturation. The proteins contained in the 80% precipitate were then fractionated by cation exchange chromatography followed by anion exchange chromatography. Purification to homogeneity was achieved by 2 step reversed phase high performance liquid chromatography (HPLC). First, HPLC fractionation was conducted on a C18 µBondapak column (30 cm x 3.9 mm) equilibrated in 0.1% trifluoroacetic acid (TFA) and eluted with a gradient of acetonitrile. Active fractions eluted from the column were pooled and rechromatographed on the same column but with a gradient of propanol in 0.9M acetic acid 0.2M pyridine (17). A third HPLC step was occasionally used to exchange the propanol solvent for the acetonitrile solvent such that the final CSF-2α sample was contained in 0.1% TFA, 48% acetonitrile.

CSF-2α was radiolabeled using the Enzymobead radioiodination reagent (Biorad) essentially following the manufacturer's specifications. Briefly, aliquots (50 µl) of CSF-2α in the acetonitrile (50 µl containing .3 µg protein) were combined with 50 µl of 0.2M sodium phosphate pH 7.2 and the acetonitrile evaporated under nitrogen. Then 50 µl of Enzymobead reagent, 20 µl ^{125}I (2 mCi) and 10 µl of 2.5% β-D-glucose were added and the mixture was incubated at 25°C for 10 min. Sodium azide (20 µl of 25 mM) and sodium metabisulphite (10 µl of 5 mg/ml) were then added and after 5 minutes at 25°C, iodinated CSF-2α was separated from unbound ^{125}I by chromatography on a 2 ml Sephadex G-25 column equilibrated in 0.05 M sodium phosphate, pH 7.2 containing 0.01% gelatin. Radiolabelled preparations had estimated specific activities in the range of 1 x 10^{16} cpm/mmole.

RESULTS

Balb/c mice were injected with CSF-2α peptides (Figure 1) that had been conjugated near their carboxy termini with palmitic acid (CDP-peptide). Beginning

TABLE 1

Peptide specificity of hybridoma culture
supernatants as assayed by Elisa.

Hybrid	CDP–CSF–$2\alpha_{1-16}$	A405[a] CDP–CSF–$2\alpha_{7-16}$	CDP–IP–1
1A8	.252	.029	.061
1H7	.164	.039	.062
2B9	.155	.035	.062
2C10	.354	.033	.030
3B10	.142	.033	.04
3F5	.219	.034	.039
4B3	.204	.034	.061
4C5	.244	.032	.052
4D3	.227	.047	.064
4D4	.417	.038	.053
4F5	.19	.034	.062
5A5	.282	.04	.069
5E2	.215	.035	.05
5E9	.285	.031	.049
6A5	.38	.034	.077
6D6	.681	.037	.084
6D11	.415	.034	.061
Controls–			
HAT medium	.049	.032	.06
PBS	.05	.034	.054
Normal serum			
1:1000	.067	.047	.078
Immune serum			
1:1000	.641	.052	.053

[a]A405 – Average absorbance at 405 nm of
triplicate points.

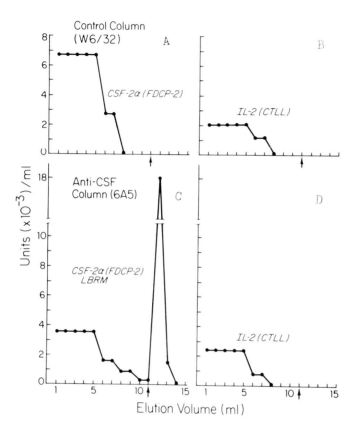

FIGURE 2. Affinity chromatography of PHA stimulated, LBRM-33-5A4 culture medium. PHA stimulated LBRM-33-5A4 culture medium was passed over a column of either W6/32 (top panels) or 6A5, anti-CSF-2α, antibody coupled to Affigel-10, fractions collected and the levels of CSF-2α and IL-2 protein determined by proliferation of factor-dependent cells. CSF-2α activity is represented in the left panel and IL-2 activity on the right. Arrow indicates elution with 0.1M glycine, pH 3.0.

6-8 weeks after immunization, high antibody titers to
the immunizing synthetic peptide were found only
inanimals receiving CDP-CSF-$2a_{1-14}$ (> 1:2560 dilution
by Elisa) but not in animals receiving the CDP-CSF-$2a_{7-16}$
synthetic peptides. Furthermore, immune sera from
CDP-CSF-$2a_{1-14}$ peptide challenged animals were capable
of specifically removing CSF-$2a$ activity from
PHA-stimulated LBRM-33-5A4 cell line conditioned
medium. However, use of immune sera in such
immunoprecipitation experiments did not alter the
level of IL-2 activity in identical CSF-$2a$ containing
medium (data not shown).

Spleens from CDP-CSF-$2a_{1-14}$ peptide immune animals
were then removed and fused to NS-1 myeloma cells
(22). Seven to ten days later, the cultures were
screened for antibodies to CDP-CSF-$2a_{1-14}$ as well as
CDP-CSF-$2a_{7-16}$ and an irrelevant peptide, IP-1 (specific
for a sequence in the human IL-2 protein). As seen in
Table 1, 17 hybridoma supernatants (out of 300 tested)
reacted specifically to CDP-CSF-$2a_{1-14}$ and not to the
other peptides when assayed by Elisa.

Two hybridomas, 6A5 and 4D4, were selected for
further characterization based on their reproducible
reactivity by Elisa assay to CDP-CSF-$2a_{1-14}$. Both 6A5
and 4D4 monoclonal antibodies were isotyped as IgG 2A,
and thus were easily purified from ascites by affinity
chromatography to Protein-A sepharose columns. The
purified anti-CSF-$2a_{1-14}$ antibodies, 6A5 and 4D4, as
well as an isotype control antibody, W6/32, were then
coupled to Affigel-10 beads. LBRM-33-5A4 culture
conditioned medium was then passed through either the
6A5-, 4D4-, or W6/32-Affigel-10 column, fractions
collected, and CSF-$2a$ and IL-2 activity measured. As
shown in Figure 2B and 2D, IL-2 contained in the
LBRM-33-5A4 medium passed directly through
both the W6/32 Affigel column and the 6A5 Affigel
column. Similarly, CSF-$2a$ did not bind to the W6/32
Affigel column (Figure 2A). In contrast, 70-90% of
the CSF-$2a$ activity present in the LBRM-33-5A4 medium
was bound by the 6A5 Affigel column and could be
eluted by a low pH wash of the column (Figure 2C).
Similar results were obtained when the monoclonal
antibody 4D4 was coupled to Affigel.

Further evidence to support the contention that
the monoclonal antibody 6A5 recognized the mature
CSF-$2a$ protein was obtained by immunoprecipitation

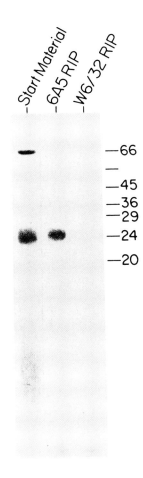

FIGURE 3. Radioimmunoprecipitation of ^{125}I labeled CSF-2α by anti-peptide antibody 6A5 and the isotype control, W6/32 coupled to Affigel-10.

of ^{125}I-labeled CSF-2α as shown in Figure 3. The anti-CSF-2α_{1-14} antibody 6A5 immunoprecipitated a single protein species with a relative molecular mass of 24,500. W6/32, on the other hand, did not precipitate any radiolabeled proteins. Similarly, 4D4-antibody precipitated the same 24,500 dalton molecular weight protein (data not shown).

DISCUSSION

The peptide CSF-2α_{1-14}, corresponding to the N terminus of CSF-2α (18), conjugated to palmitic acid was found to be highly immunogenic in mice. Serum from mice immunized with this peptide also reacted with the mature CSF-2α protein. Two hybridomas, secreting monoclonal antibodies of the IgG 2A isotype, were isolated from the fusion of spleen cells from these animals. Both monoclonal antibodies recognized CDP-CSF-2α_{1-14} peptide and the CSF-2α protein.

The use of synthetic peptide immunogens has been extensively documented, particularly in antibody responses to whole virus or their products (Rev. 25). While a number of reports of monoclonal antibodies to lymphokines have been made in the literature (22,26), few have been generated using synthetic peptides (27). Altman, et al. (28) recently reported that synthetic peptides, corresponding to several regions in the IL-2 molecule, could elicit a polyclonal antibody response in rabbits and mice that recognized both immunizing peptide and to a lesser extent the IL-2 protein. However, they were unable to demonstrate that monoclonal antibodies of similar specificity could also be generated.

Conjugation of the synthetic peptide to palmitic acid residues via the carboxy terminus has been found by our laboratory to be an alternative strategy to the traditional protein carrier method (28). The CDP-peptide has been shown to elicit good antibody formation in rabbits (T. Hopp and P. Conlon, personal observation) and with CDP-CSF-2α_{1-14}, in mice. It is not clear however why CDP-CSF-2α_{7-16} was nonimmunogenic in mice, although we have generated antibodies to the peptide in rabbits. The monoclonal antibodies, 6A5 and 4D4, appeared to require the presence of the first six amino acids in the CSF-2α peptide in order to be recognized. Whether the amino acid residues are actually involved in binding the antibody molecule, either alone or in the context of the neighboring residues, or in conferring some tertiary structure to the protein or peptides is uncertain. However, the CDP moiety probably causes a preferential recognition of the N terminus, because this end of the peptide should project out from the micellular aggregate.

CSF-2α has been purified to homogeneity (17), the NH_2-terminal amino acid sequence obtained (18), and the cDNA encoding the lymphokines cloned (30,31, unpublished observations). We found the NH_2-terminal amino acid sequence of this lymphokine to be Ala-Ser-Ile-Ser-Gly-Arg-Asp-Thr-His-Arg-Leu-Thr-Arg-Thr (18). Similarly, persisting cell factor was found to have the same NH_2-terminal sequence (32). In contrast, purified IL-3 has been reported (13) to start at position 7 of our sequence (Asp). The observation that monoclonals directed against synthetic peptides corresponding to residues 1-14 of the CSF-2α sequence can absorb CSF-2α activity from PHA-stimulated medium of LBRM-33-5A4 cells reinforces the notion that our NH_2-terminal protein sequence is correct. Similarly, using the 6A5 and 4D4 monoclonal antibodies coupled to the Affigel-10 matrix, we also observed that WEHI-3 derived CSF-2α (IL-3) bound to the column and was eluted off with low pH exactly as LBRM-33-5A4 derived factor (P. Conlon and D. Urdal, personal observation). Thus, our biochemical and immunochemical evidence would argue that CSF-2α (IL-3) has as its N-terminal residue alanine, and not the Asp residue seen by Ihle. Whether this difference between the amino-termini of the factors might be due to proteolysis during purification of IL-3 or to differential processing of IL-3 by the different clones of WEHI-3 cell is uncertain.

The anti-CSF-2α monoclonal antibodies 6A5 and 4D4 will not only prove useful in purification of the protein, but more importantly, may enable us to begin to understand the role of CSF-2α in vivo in hematopoiesis. Further efforts are underway in our laboratory to explore this possibility.

ACKNOWLEDGEMENTS

We thank Dr. T.M. Dexter for providing us with
the cell line FDC-P2. The authors also acknowledge
the excellent technical skills of Ms. Theresa Washkewicz,
Janet Merriam, and Della Friend. We wish to thank
Judy Byce for her help in the preparation of the
manuscript.
The work presented here was carried out in
collaboration with scientists from Behringwerke AG,
West Germany, F. Seiler, Director. This collaboration
is gratefully acknowledged.

REFERENCES

1. Bradley TR, Metcalf D (1966). The growth of bone
   marrow cells in vitro. Aust J Exp Biol Med Sci
   44:287.
2. Stanley ER, Heard PM (1977). Factors regulating
   macrophage production and growth. Purification
   and some properties of the colony stimulating
   factor from medium conditioned by mouse L cells. J
   Biol Chem 252:4305.
3. Burgess AW, Wilson EMA, Metcalf D (1977).
   Granulocyte/macrophage-, megakaryocyte-, eosinophil-
   and erythroid- colony stimulating factors produced
   by mouse spleen cells. Biochem J 185:301.
4. Johnson GR, Metcalf D (1980). Detection of a new
   type of mouse eosinophil colony by Luxol-Fast-Blue
   staining. Exp Hematol 8:549.
5. Williams N, Eger RR, Moore MAS, Mendelsohn N
   (1978). Differentiation of mouse bone marrow
   precursor cells into neutrophil granulocytes by
   an activity separated from WEHI-3 cell conditioned
   medium. Differentiation 11:59.
6. Stanley ER, Chen DM, Lin HS (1978). Induction of
   macrophage production and proliferation by a
   purified colony stimulating factor. Nature 274:168.
7. Schrader JW, Arnold B, Clark-Lewis I (1980). A
   Con A-stimulated T-cell hybridoma releases factors
   affecting the hematopoietic colony-forming cells
   and B-cell antibody responses. Nature 283:197.

8. Schrader JW, Clark-Lewis I (1982). A T cell-derived factor stimulating multipotential hemopoietic stem cells: molecular weight and distinction from T cell growth factor and T cell-derived granulocyte macrophage colony-stimulating factor. J. Immunol 129:30.

9. Watson J, Frank MB, Mochizuki D, Gillis S (1982). In Pick E, (ed): "Lymphokines," New York: Academic Press, p. 95.

10. Prestidge RL, Watson JD, Urdal DL, Mochizuki D, Conlon P, Gillis S (1984). Biochemical comparison of murine colony-stimulating factors secreted by a T cell lymphoma and a myelomonocytic leukemia. J Immunol 133:293.

11. Lee JC, Hapel AJ, Ihle JN (1982). Constitutive production of a unique lymphokine (IL 3) by the WEHI-3 cell line. J Immunol 128:2393.

12. Ihle JN, Rebar, L, Keller J, Lee JC, Hapel A (1981). Interleukin 3: possible roles in the regulation of lymphocyte differentiation and growth. Immunol Rev 98:101.

13. Ihle JN, et al (1983). Biologic properties of homogeneous interleukin 3. I. Demonstration of Wehi-3 growth factor activity, mast cell growth factor activity, P cell stimulating factor activity, colony-stimulating factor activity and histamine-producing cell-stimulating factor activity. J Immunol 131:282.

14. Brazill CW, Haynes M, Garland J, Dexter TM (1983). Procedures for the purification of interleukin 3 to homogeneity. J Biochem 210:747.

15. Garland JM, Dexter TH (1983). Relationship of hemopoietic growth factor to lymphocytes and interleukin 3: a short review. Lymphokine Res 2:13.

16. Yung YP, Eger R, Tertain G, Moore MAS (1981). Long-term in vitro culture of murine mast cells. II. Purification of a mast cell growth factor and its dissociation from TCGF. J Immunol 127:794.

17. Urdal DL, Mochizuki D, Conlon PJ, March CJ, Remerowski ML, Eisenman J, Ramthun C, Gillis S (1984). Lymphokine purification by reversed-phase high performance liquid chromatography. J Chromatography 296:171.

428   Conlon et al

18. Watson JD, Prestidge RL, Booth RJ, Urdal DL,
     Mochizuki DY, Conlon PJ, Gillis S (1985).
     Differentiation factors from cell lines. In
     Maizel A, Ford R (eds): "Mediators in Cell Growth
     and Differentiation," New York: Raven Press, in
     press.
19. Gillis S, Scheid M, Watson J (1980). Biochemical
     and biologic characterization of lymphocyte
     regulatory molecules. III. The isolation and
     phenotypic characterization of interleukin
     2-producing T cell lymphomas. J Immunol 125:2570.
20. Barnstable CJ, et al (1978). Production of
     monoclonal antibodies to group A erythrocytes,
     HLA, and other human cell surface antigens - new
     tools for genetic analysis. Cell 14:9.
21. Barany G, Merrifield RB (1979). In Gross E,
     Meienhofer J (eds): "The Peptides Vol 2," New
     York: Academic Press, p 1.
22. Gillis S, Henney CS (1981). Biochemical and
     biological characterization of lymphocyte regulatory
     molecules. VI. Generation of a B cell hybridoma
     whose antibody product inhibit Interleukin 2
     activity. J Immunol 126:1978.
23. Ey PL, Prowse SJ, Jenkin CR 1978). Isolation of
     pure IgG, IgG_{2a}, and IgG_{2b} immunoglobulins from
     mouse serum using
     Protein-A-sepharose. Immunochemistry 15:429.
24. Laemmli UK (1970). Cleavage of structural proteins
     during the assembly of the head of bacteriophage
     T-4. Nature (London) 227:680.
25. Lerner RA (1982). Tapping the immunological
     repertoire to produce antibodies of predetermined
     specificity. Nature (London) 299:592.
26. Stadler BM, Berenstein EH, Siraganian RP, Oppenheim
     JJ (1982). Monoclonal antibody against human
     Interleukin 2 (IL-2). I. Purification of iL-2
     for the production of monoclonal antibodies. J
     Immunol 128:1620.
27. Arnheiter H, Ohno M, Smith M, Gutte B, Zoon KC
     (1983). Orientation of a human leukocyte interferon
     molecule on its cell surface receptor: Carboxyl
     terminus remains accessible to a monoclonal
     antibody made against a synthetic interferon
     fragment. Proc Natl Acad Sci USA 80:2539.

28. Altman A, Cardenas JM, Houghten RA, Dixon FJ, Theofilopoulos AN (1984). Antibodies of predetermined specificity against chemically synthesized peptides of human interleukin-2. Proc Natl Acad Sci USA 81:2176.

29. Warner NL, Moore MAS, Metcalf D (1969). A transplantable myelomonocytic leukemia in BALB/c mice: cytology, karyotype and muramidase content. J Nat Cancer Inst 43:963.

30. Fung MC, Hapel AJ, Ymer S, Cohen DR, Johnson RM, Campbell HD, Young IG (1984). Molecular cloning of cDNA for murine interleukin-3. Nature 307:233.

31. Yokata T, Lee F, Rennick D, Hall C, Arai N, Mosmann T, Nabel G, Cantor H, Arai K-I (1984). Isolation and characterization of a mouse cDNA clone that expresses mast cell growth factor activity in monkey cells. Proc Natl Acad Sci USA 81:1070.

32. Clark-Lewis I, Kent SBH, Schrader JW (1984). Purification to apparent homogeneity of a factor stimulating the growth of multiple lineage of hematopoietic cells. J Biol Chem 259:7488.

Monoclonal Antibodies and Cancer Therapy, pages 431–440
© 1985 Alan R. Liss, Inc.

REGULATORY ISSUES SURROUNDING THERAPEUTIC USE OF
MONOCLONAL ANTIBODIES: POINTS TO CONSIDER IN THE
MANUFACTURE OF INJECTABLE PRODUCTS INTENDED FOR
HUMAN USE

Thomas Hoffman, James Kenimer, and Kathryn E. Stein

Division of Blood and Blood Products, and Division of
Bacterial Products, Food and Drug Administration,
Bethesda, MD   20205

ABSTRACT The Office of Biologics Research and
Review, FDA is responsible for regulating monoclonal
antibodies used in humans. In the absence of
long-standing experience with these agents, a set of
"Points to Consider" has evolved which represents
concerns over potential hazards associated with
widespread use of monoclonal antibodies. Here some
of the issues are highlighted, including information
needed about the hybridoma itself, manufacturing
practices, quality control, and preclinical testing.
Means for detecting and controlling contamination are
detailed. Special considerations with respect to
human-human hybrids are discussed.

INTRODUCTION

    The therapeutic use of monoclonal antibodies offers
virtually unlimited possibilities in situations where
currently available treatments are ineffective. Yet, with
this promise come new special public health concerns.
Particular problems stem from the introduction into
individuals with a variety of diseases, materials produced
by an immortal, often xenogeneic cell line grown in tissue
culture or mouse ascites. In addition, by definition, the
material reacts with components of human tissues with
potential for undesired cross-reactivity. Our office has,
therefore, attempted to compile a list of problems, side
effects, toxicities and untoward reactions of which
investigators and clinicians should be cognizant.

In addition, we have taken a multidisciplinary approach to
devising strategies which could identify the problems and
procedures designed to minimize them.

Over the last four years, internal documents within
the Office of Biologics Research and Review have evolved
to serve as an in-house manual for individuals reviewing
notices of claimed investigational exemption for new drugs
(IND) or license applications. At this writing, there
exist no formal published guidelines which, if adhered to,
would ensure a product's approval or licensure.
Nonetheless, a document called, "Points to Consider in the
Manufacture of Injectable Monoclonal Antibody Products
Intended for Human Use In Vivo" has been disseminated to
manufacturers, institutions, individual clinicians, and
investigators involved in the development of monoclonal
antibodies. These were intended to serve as departure
points for discussion in an attempt to have regulators and
manufacturers addressing the same set of issues.

Because the technology for hybridoma production is
rapidly evolving, the information in that document and in
this presentation is subject to change. Every effort will
be made to have the content be up to date and consistent
with the state of scientific knowledge in this area, and
each submission will continue to be reviewed on a case-
by-case basis. It should be borne in mind that all
material submitted to the FDA under IND is confidential
and is not subject to "freedom of information (FOI)"
requests. Therefore, all pertinent information which may
be helpful in evaluating the safety of a product should be
submitted.

DEVELOPMENT AND CHARACTERIZATION OF HYBRIDOMA CELL LINES

Many satisfactory technical approaches to hybridoma
establishment and propagation exist. At present, the vast
majority involve immortalization of antibody-producing
cells by chemically-induced fusion with myeloma cells.
Major emphasis has, therefore, been placed on
considerations relevant to murine systems. It is hoped
that principles discussed here may be applied to other
species and to interspecies hybrids as well. With most
applications, certain elementary data (described and
listed in Table 1) are helpful in orienting reviewers to
the monoclonal. Obviously the source and type of parent
myeloma is of importance. Its characterization with
respect to any heavy or light chains which it synthesizes

TABLE 1

DEVELOPMENT AND CHARACTERIZATION OF CELL LINES

1. Source, name, and characterization of parent immunoglobulin.
2. Strain and tissue origin of the immune cell.
3. Identification and characterization of the immunogen.
4. Description of the immunization scheme.
5. Description of the screening procedure used.
6. Description of cell cloning procedures.
7. Description of the seed lot system.

or secretes is useful. Similarly, the strain and tissue origin of the immune cell used for fusion, identification and characterization of the immunogen, description of the scheme for immunization, and screening and cell cloning procedures need to be described. Of particular importance is the description of the seed lot system used for establishing the primary and secondary lots. These seed cultures should be particularly well-characterized with respect to identity, stability, and known microbial contaminants and a description of how these seed cultures will be maintained should be included. It is thought that the presence of certain viral contamination, particularly with lymphocytic chorio-meningitis virus, reovirus, polyoma, or murine leukemia virus should disqualify the subsequent use of the seed lot for making monoclonal antibodies, but, in the absence of definitive data, controversy exists on this point.

With regard to the production procedure, a full description of the tissue culture facilities is in order as is a description of the supplier, genotype and husbandry of any animals used. In addition, the procedures used to control contamination, the acceptance criteria for cells, tissue culture supernatants, or ascites, and the procedures used to purify the final product are important. Purification steps beyond simple salt fractionation are recommended. Such steps might include size-exclusion, affinity, or ion exchange chromatography and/or ultracentrifugation. Other physical or chemical treatments which could substantially reduce problem contamination are useful if they do not interfere with the specificity of the monoclonal product. A list of desired production procedure information is given in Table 2.

TABLE 2

PRODUCTION PROCEDURES

1. Tissue culture procedure.
2. Supplier, genotype, husbandry of animals used.
3. Steps taken to control viral, bacterial, mycoplasma contamination.
4. Acceptance criteria for cells, tissue culture supernatants, or ascites.
5. Procedures used to purify the final product.
6. Procedure used to prepare and fill final containers.

QUALITY CONTROL TESTS

Monoclonal antibodies intended for in vivo use should be as free as possible of non-immunoglobulin contaminants. A definition of the measure of potency for each monoclonal antibody should be established. Steps should be taken to establish that the hybridoma secretion product remains unchanged; for example, biochemical and biophysical studies comparing the product to a retained sample of an initially well-characterized lot designated as an in-house reference standard is quite useful. An outline of quality controls which could be useful are given in Table 3. Principal among these is rigorous testing of immunologic

TABLE 3

QUALITY CONTROL TESTS

1. Immunologic specificity.
2. Stability.
3. Ig class, and subclass.
4. Isoelectric focusing.
5. Sterility.
6. Polynucleotide contamination.
7. Viruses.

specificity. Specificity should be tested after any chemical modification. Tests designed to test aggregation, denaturation and fragmentation of the immunoglobulin product should be performed. The degree of homogeneity should be established by appropriate tests. The immunoglobulin class, and when appropriate, the subclass should be determined and the isoelectric focusing pattern of the antibody in each bulk lot should be

directly compared with that of an in-house standard. The
material used should be tested for sterility and should be
free of mycoplasma. Since monoclonal products are the
products of malignant hybridoma cells and may have been
cultivated in ascites fluids, they may contain viruses
which could adversely affect human recipients. Among
the viruses which could present potential contamination
are lymphocytic choriomeningitis virus which should be
tested for by intracerebral inoculation into healthy
weanling LCM-negative mice or by isolation in cell
cultures combined with immunofluorescence. In addition,
the mouse antibody production (MAP test) should be
performed. This screening test provides information on
the presence of contamination with LCM, reovirus type III,
polyoma, Pneumonia virus of mice, Mouse adenovirus, Minute
viruses of mice, mouse hepatitis, K, Ectromelia, Sendai
and GD VII viruses. Other assay procedures which can
detect the mouse salivary gland (murine CMV), EDIM, Thymic
and LDH viruses should be performed. When these tests are
positive in the initial screening, confirmation may be
accomplished by additional approaches including complement
fixation, immunofluorescence, hemagglutination inhibition,
or enzyme-linked immunosorbant assay. Appropriately
controlled tests for murine leukemia viruses using the MCF
assay, the XC test, the S + L - test and reverse
transcriptase utilizing both Mg^{++} and Mn^{++} should be
performed. The product should be free of polynucleotides
at the lowest limit of detection currently available.
Considering that the major concerns of monoclonal antibody
products come from the transformed cell line,
hybridization analysis using nick-translated hybridoma
cell DNA seems to be particularly in order. This would
allow sensitivity on the order of 10 picograms DNA per
ml.

Validation procedures may establish that viral or
nucleic acid contaminants have been effectively excluded
from each bulk lot by the manufacturing process employed.
Spiking experiments with appropriately labeled viruses and
nucleic acids may be useful in this regard.

For the final filled product (defined as: a group of
final containers identical in all respects which have been
filled with the same product from the same bulk lot
without any change that will effect the integrity of
filling assembly) the tests listed in Table 4 should be
performed. Principally, the product should be tested for
potency and should meet established specifications. The

TABLE 4

TESTS ON FINAL FILLING

1. Potency and stability.
2. Electrophoretic migration.
3. Protein concentration.
4. Sterility.
5. General Safety.
6. Pyrogenicity (rabbit, limulus).
7. Identity.

electrophoretic migration of the product in both the native and reduced state should be measured relative to the in-house reference standard and the protein concentration should be determined by a suitable assay. The product material should pass sterility tests, general safety tests, and the rabbit pyrogen or limulus amebocyte lysate assay for the detection of pyrogens. Finally, an appropriate identity test should be designed and employed.

In addition, tests designed to detect and quantify potential contaminants such as hypotensive substances or additives (antibiotics, chromatography reagents, leachable components, preservatives) should be performed. Penicillin should not be present, but minimal concentrations of other antibiotics may be acceptable.

Pristane, if used in the preparation of ascites fluid, should be shown to be absent.

For products being investigated under IND, stability need only meet the demands imposed by the clinical protocol. In the case of product license applications, studies to support the proposed dating period should be performed on the final product. The tests should establish a valid dating period under realistic field conditions.

The extensive testing designed above is intended for patient populations that do not have life-threatening disease. In cases of life-threatening disease or in other special circumstances, less extensive testing may be justifiable. Even in patient populations with life-threatening disease, LCM virus, reovirus III, and polyoma should be absent from the final bulk lot. Special caution should be exercised when dealing with immuno-compromised patients since no data are available concerning the effects of injection of murine viruses into humans. In addition, immunosuppressive murine monoclonal antibodies

administered to heavily immunosuppressed patients may
predispose to fatal lymphoproliferative disorders and
other clinical complications.

PRECLINICAL ANIMAL TESTING

As with most injectable substances, the toxicity of
monoclonal antibodies may ordinarily be evaluated in
laboratory animals. However, anaphylaxis and other
allergic reactions may occur with xenogenic monoclonal
antibodies, as with most heterologous proteins, but no
available animal test system will adequately define these
products as non-allergenic in humans. Hence, the risk of
these reactions is best minimized by the use of well-
characterized, non-aggregated products in carefully-
designed and cautiously-implemented clinical protocols.
Toxicity studies should generally be performed on the
hybridoma product using a limited number of animals in at
least one species other than mice. The product should be
administered in the manner which gives proper attention to
the conditions of the proposed clinical testing and, where
feasible, at the actual human dose (or multiple thereof
per unit weight of the experimental animal), by the same
route, and with the same frequency. Appropriate
observations should be made that would be applicable to
the particular product.
Additional pharmacologic studies would appear useful
whenever they can be performed. Because of the peculiar
nature of some monoclonal antibody products, certain
pharmacological kinetic parameters may at times have to be
determined by human clinical studies.

PRECLINICAL LABORATORY TESTING

Monoclonal antibodies are homogeneous populations of
immunoglobulin molecules having antibody combining sites
which bind uniformly to discrete antigenic determinants.
They may be prepared in very concentrated form and may
exert highly potent effects. In some instances, the
antigenic determinant may be expressed in human cells or
tissues other than the intended target tissue, resulting
in undesirable cross reactions. Accordingly, laboratory
tests should be conducted to assess this possibility, and
when cross reactions are encountered, to evaluate the
resultant risk or hazard to potential recipients. One
approach to testing for cross reactivity is an immuno-

histological survey of human vital organs, blood
components, and target cells or tissues which can be
carried out using both frozen and chemically-fixed adult
or fetal tissue. Cross-reactivity may also be assessed in
blood cells or representative cultured cell lines by
clonogenic assays, microcytotoxicity testing, fluorescent
antibody methods, radioautography or other techniques.
When cross reactions are encountered, they should be
further studied to ascertain both their frequency and
their intensity in tissue samples in a relevant human
population.

If available, testing for <u>in vivo</u> cross reactivity
should be done in an animal system which shares the same
cross-reactive antigen or in an isolated human organ
perfusion system. When such systems are not available,
clinical studies may, nonetheless, be warranted. These
should involve extensive histopathologic evaluations where
possible and thorough bio-distribution studies with
reliably labeled samples of monoclonal antibody.

SPECIAL CONSIDERATIONS FOR MONOCLONAL ANTIBODIES
OF HUMAN ORIGIN

For human-human hybridomas, human antibody producing
lymphoblastoid cell lines, or mouse-human hybridomas it
is strongly recommended that steps which remove viruses
and DNA be taken during purification of the product. In
addition, tests should be performed at the seed lot stage
to detect the presence of viruses (Table 5). The use of a
cell line which is actively producing viruses is

TABLE 5

SPECIAL CONSIDERATIONS FOR MoAb OF HUMAN ORIGIN EBV

1. EBV
    a. EBNA, VCA.
    b. Co-cultivation with cord blood lymphocytes.
    c. DNA hybridization.
2. CMV - tissue culture assay.
3. HBV - HBsAg.
4. Retroviruses.
    a. Reverse transcriptase.
    b. Electron microscopy.
    c. HTLV (when available).
5. Tissue culture safety test.

discouraged. For Epstein-Barr (EB) virus, a serological
test for nuclear antigen (EBNA) should be done unless the
line is known to harbor EBV. If the line is positive for
EBV, tests for antigens known to be associated with virus
and, in addition, an assay of supernatants or irradiated
cells by cultivation with cord blood lymphocytes for 12
weeks are in order. Similarly, a DNA hybridization study
at a sensitivity capable of detecting at least one EBV
genome copy per cell should be performed on the
supernatant. A 6 week tissue culture assay with a blind
subpassage at 3 to 4 weeks in a human diploid fibroblast
line should be employed to exclude the presence of
cytomegaloviruses. A third generation test licensed for
HBsAg should be done. Of particular concern at present is
the possible presence of retroviruses. Currently reverse
transcriptase assays using both $Mg++$ and $Mn++$ may be in
order, along with competent electron microscopy on at
least 200 cells. A test for human retrovirus is probably
imminent and, if a licensed test becomes available, it
should be employed. Furthermore, a tissue culture safety
test to detect other contaminating viruses could be
performed with a series of established cell lines. These
cell lines should include human diploid cells, human
transformed cells such as Hela, simian cell lines such as
Vero and the monoclonal-producing cell line itself. A
culture should be observed for the presence of changes
attributable to growth of adventitious viral agents
including hemadsorbing viral agents.

SUMMARY AND CONCLUSION

The Office of Biologics Research and Review advocates
the use of monoclonal antibodies and other hybridoma-
derived products under conditions where optimal benefit
risk ratios are achievable. Addressing the points
outlined here would seem to be a rational, attainable, and
economically feasible endeavor for the vast majority of
individuals intent on employing these products in humans.
They are not intended, however, to obviate or supplant
sound scientific and ethical principles. In our opinion,
the use of highly purified products with optimal
specificity as established by rigorous and copious
experimental data represents the best possibility of
ensuring their efficacious and therapeutic use.

ACKNOWLEDGMENTS

The Hybridoma Committee of the Office of Biologics Research and Review has been instrumental in forming the considerations enumerated here. Dr. Bruce Merchant, its former chairman, provided helpful advice. Mrs. Sandra Fulmer typed the manuscript.

IX. MONOCLONAL ANTIBODY-RADIONUCLIDE CONJUGATES

Monoclonal Antibodies and Cancer Therapy, pages 443–472
© 1985 Alan R. Liss, Inc.

BIOCHEMICAL EFFECTS AND CANCER THERAPEUTIC POTENTIAL
OF TUNICAMYCIN

Kenneth Olden[1,3], Martin J. Humphries[1,3] and
Sandra L. White[1,2]

Howard University Medical School, [1]Cancer Center
and Department of Oncology, and
[2]Department of Microbiology, Washington, D.C. 20060.
[3]Membrane Biochemistry Section,
Laboratory of Molecular Biology, National Cancer Institute,
National Institutes of Health, Bethesda, MD. 20205.

ABSTRACT Tumor metastasis apparently involves a
number of distinct steps, many of which are thought to
be mediated by surface glycoconjugants, and some of
the changes in cell surface glycoconjugants that occur
in association with oncogenic transformation may be
related to the ability of tumor cells to metastasize.
Therefore, by modifying the structure or preventing
the biosynthesis of specific glycan components, it
should be possible to interfere with growth and metastasis of tumor cells. Firstly, we have examined the
effect of tunicamycin (TM), an inhibitor of the
synthesis of the glycan moiety of asparagine-linked
glycoproteins, on the viability of transformed fibroblasts in culture. Secondly, this drug has been used
to investigate the role of surface glycoconjugants in
tumorigenesis and/or metastasis using L1210 leukemic
cells and B16 melanoma. We find that TM (0.04 µg/ml)
is cytotoxic toward a variety of transformed cell
lines, including virally or chemically transformed
fibroblasts from chicken embryo, rat kidney, human lung
and mouse. The corresponding nontransformed cell lines
were resistant to the same and even a 10 fold higher
concentration of TM. The relationship between trans-

This work is supported by a grant (R01/CA-34918) from
the National Institutes of Health.

formation and TM cytotoxicity was strengthened by the
finding that chicken embryo fibroblasts, infected with
temperature-sensitive viral mutants, are killed by the
drug only at the temperature permissive for transformation. There is a direct correlation between the
susceptibility of transformed cells to TM cytotoxicity
and sensitivity to inhibition of protein glycosylation,
sugar and amino acid transport, and glucose metabolism.
For example, L-929 mouse fibroblasts are not killed by
TM (1.2-1. μ g/ml), and synthesis of glycoprotein is not
inhibited. Membrane fractions prepared from normal
and TM-sensitive transformed cells showed similar
activities with respect to formation of lipid-linked
N-acetylglucosamine per mg of protein, indicating that
this is not the molecular basis for the hypersensitivity of transformed cells. We suggest that the
selective cytotoxicity of TM for transformed cells is
related to decreased glucose metabolism due to impairment in uptake of nutrients. TM treatment altered
cell surface morphology with increased numbers of microvilli and blebs, and reduced adhesion to collagen
and fibronectin matrices. Also, transformed fibroblasts, pretreated with TM in vitro, were less
tumorigenic when implanted subcutaneously. Similarly,
mice receiving inoculations of L1210 leukemic cells
pretreated with TM (16 µg/ml) in vitro survived almost
twice (18-20 days) as long as those receiving implants
of untreated cells. Additionally, mice receiving an
initial inoculum of TM pretreated cells survived subsequent challenges with untreated L1210 ascites cells.
Similar survival results were obtained with mice
receiving intravenous implants of TM-treated B16
melanoma, consistent with the finding that their lung
colonization potential was markedly reduced. Finally,
preliminary studies suggest that TM-pretreatment of
highly metastatic tumor cell lines in vitro markedly
decreases their metastatic potential. Our results
suggest that TM may be therapeutically useful as an
anti-tumor agent to (i) selectively kill certain types
of malignant cells, (ii) to reduce tumorigenicity
possibly by enhancing the immunogenicity of the tumor
cells in vivo, or (iii) to inhibit metastasis by
impairment of recognitional events essential for this
process.

INTRODUCTION

The sugar moieties of surface glycoconjugants may play important roles in the interaction of metastatic cells with receptor proteins of the vascular endothelium and in the expression of target organ specificity. For example, alterations in the structural features of carbohydrate moieties of surface glycoconjugants are among the most consistent biochemical changes associated with oncogenic transformation (reviewed in references 1 and 2). The most prominent changes are (i) increased sialylation of oligo-saccharides, (ii) an increase in the size of glycopeptides, (iii) incomplete processing of asparagine-linked oligo-saccharides, (iv) increased activity of various glycosyl-transferases and glycosidases, and (v) a loss of certain glycoproteins. Comparison of the carbohydrate composition of membrane glycoproteins from 3T3 and SV40-transformed 3T3 cells showed that the glycoproteins from the transformed cells contained less sialic acid and galactosamine, and more glucosamine than the comparable fractions from non-transformed cells (3). Similar results were obtained when hamster cells were transformed by polyoma virus or hamster sarcoma virus (4). In contrast, Warren and coworkers (5) have reported that glycopeptides isolated from pronase digests of virally transformed cells had an increased amount of sialic acid, which they attributed to increased activity of sialyl transferase in the transformed cells. Further analyses of glycopeptides from the virally transformed hamster cells showed that they also contained increased amounts of sialic acid, galactose and mannose, suggesting that the glycoproteins were more highly glycosylated.

The occurrence of highly branched complex-type oligo-saccharides has been observed in a number of biological systems in vivo and in vitro which include solid tumors (6, 7), human leukemias (8), and cells transformed by various oncogenic agents (9-13). Recent studies on the influence of cell transformation on the glycosylation of viral enve-lope glycoproteins have shown that the major difference, attributable to transformation, was an increase in the relative amount of larger acidic-type oligosaccharides containing additional branch sugars (NeuNAc-Gal-GlcNAc-) (14). Similar results were obtained by comparing fibro-nectins from normal and virally transformed hamster cells (15). Glycosylated proteolytic fragments from transformed cell fibronectin were larger than those from normal cell fibronectin, and fibronectin from transformed cells had more branches per core and more sialic acid residues. The findings that transformed cells contained glycoproteins enriched in triantennary and/or tetrantennary structures versus biantennary structures are consistent with a transformation-associated increase in the extent of intracellular processing of a common precursor structure for the asparagine-linked oligosaccharides.

While most studies have shown that the carbohydrate moieties of glycoproteins from transformed cells are larger and more highly processed, this pattern is not always found. Specific glycoproteins from transformed cells have been identified which have more of the high-mannose type oligosaccharides than their normal counterpart and may represent less fully processed molecules than the glycoproteins from normal cells (16, 17). Because of these apparent inconsistencies, it may be that transformed cells exhibit a variety of alterations in their oligosaccharide synthesis and processing pathways, depending on the growth rate, cell type and state of differentiation. Perhaps the addition of extra sialic acid and/or more branch oligosaccharides may be an early oncogenic event, whereas the less well differentiated, more highly malignant, rapidly dividing cell types do not have time to finish the processing of their oligosaccharide chains to the complex structure. The finding that mouse embryonal teratocarcinoma cells have large fucose-containing glycopeptides which disappear during differentiation is consistent with the view that alterations in carbohydrates may be related to the state of differentiation (18).

The role of surface glycoconjugants in metastases of tumor cells is unknown, but it is thought that some of the changes in cell surface glycoconjugants that occur in association with oncogenic transformation may be involved in the formation of distant metastases. Highly metastatic tumor cells often differ from low-metastatic and benign tumors in expression of cell surface glycoconjugants. Evidence that these molecules control the expression of metastatic potential comes from the elegant experiments of Poste and Nicolson (19) in which they fused membranes originating from cells with high and low metastatic potentials. Significantly, the cells with the "hybrid" membranes were modified with respect to the formation of experimental metastasis. However, the functional significance, if any, of the alterations in carbohydrate moieties of surface glycoconjugants of transformed cells has not been widely examined. For instance, do the changes in structure of the oligosaccharides confer some selective advantage to the cell upon transformation? If altered or specific glycan structures are required for survival of transformed cells or for their invasion and metastasis, then one should be able to interfere with these processes by (i) preventing the glycosylation of glycoconjugants, and (ii) modifying the structure of the glycan moieties of these macromolecules.

Tumor cells depleted of the glycan moieties of surface glycoconjugants may be more immunogenic than unmodified transformed cells, hence may represent an experimental approach for immunization of animals against cancers. Previous attempts to potentiate the immune response, including nonspecific stimulation with a variety of biological or synthetic products (20), transfer of specific antitumor-immune lymphocytes (21), immunization with syngeneic target tumor (22), and sensitization with neuraminidase-treated syngeneic tumor cells (23) have all been generally unsuccessful.

Asparagine residues of glycoproteins are glycosylated by the en bloc transfer of $Glc_3Man_9GlcNAc_2$ from the lipid precursor to the nascent polypeptide in the rough endoplasmic reticulum (RER) (24). As the glycoproteins are transported through the ER, the glucose residues are removed by glucosidase I and II (25). Further processing can occur in the Golgi where α-mannosidase I and II exist, and in some instances high mannose oligosaccharides are converted to the complex glycan structure consisting of such peripheral sugars as GlcNAc, galactose, and sialic acid.

The studies to be described here were initiated to address three questions. We were interested in (i) whether N-linked surface glycoconjugants are required for survival of transformed cells in culture, and whether inhibition of glycosylation would (ii) affect tumorigenicity or metastasis, or (iii) enhance the immunogenicity of tumor cells in vivo. We are currently using tunicamycin, an inhibitor of protein glycosylation, to investigate these questions. Tunicamycin is a structural analog of UDP-2-acetamide-2-deoxy-D-glucose, and blocks the initial step in the glycosylation of the lipid intermediate in the assembly of core glycans linked to protein by N-glycosidic bonds (26-28).

The results described here demonstrate that N-linked surface glycoconjugants are required for the survival of transformed cells in culture, and that the decrease in

viability noted in their absence is probably due to an
impairment of nutrient uptake and metabolism. While tunicamycin administration to animals was found to be too toxic
for practical application in cancer chemotherapy, treatment
of tumor cells with this drug in vitro provides a new and
rational approach for eradication of metastasis. Furthermore, unlike most agents currently used in cancer chemotherapy, specific inhibitors of glycosylation would not
suppress the immune system. The studies with mouse tumor
models indicate that tunicamycin-treated cells are (i) less
metastatic, and (ii) more immunogenic than their untreated
counterparts when transplanted into syngeneic mice.

MATERIALS AND METHODS

Cell Culture

The nontransformed cell lines used in this study were
secondary chicken embryo fibroblasts (CEF) and permanent
tissue culture cell lines obtained from rat kidney (NRK),
mouse embryo (Balb/c 3T3), and human embryonic lung (WI-38).
CEF were transformed by infection with Bryan high-titer
(BH), Schmidt-Ruppin (SR), or temperature-sensitive mutant
strains of Rous sarcoma virus ts68 (from Drs. S. Kawai and
H. Hanafusa) (29) or T5 (from Dr. G. Martin) (30). Rat
kidney fibroblasts were transformed with murine sarcoma
(Kirsten-KNRK) and Moloney (MNRK) virus (obtained from
Dr. E. Scolnick). The VA-13 subline of human WI-38 cells,
transformed by SV40, was obtained from Dr. M. Bradley.
Balb/c 3T3 cells, transformed by radiation (R_1Cl_3), methyl-
cholanthrene (MC5-5) and viruses (Kirsten, KA_3Cl_3; Moloney,
Mol/Balb) were obtained from Dr. G. Todaro. The SV_1 tumor
cell line was obtained as previously described (31). All
cells were grown with or without TM (0.04-1.6 μ g/ml) in
Dulbecco-Vogt modified Eagle's minimal essential medium
(DMEM) or in Hams F10 medium supplemented with 10% tryptose
phosphate broth, 5% heat-inactivated calf serum, and 0.05%
sodium bicarbonate. Both media contained 50 IU/ml penicillin, 50 μ g/ml streptomycin and 2 mM glutamine, and cells
were cultured in 35 mm plastic tissue culture dishes
(Costar) at 37°C as described previously (32).

Transplantation of Ascites L1210 Leukemia Cells

L1210 ascites, obtained from Dr. David Cooney of the
National Cancer Institute of the NIH, were maintained in
ascites by passage in DBA/2 mice. For experiments, L1210
ascites cells were collected from mice under aseptic conditions by peritoneal lavage with cold Dulbecco's phosphate
buffered saline (DPBS), washed three times by resuspension
and centrifugation for 5 min at 800 x g. After the final
wash the cells were resuspended to a density of 10^{5-6}
cells/ml in serum free RPMI 1640 medium supplemented with
HEPES buffer (20 mM), pH 7.5, penicillin (50 units/ml) and
streptomycin (50 μ g/ml). Aliquots (2.0 ml) of the cell
suspension were added to tissue culture dishes containing
TM and incubated for varying intervals at 37°C in a humidified atmosphere of 95% air and 5% CO_2. After exposure in
vitro to TM, the L1210 cells of each dosage group were
washed three times with RPMI 1640, the percentage of
viable cells was routinely determined by trypan blue
exclusion and 0.2 ml aliquots containing 10^{5-6} viable cells
were injected into the peritoneal cavity of immunocompetent
mice. Animals were monitored for survival on a daily basis.
Those that were tumor-free 30-35 days after injection were
classified as long term survivors, and were rechallenged
with 10^{5-6} viable L1210 cells which had not been treated
with TM.

Transplantation of B16 Melanoma

Murine B16 melanoma sublines of low (B16F1) and high
(B16F10) lung colonizing potential were obtained from
Dr. I.J. Fidler of the M.D. Anderson Tumor Institute. Low
passage (fewer than 8) cells were cultured in DMEM (Grand
Island Biological Co. GIBCO, Grand Island, N.Y.) supplemented with 5% heat inactivated fetal bovine serum (Flow
laboratories, Inglewood, CA.) in a humidified atmosphere of
95% air and 5% CO_2 at 37°C. Subconfluent cell cultures
were harvested by treatment for 1.5 minutes with 2 mM EDTA
in Ca^{2+}, Mg^{2+}-free DPBS. The cells were washed twice by
alternate centrifugation and resuspension in serum-free
DMEM prior to intraperitoneal (i.p.) or intravenous (i.v.)
injection of 10^{5-6} cells. The washed cell suspensions
(10^{5-6} viable cells/ml) in DMEM were kept on ice until
injected into mice. Viability was monitored by trypan blue
exclusion, cloning efficiency, and by pulse labeling with
$[^{35}S]$-methionine (spec. act. 1000 Ci/mmol) (New England

Nuclear) after 18 hr treatment with tunicamycin. Female
C57BL/6 mice (Charles River, Kingston, MD.), 6 to 8 weeks
old, were injected i.v. or i.p. with 10^5 tunicamycin treated
or untreated viable cells. The mice were sacrificed on day
14-20 and the number of lung colonies were counted. Organs
other than lung were also monitored for metastasis.

Transplantation of Rous Sarcoma Virus Transformed Balb/c
3T3 cells

Newborn and Weanling Balb/c 3T3 mice were inoculated
subcutaneously with 0.2 ml aliquots containing 10^{5-7} TM
treated Rous sarcoma virus transformed cells, and animals
were observed at weekly intervals for the appearance of
subcutaneous tumors at the site of inoculation. Nodules of
5 mm or larger in diameter (approximately 2 weeks) were
scored as positive, and tumors of this size continued to
grow to reach a size of approximately 20 mm by 8 weeks and
eventually killed the animal. Mice without tumors by the
end of 8 weeks were scored as negative, but were monitored
for 8 more weeks.

Transport of Sugar and Amino Acid Analogues

To measure the rate of glucose uptake, the medium was
aspirated and replaced with fresh growth medium containing
0.5 uCi/ml $[^{14}C]$ 2-deoxy-D-glucose (0.25 mM) (a nonmetaboli-
zable glucose analogue). After incubation at 23°C for
5 min, the medium was decanted and cells were rapidly
washed three times with ice cold DPBS containing Ca^{2+} and
Mg^{2+}. The cells were homogenized in 2% SDS (sodium dodecyl
sulfate) prepared in 10 mM sodium phosphate, pH 7.0, and
heated for 2 min at 100°C, then total radioactivity was
determined by liquid scintillation spectrometry. Alternatively, free intracellular radiolabeled substrate was
extracted with ice-cold 10% trichloroacetic acid, neutralized and counted in Aquasol (New England Nuclear). The
results of these two procedures were identical, and uptake
was linear for at least 10 min.

Glucose Metabolism

The rate of glucose metabolism was measured by a
modification of the Umbriet procedure (33) by determining
the amount of CO_2 released in 30 min assays with $[^{14}C]$

(U)-D-glucose (0.5 uCi/ml) as substrate (34). Cultures in
fresh growth medium were placed in air-tight chambers, and
the reaction was initiated by adding radiolabeled glucose
with a 25 gauge needle through a re-sealable port. The
reaction was terminated by adding concentrated sulfuric
acid. The respiration chamber was pressurized to force the
liberated CO_2 out of the chamber into a Hyamine hydroxide
trap. The efficiency of CO_2 recovery was greater than 97%
(34).

Attachment Assay

    Cell attachment was performed according to the
procedure described by Klebe (45). Cells were labeled for
24 hr with [^{3}H]-thymidine (1 mCi/ml, spec. act. 15 Ci/mmol).
Cycloheximide (5 ug/ml) was added to the TM-treated and
untreated cultures 2 hr prior to detachment with EDTA, and
was included in both the wash buffer and cell attachment
medium (DMEM supplemented with bovine serum albumin at a
concentration of 200 ug/ml). A 1 ml suspension, containing
10^5 cells, was added to 35 mm dishes coated with a mixture
of laminin and collagen (type IV), at concentrations of
1 ug/ml and 5 ug/ml respectively, and incubated at 37°C for
up to 120 min. The medium containing the unattached cells
was removed, the attached cells were harvested by incubation
with EDTA (0.01%), and the number of cells were estimated.

Chemicals

    TM was a gift from Dr. Gakuza Tamura via the Drug
Evaluation Branch of the National Cancer Institute. The
radiochemicals [^{14}C] (U)-L-leucine (spec. act. 325 mCi/
mmol), 2,1-[^{14}C]-deoxy-D-glucose (spec. act. 212 mCi/mmol),
[^{14}C] (U)-D-glucose (spec. act. 54 mCi/mmol), [^{35}S]-
methionine (spec. act. 1000 Ci/mmol) and 2-[^{3}H](N)-D-
mannose (spec. act. 18 Ci/mmol) were obtained from New
England Nuclear.

Protein Determinations

    Protein determinations were performed according to the
procedure of Lowry et al. (35) with bovine serum albumin as
standard.

RESULTS

Effect of Tunicamycin on Cell Morphology and Viability

     To examine the cytotoxic effects of TM on normal and transformed cells, cultures were incubated for 36 hr in medium with or without 0.05 ug/ml TM. Viability was monitored (i) by the capacity of the cells to exclude trypan blue, (ii) by their plating efficiency, and (iii) by their capacity to resume normal growth following TM treatment. When treated with TM, most of the transformed cell lines acquired a more rounded morphology and subsequently detached from the culture dish (shown in figure 1). The detached cells stained with trypan blue and did not re-attach when subcultured in fresh medium without TM nor form colonies when plated at a density of 2,000 cells per 50 cm^2 dish and cultured for 10 days. The few cells remaining attached to the dish after TM pretreatment were also shown to be irreversibly damaged by trypan blue staining and absence of colony formation. Cells cannot be stained with trypan blue unless there is a complete cessation of metabolism (36, 37).

     The results shown in figure 2 indicate that the majority of the transformed cells examined were killed by TM treatment with an LD50 (not shown) of 0.02 to 0.035 ug/ml. However, four of the transformed cell lines (KNRK, L-929, and R_1Cl_3 and $KaCl_3$ Balb/c 3T3) were resistant to TM killing and inhibition of protein glycosylation at the concentration of TM used in these experiments. In fact, L-929 cells were resistant to TM killing even at a concentration of 2.0 ug/ml for 36 hr.; however, the cells acquired a rounded morphology (figure 1, Panel B). We have shown in subsequent studies that L-929 cells have an elevated level of GlcNAc transferase relative to the other cell lines used in the present survey, which might account for the apparent resistance of this cell line. Killing by TM is not due to viral infection per se since virally infected chicken embryo fibroblasts (T5-CEF and ts 68-CEF) are sensitive only at the temperature (36°C) permissive for transformation (figure 2). Also, there is no correlation between the transforming agent used (virus, chemical, or radiation) and sensitivity to TM. The nontransformed cell lines were uniformly resistant to TM killing (figures 1 and 2) even after treatment for 72 hrs. Except for 3T3 cells, the growth rate of which was markedly decreased, tunica-

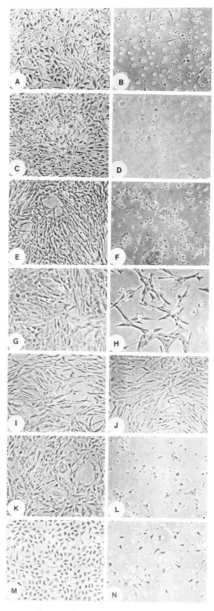

Figure 1. Effect of tunicamycin on normal and transformed
cells in culture. Shown are phase-contrast micrographs of
untreated cultures (left panels) and cultures treated with
tunicamycin (right panels). Tunicamycin concentration of
2.0 ug/ml was used in cultures shown in panels A and B, and
0.05 ug/ml was used in cultures shown in the remaining panels.

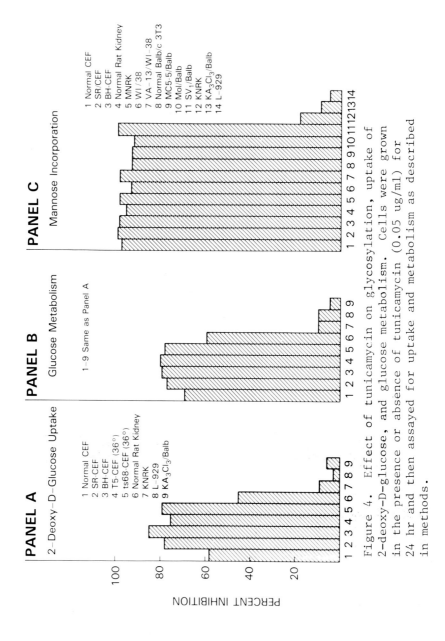

Figure 4. Effect of tunicamycin on glycosylation, uptake of 2-deoxy-D-glucose, and glucose metabolism. Cells were grown in the presence or absence of tunicamycin (0.05 ug/ml) for 24 hr and then assayed for uptake and metabolism as described in methods.

mycin only slightly inhibited (17-25%) the growth of the
non-transformed cells. However, the non-transformed cells
acquired an elongated, spindle-shaped morphology with
numerous surface blebs and microvilli after 36 h treatment
with tunicamycin (figure 3). Other non-transformed cells
examined, for which transformed counterparts were not
available (chick embryo myoblasts, myotubes, chondrocytes,
and neural crest cells) were also not killed by tunicamycin.
Nontransformed cells were also resistant to higher dosages
of TM (2 ug/ml) for up to 36 h of treatment; however, the
resistance of normal cells is not similar to that of transformed cells as glycosylation is strongly inhibited
(figure 4, Panel C).

Normal growth rate and morphology were restored in
24 h following the removal of tunicamycin (0.05 ug/ml,
24 hr pretreatment) from the medium of non-transformed CEF.
Altered levels of cAMP and/or fibronectin which are known
to affect cell adhesion (38, 39), do not appear to be
responsible for the changes induced by tunicamycin treatment since their presence in the culture medium during
incubation with the drug (36 h), at concentrations of
1.5 mM (dibutyryl cAMP) and 50 ug/ml respectively, failed
to inhibit or reverse the cytotoxic effects. All the
results reported here were obtained using subconfluent
monolayer cultures in the logarithmic phase of growth.
However, the cytotoxicity is independent of cell density
since both sparse and confluent cultures were similarly
affected by tunicamycin treatment.

In other experiments medium containing tunicamycin
was changed at 6 h intervals on normal and transformed CEF
and the glucose concentration was increased from 5 to 100
mM to test the possibility that tunicamycin cytotoxicity
was due to the accumulation of toxic metabolites, or to the
exhaustion of metabolic substrate from the media. These
alterations did not prevent the effects of tunicamycin on
the cell lines tested.

Two other inhibitors of glycosylation (D-glucosamine
and 2-deoxy-D-glucose) were tested at doses of 20 mM and
10 mM, respectively, to determine whether they were also
cytotoxic towards transformed cells. At these concentrations, treatment with both inhibitors also resulted in
a 93-99% decrease in cell viability (results not shown).
However, results with these analogues are difficult to
interpret since they affect several metabolic processes
(22, 40-42).

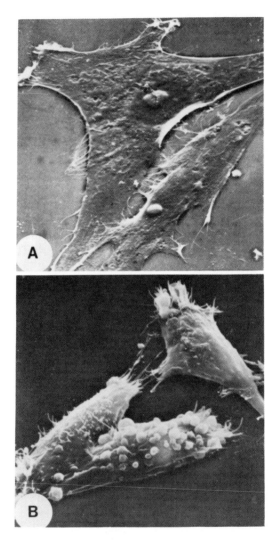

Figure 3. Effect of tunicamycin on the surface morphology
of chicken embryo fibroblasts. Shown are scanning electron
micrographs of untreated (A) and tunicamycin (0.05 ug/ml)-
treated (panel B) cells. Cells were treated with the drug
for 48 hrs. Untreated and treated cells are shown at
magnifications of 1000 and 2000 respectively.

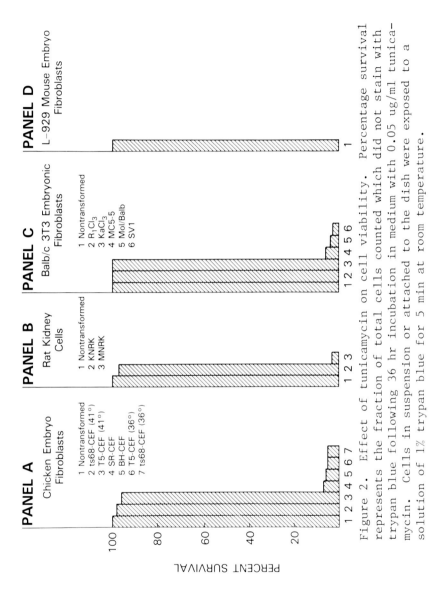

Figure 2. Effect of tunicamycin on cell viability. Percentage survival represents the fraction of total cells counted which did not stain with trypan blue following 36 hr incubation in medium with 0.05 ug/ml tunicamycin. Cells in suspension or attached to the dish were exposed to a solution of 1% trypan blue for 5 min at room temperature.

To investigate the effects of tunicamycin on protein glycosylation in normal and transformed cells, cultures were preincubated for 6 h in medium with or without 0.05 ug/ml of the drug, then 2-[^{3}H]-mannose was added and cultures were incubated for another 3 h. Cells were extracted with 10% trichloroacetic acid, homogenized in 1% SDS and amounts of radioactivity in the homogenates were determined. As shown in figure 4, there was a marked inhibition (93-99%) of incorporation of mannose into acid-precipitable macromolecules of both non-transformed and tunicamycin-sensitive transformed cells, but only a slight inhibition of protein glycosylation in the tunicamycin-resistant transformed cells (KNRK, KA$_3$Cl$_3$, and L-929). The reduction in leucine incorporation into protein ranged from 3% to 27% and did not correlate with tunicamycin cytotoxicity (result not shown). Previous studies in our laboratory have shown that TM also inhibits synthesis of sulfated proteoglycans (44). These results suggest that a marked inhibition of glycosylation is required for tunicamycin cytotoxicity towards transformed cells.

Since tunicamycin was found to be toxic to transformed cells at doses similar to those reported to inhibit protein glycosylation and nutrient uptake (34, 43), we suspected that there might be a correlation between nutrient uptake and tunicamycin cytotoxicity. Therefore, uptake of 2-deoxy-D-glucose and glucose metabolism were measured in untreated and tunicamycin treated cells to see if there was a relationship between these metabolic events and sensitivity to this drug. It is apparent from inspection of figure 4 that there is a correlation between glucose uptake and metabolism and sensitivity of the transformed cells to tunicamycin, however such a correlation is not found for nontransformed cells. The transport of 2-deoxy-D-glucose and glucose metabolism were both inhibited 2- to 4-fold in non-transformed CEF and 3- to 5-fold in the tunicamycin-sensitive transformed chick cells (figure 4). However, neither process was significantly affected in L-929 or other transformed cells, which were also resistant to tunicamycin cytotoxicity. A similar inhibition of uptake of α-amino-isobutyric acid and uridine (not shown) was observed in the tunicamycin treated cells. These results suggest that the rapid uptake and metabolism of glucose or other metabolic energy sources are critical for the survival of nontransformed cells, and the decrease in transport is somehow related to inhibition of protein glycosylation. We had previously shown by kinetic analysis

that the Km for glucose uptake was unaltered, but that the
actual number of functional carrier molecules was decreased
(43).

Lung Colonization Potential of Tunicamycin Treated B16
Melanoma

To investigate the possible involvement of carbohydrate moieties of surface glycoconjugants in the recognitional events associated with metastasis and invasion,
we chose a highly metastatic F10 variant of B16 melanoma
as it represents an animal tumor model that mimics clinical
metastatic diseases (46). We measured the capacity of TM-
treated and untreated cells to colonize the lung following
discharge into the blood vascular system. Since clearance
and accumulation of F10 cells in the lung occurs within
the first few minutes following injection (50), the cells
depleted of N-linked surface glycoconjugants may be com-
promised with respect to escape from the blood vascular
system and accumulation in the specific target organ.
For these studies monolayer cultures of B16 melanoma
were treated with various concentrations of TM for 24 hr,
detached, harvested, injected into syngeneic mice, and the
number of colonies in the lungs was scored with the aid of
a dissecting scope. It is apparent from inspection of the
data shown in figures 5 and 6 that there is a direct
relationship between tunicamycin concentration, percent
inhibition of glycosylation and lung colony formation with
almost complete inhibition of the latter two processes at
the highest concentration of the drug. The decrease in the
number of colonies was not due to the formation of extra-
pulmonary metastasis as tumor colonies were not found in
other organs. Also, the TM-modified cells still retained
the capacity of tumorigenesis as large tumor masses
developed following injection into the peritoneal cavity of
irradiated mice, and the time required for the tumor to
kill the host was not significantly different from the
control.

Adhesion of B16 Melanoma to Extracellular Matrix Proteins

Since fibronectin, laminin and collagens (types IV and
V) are major glycoproteins of the basal lamina matrix of
capillary endothelial cells (47, 48), we examined the
adhesion of TM-treated cells to matrices composed of
mixtures of these glycoproteins. TM-treated and untreated

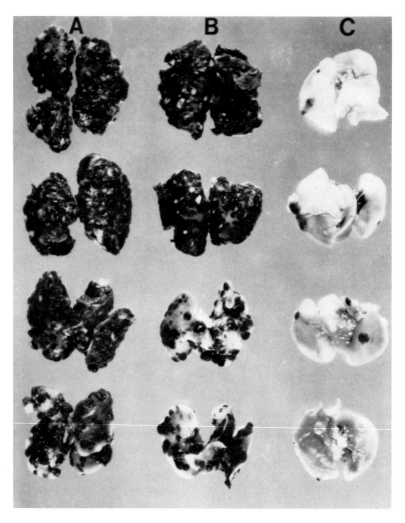

Figure 5. Effect of tunicamycin on lung colonization
potential of B16 melanoma.

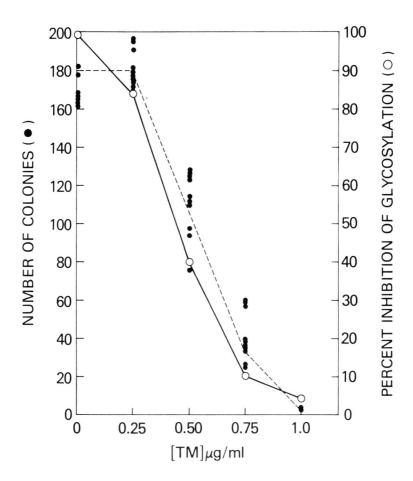

Figure 6.   Effect of tunicamycin on glycosylation and lung colonization potential of B16 melanoma.   Cells were incubated with or without tunicamycin for 18 hr in medium containing 2 uCi/ml [2-3H]-mannose, and cells, grown in a parallel experiment without 3H-mannose, were injected i.v. as described in methods.

cells were radiolabeled with ^{3}H-thymidine, and were
harvested by treatment with 2 mM EDTA prepared in Ca^{+2},
Mg^{+2}free DPBS, washed 3 times with DMEM containing 1%
bovine serum albumin, suspended in the same solution at
10^5 cells/ml, and the kinetics of adhesion was measured.
From inspection of the time course of adhesion (shown in
figure 7), it is apparent that there is as much as a 2-3
fold difference in the rate of adhesion between untreated
and TM-treated cells. This is consistent with the earlier
results reported by Irimura and coworkers (49), in which
they examined adhesion of several B16 melanoma variants to
vascular endothelial cell monolayers. These results
suggest that the TM-modified cells are less capable of
binding to specific receptor proteins than their untreated
counterparts.

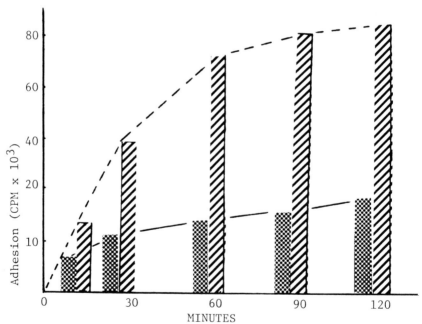

Figure 6.   Effect of tunicamycin pretreatment on cell
attachment. Procedures are described in methods.

Tumorigenicity of Tunicamycin-Modified L1210 Murine
Leukemia Cell

To examine the effect of TM-treatment on the
tumorigenicity L1210 cells were incubated with various
concentrations of the drug for 24 hr, then 10^5 viable cells
were injected into the peritoneal cavity of DBA/2 mice.
The results shown in table 1 indicates that the survival
of mice receiving implants of TM-treated cells was significantly longer than the survival of those which were
injected with an equal number of untreated cells. The
increase in survival was not due to the inability of the
TM-modified cells to form tumors as mice which received a
nonlethal dose (375 rad) of x-irradiation, prior to implantation of the TM-treated cells, developed large tumor
masses in 10-12 days and died with a mean survival time of
12-16 days (table 2). These results suggest that treatment
of the tumor cells with TM enhances their immunogenicity
without decreasing their tumorigenicity. However, the
host immune effector mechanism(s) has not been identified.

Table 1
SURVIVAL OF DBA/2 MICE FOLLOWING INJECTION
OF TUNICAMYCIN TREATED L1210 CELLS

Group	Concentration of Tunicamycin	Mean Survival (Days)
A	0	8-10
B	0.8 ug/ml	15-17
C	4 ug/ml	21-27
D	8 µ g/ml	35 (Three mice had not died when the exper- iment was terminated on day 45.)

There were 10 mice per group, and the data shown is representative of the average of three experiments. The three
survivors of group D were challenged with 10^5 viable,
untreated cells; one died on day 14, another on day 23, and
the third one day 29. TM treatment was for 24 hr.

Table 2

SURVIVAL OF IRRADIATED DBA/2 MICE FOLLOWING INJECTION OF
TUNICAMYCIN TREATED L1210 CELLS

Concentration of Tunicamycin	Mean Survival (Days)
0	8-10
0.8 μg/ml	8-10
4 ug/ml	10-14
10 ug/ml	12-18

There were 10 mice in each experimental group, and the
data represents the average of two separate experiments.
Mice were exposed to 375 rads of irradiation for 16 hr.

DISCUSSION

Transformed cells can be distinguished from nontransformed cells on the basis of the structures of their cell
surface glycoconjugants. If these alterations are involved
in metastasis and invasion of malignant cells, then agents
which modify the surface glycoconjugants of transformed
cells may be potentially useful in cancer chemotherapy.
In the present study we have used TM to prevent the glycosylation of N-linked surface glycoproteins to assess their
role in neoplastic transformation. The results presented
here suggest that carbohydrates are important for the
survival, adhesion and metastasis of transformed cells.
For example, we have shown that low concentrations of TM
are cytotoxic toward most, though not all, of the transformed cell lines tested; similar concentrations are
without effect on their nontransformed counterparts. The
effect on transformed cells is not related to the nature
of the transforming agent nor solely to the presence of
the transforming virus as cells transformed by diverse
agents (chemicals, radiation, viruses) are killed by TM,
and cells infected by the temperature-sensitive viral
mutants ts68 and T5 are subject to TM cytotoxicity only at
the temperature permissive for transformation.
Analysis of protein glycosylation, nutrient transport
and glucose metabolism reveal a correlation between inhibition of these metabolic events and sensitivity of

transformed cell to TM; that is, glycosylation and glucose
uptake and metabolism are not strongly inhibited in the
TM-resistant transformed cell lines, but are strongly
inhibited in those transformed cell lines killed by TM-
treatment. The resistance of the four transformed cell
lines (KNRK, R_1Cl_3- and Ka_3Cl_3-3T3, and L-929) is probably
a reflection of either strain specific differences in
permeability to this antibiotic or to enhanced levels of
N-acetylglucosamine glycosyltransferase as shown using
extracts of L-929 cells. However, the resistance of non-
transformed cells is not due to lack of inhibition of
glycosylation, nutrient uptake nor glucose metabolism
since these processes are strongly inhibited. The selective cytotoxicity of TM toward transformed cells suggests
that these cells cannot survive the reduced glycolytic
state brought on by the decrease in the number of functional glucose transport glycoproteins. This suggestion
is compatible with the findings that tumor cells exhibit
high aerobic glycolysis (51-54).

Following TM-treatment there is an apparent difference
in the malignancy of L1210 leukemia cells and B16 melanoma
as defined by the increased mean survival time of the
recipient hosts (DBA/2 and C57BL/6 mice). The fact that
TM-treated cells kill X-irradiated hosts with a mean
survival time similar to that found for untreated cells
suggest that exposure to the antibiotic increases the
immunogenicity of the tumor cells. This is substantiated
by the additional finding that some of the long term
survivors following injection of TM were resistant to a
subsequent challenge of untreated L-1210 cells.

The studies with B16 melanoma indicate that N-linked
oligosaccharide moieties are important in escape from the
blood vascular system, colonization of the lung, and in
adhesion to collagen/fibronectin matrix. Preliminary
results with swainsonine, an inhibitor of Golgi α-manno-
sidase II, suggest that N-linked oligosaccharides play a
direct and specific role since conversion from complex to
the hybrid-type oligosaccharide structure prevents lung
colonization of B16 melanoma (M. Humphries, S. White and
K. Olden, unpublished results). Additionally, the specific
oligosaccharide structure is apparently required for an
early step in extravasation or colonization since the
effects of TM are reversible in 24 to 36 hr. Of course,
the assumption made in the present studies with TM is that
the deglycosylated proteins are expressed on the cell
surface - a view which is consistent with our finding that

surface-labeled polypeptide band patterns of control and
TM-treated cells were similar. While we have shown that
TM-treatment has brought about a dramatic reduction in lung
colonization following intravenous injection of B16 melanoma cells, we cannot exclude the possibility that the TM-
treated tumor cells have reduced survival potential in the
blood vascular system due to turbulence or other physical
factors.

Previous studies which have emphasized the importance
of surface glycoconjugants in malignant transformation and
metastasis (1, 55, 56) are based on three kinds of observations. First, there is the strong correlation between
transformation and alterations in structure of glycoconjugants. Second, the degree of surface sialylation is known
to affect tumor metastasis. For example, treatment of
malignant cells with neuraminidase shifts the distribution
of metastatic colonization from the lungs to the liver (57).
Third, highly metastatic tumors often differ from low metastatic and benign tumors in expression of cell surface
glycoconjugants. The present study represents an attempt
to demonstrate a direct relationship between alterations
in carbohydrate structures and the pathogenesis of neoplastic transformation.

Our findings suggest a new experimental approach for a
rational chemotherapy, namely, the use of drugs that
deplete or modify the glycan moieties of surface glycoconjugants. Swainsonine and other inhibitors of glycosylation may prove useful in identification of specific
glycan interations involved in metastasis and invasion.

REFERENCES

1. Nicolson, GL (1976). Transmembrane control of the
    receptors on normal and tumor cells. II. Surface
    changes associated with transformation and malignancy.
    Biochim Biophys Acta 458:1.

2. Ruddon, RW (1981). "Cancer Biology." New York,
    Oxford University.

3. Wu, HC, Meezan, E, Black, PH and Robbins, PW (1969).
    Comparative studies on the carbohydrate-containing
    membrane components of normal versus transformed mouse
    fibroblasts. I. Glucosamine-labeling patterns of 3T3,
    spontaneously transformed 3T3, and SV-40 transformed

3T3 cells. Biochemistry 8:2509.

4.   Grimes, WJ (1973). Glycosyltransferases and sialic
     acid levels of normal and transformed cells. Bio-
     chemistry 12:990.

5.   Warren, L, Fuhrer, JP and Buck, CA (1972). Surface
     glycoproteins of normal and transformed cells: a diffe-
     rence determined by sialic acid and a growth-dependent
     sialyl transferase. Proc Natl Acad Sci 69:1838.

6.   Warren, L, Zeiden, I and Buck, CA (1975). The surface
     glycoproteins of a mouse melanoma growing in culture
     and as a solid tumor in vivo. Cancer Res 35:2186.

7.   Van Beek, WP, Smets, GA and Emmelot, P (1973).
     Increased sialic acid density in surface glycoprotein
     of transformed and malignant cells – a general pheno-
     menon? Cancer Res 33:2913.

8.   Van Beek, WP, Smets, GA and Emmelot, P (1975). Changed
     surface glycoprotein as a marker of malignancy in human
     leukaemic cells. Nature 253:457.

9.   Ruddon, RW (1978). "Biological Markers of Neoplasia:
     basic and applied aspects." Elsevier, N.Y.

10. Emmelot, P (1973). Biochemical properties of normal and
     neoplastic cell surfaces; a review. Eur J Cancer 9:319.

11. Meezan, E, Wu, HC, Black, PH and Robbins, PW (1970).
     Comparative studies on the carbohydrate-containing mem-
     brane components of normal versus-transformed mouse
     fibroblasts. II. separation of glycoproteins and glyco-
     peptides by sephadex chromatography. Biochemistry 8:
     2518.

12. Buck, CA, Glick, MC and Warren, L (1970). A comparative
     study of glycoproteins from the surface of control and
     Rous sarcoma virus transformed hamster cells. Biochem-
     istry 9:4567.

13. Glick, MC, Rabinowitz, Z and Sachs, L (1974). Surface
     membrane glycopeptides which coincide with virus trans-
     formation and tumorigenesis. J Virol 13:967.

14. Hunt, LA, Lamph, W and Wright, SE (1981). Transforma-
     tion-dependent alterations in the oligosaccharides of
     Prague C Rous sarcoma virus glycoproteins. J Virol
     37:207.

15. Wagner, DD, Ivatt, R, Destree, AT and Hynes, RO (1981).
     Similarities and differences between fibronectins of
     normal and transformed hamster cells. J Biol Chem
     256:11708.

16. Koyama, K, Nudelman, E, Fukuda, M and Hakomori, SI
     (1969). Correlation of glycosylation in a membrane
     protein with a molecular weight of 150,000 with tumori-
     genic property of rat fibrosarcoma variants. Cancer
     Res 39:3677.

17. Muramatsu, T, Koide, N, Ceccarini, C and Atkinson, P
     (1976). Characterization of mannose-labeled glyco-
     peptides from human diploid cells and their growth-
     dependent alterations. J Biol Chem 251:4673.

18. Muramatsu, T, Gachelin, G, Nicolas, JF, Condamine, H,
     Jakob, H and Jacob, J (1980). High mannose glyco-
     peptides from embryonal carcinoma cells. J Biochem
     88:685.

19. Poste, G, and Nicolson, GL (1980). Blood-Borne tumor
     cell arrest and metastasis modified by fusion of
     plasma membrane vesicles from highly metastatic cells.
     Proc Natl Acad Sci USA 77:399.

20. Mathe, G (1968). Immunotherapie active de la leucemie
     L1210 appliquee apres la greffe tumorale. Rev Fr Etud
     Clin Biol 13:881.

21. Kende, M, Lenwood, DK, Gaston, M and Goldin, A (1975).
     Immunotherapy of transplantable Moloney leukemia with
     cyclophosphamide and allogeneic spleen lymphocytes and
     reversal of graft-versus-host disease with alloanti-
     serum. Cancer Res 35:346.

22. Bekeski, JG, Roboz, JP, Zimmerman, E and Holland, JF
     (1976). Treatment of spontaneous leukemia in AKR mice
     with chemotherapy, immunotherapy, or interferon.
     Cancer Res 36:631-639.

23. Sethi, KK, Brandis, H (1973). Neuraminidase induced loss in the transplantability of murine leukemia L1210. Induction of immunoprotection and the transfer of induced immunity to normal DBA/2 mice by serum and peritoneal cells. Br J Cancer 27:106.

24. Hubbard, SC and Evatt, RJ (1981). Synthesis and processing of asparagine-linked oligosaccharides Annu Rev Biochem 50:555.

25. Grinna, LS and Robbins, PW (1979). Glycoprotein biosynthesis-rat liver microsomal glucosidases which process oligosaccharides. J Biol Chem 254:8814.

26. Takatsuki, A, Arima, K, Tamura, G (1971). Tunicamycin, a new antibiotic. I. Isolation and characterization of tunicamycin. J Antibiotics (Tokyo) 24:215.

27. Takatsuki, A, Tamura, G (1971). Effect of tunicamycin on the synthesis of new castle disease virus. J Antibiotics (Tokyo) 24:785.

28. Struck, DK, Lennarz, WJ (1977). Evidence for the participation of saccharide lipids in the synthesis of the oligosaccharide chain of ovalbumin. J Biol Chem 252:1007.

29. Kawai, S, Hanafusi, H (1971). The effects of reciprocal changes in temperature on the transformed state of cells infected by Rous sarcoma virus mutant. Virol 46:470.

30. Martin, GS (1971). Mutants of the Schmidt-Ruppin strain of Rous sarcoma virus. In: L. Silvestri (ed.) "The Biology of Oncogenic Viruses," p. 320, North Holland, Amsterdam.

31. Yamada, KM, Yamada, SS, Pastan, I (1976). Cell surface protein partially restores morphology adhesiveness, and contact inhibition of movement to transformed fibro-blasts. Proc Natl Acad Sci (Wash) 73:1217.

32. Olden, K, Yamada, KM (1977). Mechanism of the decrease in the major cell surface protein of chick embryo fibro-blasts after transformation. Cell 13:461.

33. Umbriet, WW, (1972). Manometric and Biochemical Techniques (Umbriet, WW and Burris, RH, eds) p. 1, Burgess Publishing Co., Yellow Springs, Ohio.

34. Olden, K, Pratt, RM, Jaworski, C, Yamada, KM (1979). Evidence for role of glycoprotein carbohydrates in membrane transport: specific inhibition by tunica-mycin. Proc Natl Acad Sci (Wash) 76:791.

35. Lowry, OH, Rosebrough, NJ, Farr, AL and Randall, RJ (1951). Protein measurement with the Folin phenol reagent. J Biol Chem 193:265.

36. Eaton, MD, Scala, AR, Jewell, M (1959). Methods for measuring viability of ascites cells by dye exclusion and respiration as affected by depletion, poisons and viruses. Cancer Res 19:945.

37. King, DW, Paulson, MS, Pucket, BS, Krebs, AT (1959). Cell death. IV. The effect of injury on the entrance of vital dye in Ehrlich tumor cells. Amer J Path 35:1067.

38. Willingham, MC, Carchman, RA, Pastan, I (1974). A mutant of 3T3 cells with cyclic AMP metabolism sensitive to temperature change. Proc Natl Acad Sci (Wash) 70:2906.

39. Bekesi, JG, Ameault, G, Walter, L, Holland, JF (1976). Immunogenicity of leukemia L1210 cells after neura-minidase treatment. J Natl Cancer Inst 49:107.

40. Molnar, Z, Bekesi, JG (1972). Effects of D-glucosamine, D-mannosamine, and 2-deoxy-D-glucose on the ultrastruc-ture of ascites tumor cells in vitro. Cancer Res 32:380.

41. Myers, MW, Sartorelli, AC (1975). The effects of low concentrations of 2-deoxy-D-glucose on the growth, surface architecture, and glycoprotein metabolism of p388 lymphoma cells. Biochem Biophys Res Commun 63:164.

42. Olden, K, Pratt, RM, Yamada, KM (1978). Role of carbo-hydrates in protein secretion and turnover: effects of tunicamycin on the major cell surface glycoprotein of chick embryo fibroblasts. Cell 13:461.

43. Olden, K, Pratt, RM, Yamada, KM (1979). Selective cytotoxicity of tunicamycin for transformed cells. Int J Cancer 24:60.

44. Pratt, RM, Yamada, KM, Olden, K, Ohanian SH, Hascall, VC (1979). Exp Cell Res 118:245.

45. Klebe, R (1974). Isolation of a collagen-dependent cell attachment factor. Nature 250:248.

46. Fidler , IJ, Gersten, DM and Hart, IR (1978). Biology of cancer invasion and metastasis. Adv Cancer Res 28:149.

47. Liotta, L, Rao, CN, Barsky, SH (1983). Tumor invasion and the extracellular matrix. Lab Invest 49:636.

48. Liotta, LA, Goldfarb, RH (1984). Interactions of tumor cells with the basement membrane of endothelium: In (Horn, KV and Sloane, BF, eds) "Hemostatic Mechanisms and Metastasis." Martinus Nijhoff. The Hogue, p. 319.

49. Irimura, T, Gonzalez, R, Nicolson, GL (1981). Effects of tunicamycin on B16 metastatic melanoma cell surface glycoproteins and blood-Borne arrest and survival properties. Cancer Res 41:3411.

50. Fidler, IJ, Gersten, DM, Hart, IR (1978). The biology of cancer invasion and metastasis. Adv Cancer Res 28:149.

51. Warburg, O (1956). On the origin of cancer cells. Science 123:309.

52. Fagen, J, Racker, E (1978). Determinants of glycolytic rate in normal and transformed chick embryo fibroblasts. Cancer Res 38:749.

53. Hatanaka, M (1974). Transport of sugars in tumor cell membranes. Biochim Biophys Acta 355:77.

54. Criss, WE (1973). Control of the adenylate charge in Novikoff ascites cells. Cancer Res 33:57.

55. Smith, DF, Walborg, EF (1977). The tumor cell periphery: carbohydrate components. In: "mammalian cell membranes;

surface membrane of specific cell types," GA Jamieson
and DM Robinson (eds) vol 3 p. 115 London, Butter-
worths.

56. Warren, L, Buck, CA, Tuszynski, GP (1978).   Glycopep-
     tide changes and malignant transformation: a
     possible role for carbohydrate in malignant behavior.
     Biochim Biophys Acta 516:97.

57. Sinha, BK, Goldenberg, GJ (1974).   The effect of
     trypsin and neurominidase on the circulation and
     organ distribution of tumor cells.   Cancer 34:1956.

Monoclonal Antibodies and Cancer Therapy, pages 473–488
© 1985 Alan R. Liss, Inc.

USE OF MONOCLONAL ANTIBODIES FOR DETECTION
OF LYMPH NODE METASTASES

John N. Weinstein[1], Christopher D.V. Black[1], Andrew M. Keenan[2], Oscar D. Holton, III[1], Steven M. Larson[2], Susan M. Sieber[3], David G. Covell[1], Jorge Carrasquillo[2], Jacques Barbet[1], and Robert J. Parker[3]

1. Laboratory of Mathematical Biology, National Cancer Institute (NCI), National Institutes of Health (NIH), Bethesda, MD 20205, U.S.A.

2. Nuclear Medicine Department, Clinical Center, NIH.

3. Office of the Director, Division of Cancer Etiology, NCI.

ABSTRACT As an alternative to the more usual i.v. route for administration of monoclonal antibodies, we have been developing techniques for immunolymphoscintigraphy — delivery of radiolabeled antibody via lymphatic vessels for detection of tumor in lymph nodes. Using a metastatic hepatocarcinoma in guinea pigs, we find that subcutaneous injection leads to specific localization of antibody in lymph node metastases, as indicated by gamma camera imaging, double-label isotopic tracers, and autoradiography. We have also defined three types of dual-antibody technique which may usefully increase the power of immunolymphoscintigraphy.

When lymph nodes are the target, the lymphatic route can offer greater efficiency, faster localization, and less systemic toxicity than does the i.v. route. In addition, there may be less cross-reaction with antigen expressed on normal cells. Clinical protocols have been initiated at the National Institutes of Health for immunolymphoscintigraphy in melanoma, lymphoma, and mammary carcinoma.

INTRODUCTION

The status of regional lymph nodes is an important element in the staging of almost all tumors, but assessment of the nodes can be difficult. Clinical examination is notoriously unreliable, as indicated by the large false-positive and false-negative rates quoted in various clinical series (e.g., 27 and 34%, respectively for axillary nodes in breast cancer (1)). Prognosis is usually better correlated with histopathology than with clinical examination, but some degree of morbidity is associated with surgical lymph node dissections.

Non-invasive imaging techniques, if sufficiently reliable, would complement or replace surgical dissection. However, most of the imaging techniques in current practice — X-ray, computerized tomography, nuclear magnetic resonance imaging — are not reliable for detection of metastases much smaller than a centimeter in diameter (i.e., 1 gram, or approximately 1 billion cells). Hence, surgical lymph node exploration remains a central feature of many staging protocols, even when available evidence indicates no increase in survival as a consequence of the procedure.

In principle, imaging with monoclonal antibodies can be much more sensitive than the current techniques, as the following calculation (2) makes clear. Consider an antigenic tumor whose cells can bind an average of 500,000 antibody molecules at saturation. If the antibody were labeled with ^{131}I to a specific activity of 10 mCi/mg, there would be 1.25×10^{-9} mCi (2.75 disintegrations per minute) per cell. For ^{131}I the practical lower limit for detection of a point source using a standard gamma camera is on the order of 100,000 disintegrations per minute (assuming a reasonable imaging time and only spontaneous background). According to this calculation, approximately 40,000 antibody-labeled cells (i.e., 0.04 mg) could, in principle, be detected. That represents an improvement of several orders of magnitude over imaging techniques in current use.

Detection of 40,000 cells is probably not a realistic goal, but this number suggests that diagnostic imaging with monoclonal antibodies will not be limited by intrinsic sensitivity. Rather, the practical limits of sensitivity will be determined by the pharmacology — that is, by such factors as the amount of antibody that can be delivered and bound selectively to the tumor, the nonspecific background, and the rate at which antibody is catabolized.

Monoclonal antibodies have generally been administered intravenously. However, only a small portion of blood flow passes through a small tumor in each circulation time, so delivery by that route is inefficient. As an alternative to i.v. injection, we (2-6) and others (7) have been studying the delivery of monoclonal antibodies via the regional lymphatics from a subcutaneous injection site. Similar studies have also been done with polyclonal preparations (8,9). If regional lymph nodes are the target, this approach should be more efficient than the i.v. route. A major physiologic function of the lymphatic system is to scavenge proteins (including immunoglobulin molecules) that have leaked out of the local capillaries, filter those proteins through lymph nodes, and return them to the general circulation.

The lymphatic route of administration is one instance of regional delivery, — as distinct from the i.v. route, which reaches almost all parts of the body. Other types of regional administration include intraarterial, intraperitoneal, intranpleural, intrabronchial, and cerebrospinal injections.

PHARMACOLOGY OF THE LYMPHATICS

Figure 1 shows a fine rendering by the French anatomist Sappey of the lymphatics serving the torso. Lymph flows from lymphatic capillaries through larger and larger vessels to lymph nodes in the axilla and groin.

The lymphatic system is shown more schematically in Figure 2. If a low molecular weight, water soluble substance is injected subcutaneously, almost all of it passes directly into blood capillaries. Macromolecules do not readily pass into blood vessels, probably because of hindrance by the basement membrane and endothelial cell layer. Terminal lymph capillaries, on the other hand, are specialized for uptake of macromolecules, particles, and cells. They lack a formed basement membrane (10) and have openings in their endothelial walls (11). We find that most of the IgG molecules injected subcutaneously pass into the lymphatics rather than the blood capillaries (unpublished data).

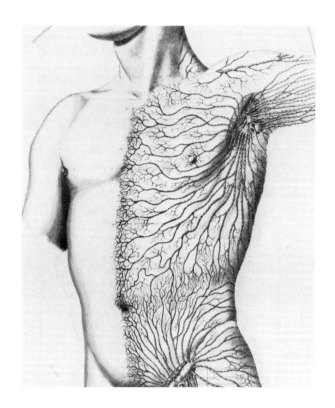

FIGURE 1. Nineteenth century drawing (by Sappey) of
the lymphatics of the torso. As if in two river systems,
lymph drains into larger and larger tributaries, finally
emptying into the axillary lymph nodes above and the nodes
of the groin below (15). "Sappey's line," which is
variable in placement but at about the level of the
umbilicus, divides the two watershed regions.

Once lymph has formed in terminal capillaries, it
flows into larger and larger vessels, propelled by
hydrostatic pressure, extrinsic skeletal muscle action, and
rhythmic contraction of smooth muscle in the vessel walls.
Retrograde flow is prevented by a system of valves. Upon

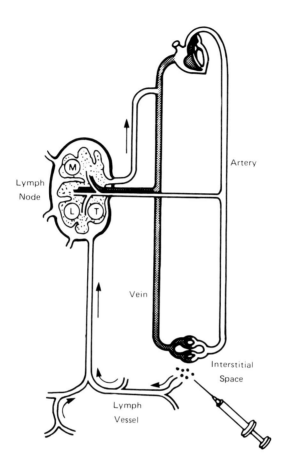

FIGURE 2. Schematic view of subcutaneous antibody administration. Immunoglobulin molecules pass through endothelial clefts into a terminal lymphatic vessel and flow with the lymph toward regional lymph nodes. In the first node encountered, or in more distant nodes of the chain, antibody may bind to normal cells such as the macrophages (M) and lymphocytes (L), or to tumor cells (T). Antibody not cleared from the lymph flow finally passes into the bloodstream, largely via the thoracic duct. Modified from Ref. 3.

reaching a lymph node, lymph flows into the subcapsular sinus, then through sinusoids into the medulla. Immunoglobulin in the lymph may bind specifically or nonspecifically to the various cell types and/or to stromal elements in the node. If not retained by the first node encountered, the immunoglobulin passes to others in the chain. If still not removed from lymph flow, it passes into the bloodstream, largely via the thoracic duct.

MONOCLONAL ANTIBODIES DIRECTED AGAINST NORMAL LYMPH NODE CELLS

Exploratory experiments are difficult to do in the clinical setting, hence we initially studied lymphatic delivery of monoclonal antibodies in vitro and in animals. To simplify the task even further, we began with antibodies directed against normal cells in the lymph node, not against cancer cells.

Our studies of antibodies directed against H-2K determinants (12) and T-cell antigens are described elsewhere (2,3). Figure 3 shows the first pair of animals imaged with a gamma camera after subcutaneous injection (in the footpads) of an I^{125} labeled anti-K^k antibody. Two hours after injection the popliteal and lumbar lymph nodes were well visualized in the K^k-positive mouse but not in the K^k-negative one. Each popliteal node weighed, on average, 0.8 mg. Hence, good images were obtained from about a million cells. In concentration units, the uptake in popliteal nodes exceeded 10,000 percent of dose per gram.

The following briefly summarizes our findings after injection of IgG into the hind footpads of mice: (i) Both specific and nonspecific IgG's pass efficiently to the popliteal and lumbar nodes, principally during the first 2 to 3 hours after injection. (ii) Accumulation of radioiodine label in popliteal nodes reaches a plateau within 2 to 4 hours and then declines. The mechanisms by which radioisotope is eliminated from the node probably include dissociation of bound antibody, catabolism of antibody, and cell migration. (iii) For irrelevant control IgG, the percent of dose appearing in lymph nodes and in systemic organs is essentially independent of the dose administered. That is, the kinetics of distribution are linear. (iv) In contrast, the percentages of specific antibody found in various organs are strongly dependent on

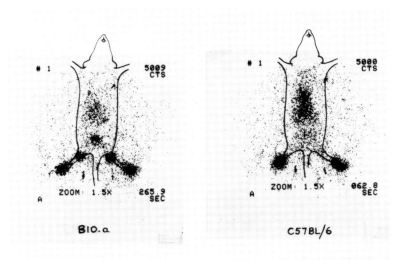

FIGURE 3. Gamma camera images of H-2K^k-positive (left) and H-2K^k-negative (right) mice 2 hours after injection in both hind footpads with ^{125}I-labeled anti-H-2K^k IgG (approx. 0.25 µCi/foot). The most prominent foci are the injections sites. Popliteal nodes (behind the knees) and lumbar nodes (in the lower abdomen) are also prominent in the antigen-positive mouse. Body background is more pronounced in the negative animal because more antibody has spilled over into the systemic circulation. (From ref. 2).

the absolute dose. In the case of antibody directed against H-2K^k, binding sites proximal to the point of injection appeared to saturate first. Antibody then "overflowed" to more distant lymph nodes along the chain, and finally into the bloodstream for systemic distribution. (v) At appropriately chosen doses, the selectivity ratio (specific/nonspecific) in the target lymph nodes exceeded 50:1 as early as 2 hours after injection. More than 20% of the injected dose could be bound in the nodes. (vi) Antibody directed against a subset of T-cells in the lymph node (i.e., Lyt 2) appeared to label all cells of that subset in the popliteal nodes. (vi) Delivery of antibody to regional nodes was faster and more efficient after injection in the footpads than in other subcutaneous sites tested.

These studies with anti-H-2K^k and anti-Lyt 2 provide an experimental basis for imaging of radiolabeled monoclonals directed against normal cell types in human nodes. Such antibodies may provide an alternative to [99]technetium-labeled colloids for use in "nonspecific" lymphoscintigraphy. More speculatively, they might provide a non-invasive way to assess or modulate the immune status of regional lymph nodes.

MONOCLONAL ANTITUMOR ANTIBODIES

Studies with antibody to normal cell types also contributed to the design of protocols for lymphatic delivery of an antitumor monoclonal antibody to lymph node metastases of line 10 (L10) hepatocarcinoma in guinea pigs. If 10^6 L10 cells are implanted intradermally in the flank, metastasis takes place within 1 week to the ipsilateral superficial distal axillary (SDA) lymph node.

D3 is a murine IgG_1 directed against a 290,000 dalton dimer on L10 cells. It localizes selectively in L10 tumors after i.v. administration (13,14). We injected the antibody either in the forepaw or in the flank near the tumor. The gamma camera image in Fig. 4 (lefthand panel) suggests accumulation of D3 in cancerous SDA nodes after injection in the flank. Without moving the (anaesthetized) animal from its position under the gamma camera, we dissected out the SDA node and imaged again. As indicated in Fig. 4 (right-hand panel), the focus of activity disappeared, substantiating that it had represented the lymph node. At the same dose, normal nodes were not visualized.

However, lymph node uptake did not prove specificity of binding. Antibody could have been accumulating nonspecifically, either in reactive nodes or in tumor substance within the nodes. We demonstrated the specificity of binding by double-label experiments with ^{125}I-labeled D3 and ^{131}I-labeled MOPC 21 (an isotype-matched control). The specific/nonspecific ratio of accumulation in lymph node tumor was approximately 100 to 1. Normal nodes and other organs showed no appreciable selectivity. As expected if antibody were reaching the

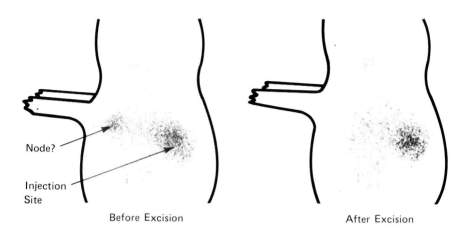

Before Excision   After Excision

FIGURE 4. Gamma camera images of a guinea pig bearing L10 hepatocarcinoma in the flank. The animal was imaged 27 hours after subcutaneous injection of ^{125}I-labeled D3 antibody in the flank. The left-hand panel shows the injection site and a focus thought to represent a cancerous lymph node. Upon excision of the node under anaesthesia, the focus of radioactivity disappeared. From ref. 6.

nodes principally by local lymphatic flow, nodes outside of the regional drainage system contained very little radioactivity, even when they contained metastases.

Proof of specificity did not, however, indicate that antibody delivered via the lymphatics was indeed bound to metastatic cells. It might instead have been bound to antigen shed from the primary tumor into lymphatic vessels and deposited in the lymph nodes. This was thought to be the case in clinical studies with a polyclonal antibody directed against carcinoembryonic antigen (15,16). Such interference by shed antigen would tend to produce false positives whatever the route of administration. To investigate the possibility of binding to shed antigen, we did two types of experiment.

In the first (6), guinea pigs were injected with L10 cells in each flank. Nine days later, after metastasis to the nodes had taken place, the primary tumor was excised from one flank under anaesthesia. On day 18 the animals were injected in both flanks with ^{125}I-D3 and ^{131}I-MOPC 21. The lymph node metastases on the two sides showed equivalent selective D3 uptake. Therefore, selective binding in the node could not have been a result of antigen-shedding by the primary tumor (unless the antigen had been shed 9 days prior to injection).

In the second type of experiment, localization in tumor itself was demonstrated by autoradiography. L10 cells reach the lymph node via afferent lymphatic vessels and proliferate along the subcapsular space before infiltrating the parenchyma of the node. When ^{125}I-D3 was injected into the flanks of animals with tumor, localization of radioactivity corresponded closely to the histologic location of metastatic tumor (Figure 5). There was no evidence of binding to antigen within normal node parenchyma.

DUAL-ANTIBODY IMAGING TECHNIQUES

Table 1 lists several dual antibody techniques which might be clinically useful. The simplest involves tandem use of anti-tumor antibody and irrelevant isotype-matched reagent to assess the specificity of tumor localization.

A second approach uses anti-tumor antibody together with an antibody directed against lymphoid cells, lymphoid subsets, macrophages, or any other component of the node. The anti-tumor reagent is intended to detect (or treat) tumor directly; the companion antibody assesses integrity of the lymph node chains and, speculatively, the immune status of the node.

In a third type of dual antibody technique, lymphatic delivery can be combined with i.v. administration of the same antibody. Since large tumors distort or block lymph flow, the lymphatic route is likely to be most discerning for small metastases. The i.v. injection would be used to detect or treat larger lymph node masses as well as tumor in other organs.

For detection techniques, two antibodies labeled with different isotopes can be co-injected, as we have done using I^{125} labeled D3 and I^{131} labeled antibody (8BE6) directed against guinea pig T-cells (data not shown). Alternatively, two antibodies labeled with the same isotope can be administered sequentially, as demonstrated in Figure 6. In this case, I^{125} labeled D3 was injected s.c. in guinea pigs to image lymph node metastases of L10 tumor,

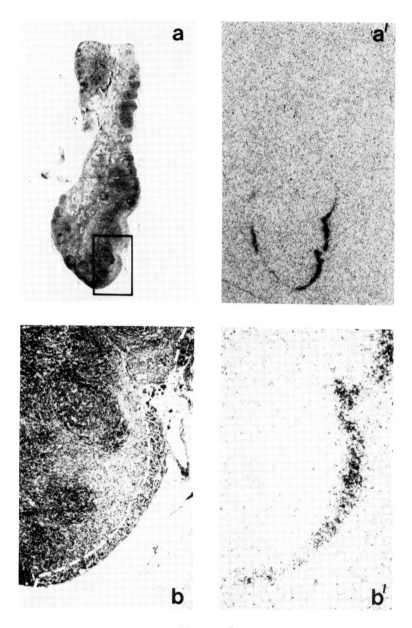

Figure 5

FIGURE 5. Autoradiographic study of a cancerous superficial distal axillary node 24 hours after ipsilateral s.c. injection of ^{125}I-D3. The guinea pig was injected with 34 µg D3 (3.4 µCi) on day 21 after implantation of 106 L10 cells. (a) Stained section. Tumor occupied approximately 2% of the node. (a') Autoradiogram of 6-µm section cut adjacent to that in (a). Grains representing ^{125}I-labeled IgG are seen along the rim of the node at one end. (b) Higher magnification corresponding to the inset box in (a). Tumor cells occupy the area demarcated by white dashed line. (b') Autoradiogram of section adjacent to that in (b). From Ref. 4.

TABLE 1.
DUAL-ANTIBODY TECHNIQUES

Antibodies	Aims
Anti-tumor + Irrelevant	To assess specificity
Anti-tumor + Anti-(lymph node cell)	To detect or treat tumor while assessing gross integrity of node chains
Anti-tumor s.c. + Anti-tumor i.v.	To detect or treat both small and large

and I^{125} 8BE6 was later injected to show the location of (and access to) the nodes.

DISCUSSION

Clinical studies on lymphatic delivery of monoclonal antibodies have begun, both at the National Institutes of Health and elsewhere. While it is not possible yet to say whether the positive results in animals and initial results in humans will lead to effective clinical use, we can

SEQUENTIAL DUAL-ANTIBODY IMAGING WITH
ANTI-TUMOR AND ANTI-T CELL MoAbs

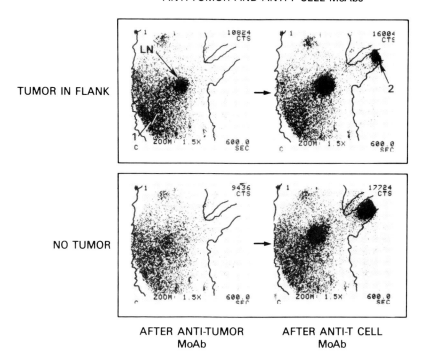

TUMOR IN FLANK

NO TUMOR

AFTER ANTI-TUMOR
MoAb

AFTER ANTI-T CELL
MoAb

FIGURE 6. Dual-antibody immunolymphoscintigraphy. L10 tumor was injected intradermally in the flank of a guinea pig and allowed to metastasize to the superficial distal axillary lymph node. The animal was injected s.c. in the flank with I^{125} labeled D3 antibody. The lymph node metastasis was visualized 24 hours later (top left-hand panel). I^{125} labeled 8BE6 anti-T cell antibody was then injected in the forepaw and the top right-hand image recorded 2 hours later. Both antibodies contributed in measurable amounts to the final focus of gamma radioactivity representing the node. The lower panels show images of a normal guinea pig injected in the same sequence.

identify some of the possible advantages and limitations of this approach vis a vis i.v. administration.

Lymphatic delivery is clearly limited to regional lymph nodes. Metastases in the liver, lung, bone, brain, and other common sites will not be detected (except in so far as antibody escapes the lymphatics and distributes via the bloodstream). Since the lymphatic vessels must be patent if antibody is to reach its target, large masses may prevent access or distort lymph flow. Lymphatic delivery is therefore best suited for small metastases. As indicated in the description of dual-antibody techniques, the lymphatic route will probably be used in combination with i.v. injection, the former to detect small masses, the latter to detect large, well-vascularized ones. As suggested by Figure 6, it may also be helpful to use the antitumor antibody in tandem with an antibody directed against normal lymph node cells, the latter to show the location of nodes and to signal disruption of the lymphatic chains.

Radiation toxicity at the injection site appears not to be a serious problem for diagnostic studies (unpublished observations). However, for therapy with drugs, toxins, or radionuclides conjugated to antibodies, local toxicity may be a major limitation. Direct injection into a cannulated lymphatic vessel may be preferable.

The principal advantage of the lymphatic route is its efficiency. Much smaller doses can be used to image smaller amounts of tumor. The mouse popliteal nodes weighed less than 1 mg, but they were imaged within a few minutes at doses of less than 1 μCi of ^{125}I (3). As little as 3 mg of metastatic tumor was imaged in the guinea pig (4). However, for therapy with antibody conjugates, the lower dose and compartmentation in the lymphatics would presumably decrease systemic toxicity.

As has been discussed previously (3), regional localization in the lymphatics should reduce cross-reactive binding of antibody to antigen on normal cells (unless those cells were located in the lymphatics). Cross-reaction could even be an advantage with respect to diagnostic studies, clearing the circulation of radioactivity which would otherwise appear as background superimposed on images of the nodes. Shedding of antigen into regional nodes from the primary tumor would tend to interfere with identification of lymph node metastases regardless of how the antibody was administered.

"Immunolymphotherapy" with antibody alone or antibody conjugates may prove useful for regional control of lymph node metastases, though its range of application is expected to be much more limited than that of immunolympho-scintigraphy.

ACKNOWLEDGEMENTS

We are grateful to E. Shevach, D. Sachs, J. Bluestone, and H.C. Morse, III for antibodies used in these studies. We thank M.J. Talley for excellent technical assistance and K. Marconi for help in preparation of the manuscript.

REFERENCES

1. Hellman S, Harris JR, Canellos GP, and Fisher B (1982). Cancer of the Breast. In De Vita VT, Hellman s, and Rosenberg SA (eds): "Cancer. Principles and Practice of Oncology," Philadelphia: Lippincott, pp. 914-970 (see Table 27-4).
2. Weinstein JN, Parker RJ, Holton OD, III, Keenan AM, Covell DG, Black CDV, and Sieber SM (1985). Lymphatic delivery of monoclonal antibodies: Potential for detection and treatment of lymph node metastases. Cancer Investigation 3:85-95.
3. Weinstein JN, Parker RJ, Keenan AM, Dower SK, Morse HC, III and Sieber SM (1982). Monoclonal antibodies in the lymphatics: Toward the diagnosis and therapy of tumor metastases. Science 218:1334-1337.
4. Weinstein JN, Steller MA, Keenan AM, Covell DG, Key ME, Sieber SM, Oldham RK, Hwang KM, and Parker RJ (1983). Monoclonal antibodies in the lymphatics: Selective delivery to lymph node metastases of a solid tumor. Science 222:423-426.
5. Weinstein JN, Steller MA, Covell DG, Holton OD, III, Keenan AM, Sieber SM, and Parker RJ (1984). Monoclonal antitumor antibodies in the lymphatics. Cancer Treat. Rep. 68:257-264.
6. Weinstein JN, Keenan AM, Holton OD, III, Covell DG, Sieber SM, Black CDV, Barbet J, Talley MJ, and Parker RJ (1985). Use of monoclonal antibodies to detect metastases of solid tumors in lymph nodes. Symposium of the International Workshop on Monoclonal Antibodies and Breast Cancer, in press.

7. Thompson CH, Stacker SA, Salehi N, Lichtenstein M, Leyden MJ, Andrews JT, and McKenzie IFC (1984). Immunoscintigraphy for detection of lymph node metastases from breast cancer. Lancet, Dec. 1, pp. 1245-1247.

8. DeLand FH, Kim EE, Corgan RL, Casper S, Primus FJ, Spremulli E, Estes N, and Goldenberg DM (1979). Axillary lymphoscintigraphy by radioimmunodetection of carcinoembryonic antigen in breast cancer. J. Nucl. Med 20:1243-1250.

9. DeLand FH, Kim EE, and Goldenberg DM (1980). Lymphoscintigraphy with radionuclide-labeled antibodies to carcinoembryonic antigen. Cancer Res. 40:2997-3000.

10. Barsky SH, Baker A, Siegal GP, Togo S, and Liotta LA (1983). Use of anti-basement membrane antibodies to distinguish blood vessel capillaries from lymphatic capillaries. Am. J. Surg. Pathol. 7:667-677.

11. Leak LV (1971). Studies on the permeability of lymphatic capillaries. J. Cell Biol. 50:300-323.

12. Sachs DH, Mayer N, Ozato K (1981). Hybridoma antibodies directed toward murine H-2 and Ia antigens. In "Monoclonal Antibodies and T-Cell Hybridomas," Eds. Hammerling U and Kearney JF, Amsterdam, Elsevier, pp. 95-101.

13. Key ME, Bernhard MI, Hoyer LC, et al. (1983). Guinea pig line 10 hepatocarcinoma model for monoclonal antibody serotherapy II. In vivo localization of a monoclonal antibody in normal and malignant tissues. J. Immunol. 130:1451-1457.

14. Bernhard MI, Hwang KM, Foon KA, Keenan AM, Kessler RM, Frincke JM, Tallam DJ, Hanna MG, Jr, Peters L, and Oldham RK (1983). Localization of indium[111] and iodine[131] labeled monoclonal antibody in guinea pigs bearing line 10 hepatocarcinoma tumors. Cancer Res. 43:4429-4433.

15. Sappey MPC (1885). "Anatomie, Physiologie, Pathologie des Vaisseaux Lymphatiques," Paris, A. Delahaye and E. Lecrosnier.

Monoclonal Antibodies and Cancer Therapy, pages 489–492
© **1985 Alan R. Liss, Inc.**

WORKSHOP SUMMARY: MONOCLONAL ANTIBODIES TO EXTRACELLULAR
MATRIX AND CYTOSKELETAL COMPONENTS

Michael D. Pierschbacher

Cancer Research Center
La Jolla Cancer Research Foundation
10901 North Torrey Pines Road
La Jolla, CA 92037

Dr. Pierschbacher opened the workshop by presenting a
paper entitled "Monoclonal Antibodies and Synthetic
Peptides Reveal a Family of Cell Adhesion Molecules"
(Michael D. Pierschbacher, Robert Pytela, Edward G.
Hayman, Shintaro Suzuki, and Erkki Ruoslahti, LA Jolla
Cancer Research Foundation, La Jolla, CA 92037)
Fibronectin contains a domain which interacts with
cell surfaces. The cell attachment activity of fibronectin can be duplicated with short synthetic peptides having
the amino acid sequence glycyl-L-arginyl-glycyl-L-aspar-
tyl-L-serine that is present in that domain. Each of the
amino acids Arg-Gly-Asp appears to be necessary for
maintenance of the activity of this peptide, while the
serine residue can be replaced with some, but apparently
not all, possible residues. This recognition sequence is
present in a number of proteins other than fibronectin
which interacts with cells. These proteins include
collagens, fibrinogen, vitronectin, thrombin, a bacterial
surface protein and two viral proteins, as well as
discoidin-I, a protein implicated in the aggregation of
Dictyostelium discoideum. A similar sequence is also
repeated in some fibronectin molecules, suggesting that
fibronectin molecules can have more than a single cell
attachment site. Synthetic peptides constructed from
sequences taken from several of these other protein, as
well as some of the proteins themselves, have been shown
to promote cell attachment. At least two different cell
surface receptors exist which recognize the Arg-Gly-Asp
sequence. One of them recognizes it in the unique context
of fibronectin and the other in vitronectin. This
tripeptide sequence may, therefore, constitute an ancient
cellular recognition mechanism common to many proteins.
Dr. Reisfeld presented the paper "Biosynthesis of a
Melanoma-Associated Chondroitin Sulfate Proteoglycan"

(Ralph A. Reisfel, John Harper, and Vito Quaranta, Scripps Clinic and Research Foundation, La Jolla, CA).

This work concerns the fact that human melanoma cells express a cell bound chondroitin sulfate proteoglycan (MPG) that represents an excellent target for tumor cell destruction by monoclonal antibody (Mab) 9.2.27 in combination with immunological effector cells. Pulse-chase analyses with 9.2.27 indicated that biosynthesis of MPG proceeds through a 240 kDa component having N-linked, high mannose oligosaccharides whose molecular mass decreases to 235 kDa following digestion with endo-β-N-acetylglucos- aminidase H. Almost immediately following processing of high mannose oligosaccharides to the complex type and addition of o-linked oligosaccharides forming a core protein of 250 kDa, chondroitin 4- and/or 6-sulfate chains are initiated and elongated into glycosaminoglycan chains. MPG synthesis in human melanoma cells was found to be regulated by acid compartments involved in certain Golgi-related functions where a low pH mechanism appears responsible for delivery of mature glycoprotein to the site of glycosaminoglycan synthesis in Golgi-related vesicles. MPG core protein was found to be expressed at the cell surface in two forms, either free or as a part of MPG, apparently through alternate processing pathways. Changes in intracellular pH induced by addition of NHCL (15 mM) drastically shifted the balance of surface core proteins towards the free form, possibly by inhibiting access of core protein to the intracellular site of MPG maturation. These data suggest a regulatory mechanism by which human melanoma cells may control proteoglycan levels in their extracellular matrix, possibly for their adhesive properties.

Dr. Thomas F. Bumol (Lilly Research Laboratories, Indianapolis, IN) described several studies employing monoclonal antibodies to study extracellular matrix molecules in human tumor cells. Studies were described with monoclonal antibody 9.2.27, directed at human melanoma cells, which demonstrated that this antibody is directed at the 250 kDa core glycoprotein of chondoritin sulfate proteoglycan in these cells. This antibody was utilized to study the biosynthesis and cellular topography of these proteoglycans in melanoma and continues to be a probe for glycoconjugate biosynthesis in conjunction with several novel monovalent ionophores. Several additional matrix molecules were examined in similar fashion with monoclonal antibody probes for fibronectin (supplied by

Drs. Pierschbacher and Ruoslahti) and thombospondin (supplied by Dr. Mark Ginsberg, Scripps Clinic). Dr. Bumol documented by pulse-chase immunoprecipitation experiments that melanoma cells synthesized and actively secreted these matrix glycoproteins. Further monoclonal antibody probes are being developed to study the basis of the lack of an organized matrix in these metastatic human cells in the presence of active biosynthesis of extracellular matrix molecules. Dr. Bumol concluded his talk by presenting some preliminary data demonstrating that the 9.2.27 monoclonal antibody could also be utilized to potentially target oncolytic drugs (vinblastine) to melanoma cells, even if its target antigen is a pericellular matrix molecule.

Dr. Hsu then followed with the paper "Enrichment of a Chondroitin Sulfate Proteoglycan on a Metastatic Melanoma Cell Line" (Daniel K. Hsu, David A. Cheresh, Ralph A. Reisfeld, Scripps Clinic and Research Foundation, La Jolla, CA) describing how the identification of cell surface changes associated with the metastatic phenotype of tumor cells may aid in understanding their invasive properties. In this regard, the cell surface proteoglycan variant A3750M (Kozlowski, J.M. et al., 1984, Cancer Res. 44, 3522-3529) was examined. These researchers observed a two-fold enrichment of a cell surface proteoglycan defining monoclonal antibodies (Mabs) 9.2.27 and 155.8 with fluorescence activated cell sorter (FACS) analysis; however no difference was observed in the expression of HLA-A,B,C between the two cell lines, indicating that the elevated proteoglycan level is not simply due to increased total protein synthesis. Both parent and metastatic cell lines exhibited identical forward-angle light scatter by FACS, suggesting that the change in the two cell lines had similar growth rates and the observed change in the two cell lines had similar growth rates and the observed differential antigen expression was consistent through the cell cycle. Competitive antigen assays of cell lysates and culture media using the Mab 9.2.27-horseradish peroxidase conjugate showed similar increases of the total cell-associated 9.2.27-antigen and antigen shed into the culture media, respectively, in the metastatic variant over the parent line. This finding was confirmed by Western blots with Mab 9.2.27. Use of the lysosomotropic agent NH_4-Cl in pulse-chase studies with ^{35}S-methionine suggests that the mature 250 kilodalton antigen is degraded at a lower rate in A375-M cells than in A375-P

cells. These results suggest the following: 1) highly
metastatic A375-M melanoma cells express larger quantities
of the cell surface antigen defined by Mab 9.2.27 than the
parent A375-P; 2) the difference in expression of the
9.2.27 antigen on A375-M and A375-P cells is not caused by
a general increase in protein synthesis; 3) in A375-M
cells higher expression of the 9.2.27 antigen results from
lowered regulation by low pH compartments during biosynthesis and not from higher rates of translation or
transport to the cell surface.

X. CANCER VACCINES

Monoclonal Antibodies and Cancer Therapy, pages 495–503
© 1985 Alan R. Liss, Inc.

APPLICATIONS OF MONOCLONAL ANTIBODIES TO ACTIVE
SPECIFIC IMMUNOTHERAPY [1]

Malcolm S. Mitchell, M.D.

Departments of Medicine and Microbiology
University of Southern California
School of Medicine
and
Comprehensive Cancer Center
Los Angeles California, 90033

ABSTRACT   Monoclonal antibodies have several
potentially important roles to play in the
development of active specific immunotherapy.
Principal among these is the determination of the
antigenic content of the tumor vaccines, either
absolutely or relatively depending upon the purity
of the antigenic standard. Monitoring the course of
disease in patients with detectable serum levels of
antigen might be accomplished by analogous methods
with monoclonal antibodies. An improved
determination of antibody responses to the specific
antigens administered is at least potentially
possible, through the use of panels of monoclonal
antibodies. Human monoclonal antibodies may be of
particular importance in determining the presence
and concentration of "relevant" immunogens.
Conversely, useful human monoclonal antibodies may
be important by-products of successful vaccinations
with tumor-associated antigens.

[1]Supported by grants from the National Cancer
Institute, CA 36233, the Concern Foundation, the Eckstrom
Trust and the Mirkin Foundation.

INTRODUCTION

The development of methods for producing monoclonal antibodies to human tumor-associated antigens has had far-reaching consequences in every area of tumor immunology. The effort to devise reproducible procedures for active specific immunotherapy of cancer patients is certainly no exception to this statement. Active specific immunotherapy can be defined as the attempt to stimulate the tumor-bearing host directly with tumor-associated antigens, either with whole tumor cells, usually irradiated or otherwise killed, or with nonviable lysates or extracts made from those cells. The procedure is often referred to as "vaccination". Monoclonal antibodies have a number of important roles to play in the development of "vaccines", whether of tumor cells or tumor-associated antigenic materials. Several of these applications have already been made, while others have considerable potential for the future. I would like to discuss these in outline, with some specific examples drawn from our own work and from the literature. More detail on our own particular applications of monoclonal antibodies will be given in the paper by Kan-Mitchell et al. later in this volume (1).

DETERMINATION OF THE ANTIGENS IN THE VACCINE

In the past, most clinical trials of tumor vaccines have not attempted to determine the content of immunogenic materials in the preparations that were administered. Perhaps with autologous immunizations it is possible to justify this omission, since one is limited in the range of antigens that can be administered to those that are expressed in the patient's own tumor. But even there it is desirable to know which antigens are present. It is now possible with an increasing number of human tumors to determine specifically which antigens are present on the tumor cells, or in the lysates or extracts, that are to be used for the immunization. Murine monoclonal antibodies are now available that can identify antigens on the surface of a variety of tumors: including melanoma, neuroblastoma, and acute myelocytic leukemias, and carcinomas of the colon, breast, ovary, pancreas, and lung, to name just a few (2). A variety of methods might be applied with these antibodies, depending upon the state of the tumor antigens.

Soluble extracts or lysates are most easily amenable to a
quantitation of their content of antigens. A binding
inhibition enzyme immunoassay (1) may be utilized for the
determination of soluble antigens in tumor lysates or
extracts. In this procedure, the material containing the
putative antigens is first reacted with a peroxidase-
labeled monoclonal antibody directed against an epitope of
the tumor antigen in question. The labeled antibody is
then added to plastic microwells containing tumor cells
bearing the target antigen.   If the same epitope to which
the monoclonal antibody is directed is present in the
putatively antigenic extract, the binding of the antibody
to its target cells will be inhibited. The degree of
inhibition is directly proportional to the representation
of the antigen in the extract. A standard curve is first
established with dilutions of purified antigen, if
available, or with an extract known to contain a
significant concentration of the target antigen---an
extract that must be available in sufficient quantity for
use in a large number of assays. The latter situation
allows only the calculation of arbitrary "antigenic units"
rather than milligrams of antigen but permits the
administration of a predetermined relative dosage among
several treatment groups. After an "antigenic unit" is
defined, such as the amount of binding inhibitory activity
contained in 10 ul of undiluted standard antigen, the
determination of the antigenic content of an unknown
preparation is relatively simple. Ten ul of one or two
dilutions of unknown can be incubated with the monoclonal
antibody and the content of antigen is determined through
reference to the linear portion of the standard curve.
This value can be determined equally well with the
regression equation describing the "best-fit" curve or
interpolation from the drawn standard curve. By our
methods, we can accurately identify as little as few as
0.031 antigenic units in 10 ul, or 3.1 antigenic units per
ml (1). If several monoclonal antibodies to different
important epitopes are available, this procedure can be
repeated with each, to quantitate the content of a spectrum
of tumor-associated antigens.

    An alternative method for quantitating the
concentration of an antigen in vaccines is possible when
the epitope identified by the monoclonal antibody is
expressed repeatedly on an antigen in the vaccine. Bast et
al. (3) used their anti-ovarian carcinoma monoclonal

antibody OC-125 in a direct solid phase radioimmunoassay
with antibody-coated beads as the probe for the
corresponding antigen, CA-125 . Unlabeled OC-125 on
polystyrene beads was used to trap the antigen, and
radiolabeled OC-125 was used to identify the bound antigen
on the beads.   This is in effect a "double determinant
immunoassay ", since attachment of antibody to the repeated
epitope serves both as a means of trapping and detecting
the antigen, much as in a true double determinant
immunoassay. The latter, as reported by several groups (4-
6), is more generally applicable. In one variety of double
determinant assay described by Koprowski and associates
(5,6), polyclonal IgG was first generated in rabbits
immunized with the immunoaffinity-purified antigenic target
of a monoclonal antibody. This polyclonal antibody was
used with the orginal monoclonal to identify the same
antigen in a solid-phase radioimmunoassay. The assay
depends upon the polyclonal antibody's binding at multiple
sites, entrapping the antigen, and preventing loss of the
antigen throughout the assay, which entails several washes.
The major theoretical advantage to this type of method,
which takes advantage of more than one determinant
simultaneously or sequentially, is the more specific
identification of an antigen, particularly in complex
mixtures such as serum. With tumor extracts, if care is
first taken to use only the tumor and not a great deal of
surrounding normal tissues, a binding inhibition method
depending upon a single epitope may be sufficient. The
immunosorbent column to which a monoclonal antibody is
bound is an excellent way to purify a specific antigen for
use in active immunization. It is a good preparative
procedure for concentrating an important, but relatively
poorly represented, antigenic component of an extract for
use in a vaccine, but is obviously not an efficient
analytical method.

     As we have mentioned several times in passing, antigens
in the sera of patients with a particular tumor can be
identified by the same procedures outlined here for
detection of the antigens in an extract or lysate of tumor
cells. In fact, many monoclonal antibodies have been used
for this purpose in melanoma and ovarian cancer (1,3,5-7).
The analysis of a serum for its content of a low level of
antigens has several problems that are less likely with
antigenic extracts. The presence of nonspecific reactivity
in serum with an indicator antibody is frequently a problem

with such a   complex mixture of proteins. Nevertheless,
these technical problems are more vexing than insoluble.
Most vaccines will not elevate the level of serum antigens,
since most are given intradermally or subcutaneously rather
than intravenously. Nevertheless, the level of serum
antigens may prove useful in following the course of a
patient's disease, i.e., searching for a relapse despite
the vaccination, in much the same way as carcinoembryonic
antigen (CEA) levels are useful for monitoring patients
whose tumors shed this antigen.

USEFULNESS OF HUMAN MONOCLONAL ANTIBODIES

Human monoclonal antibodies have several very
desirable attributes for studies on immunization of human
beings. First is their intrinsic ability to detect
relevant antigens, i.e. antigens that are immunogenic to
patients. This is not to imply that mouse antibodies
necessarily identify irrelevant molecules, but one would
cerrtainly expect that those antigens that have been
immunogenic in one patient might be appropriate to include
in a vaccine designed to boost the immunity of another with
a similar tumor. It is disconcerting, however, that
usually we do not know whether the individual from whose
cells we generate a monoclonal antibody will later develop
recurrent disease or will be cured by the surgery at which
his nodes were obtained. (By our strategy the donor of
lymphocytes is always one from whom a primary tumor has
just been resected and whose lymph node used for the fusion
is free of tumor cells.) This information could tell us
whether the humoral immunity developed in the B cells of
that fused node was of any benefit to the autologous host,
and by extension whether the antigens immunogenic for him
might really be the most appropriate immunogens to be
administered to others.   Human monoclonal antibodies, have
been produced mainly through the fusion of mouse myeloma
cells with human lymphocytes from the lymph node draining
the site of the primary tumor, since human fusion partners
have been generally unavailable. Although stability of
these hybridomas has been a significant problem, technology
is now advanced to permit their survival for many months
with careful handling. Of considerable interest is that the
human antibodies that have been produced thus far have
almost entirely detected cytoplasmic antigens rather than
the surface antigens identified with mouse monoclonals

(8,9). The nature of the antigens detected is uncertain for the most part, although cytoskeletal elements are a prominent target (8,10). This raises the obvious question of whether surface antigens should be included as prominently, or at all, in vaccines. Our own vaccination trial was based originally on the premise that selective removal of surface antigens, as in murine model systems (11,12) with 1-butanol or octylglucoside, was the most desirable approach. The data with human monoclonal antibodies suggest at the very least that cytoplasmic constituents should not be excluded from vaccines, and perhaps should even be the predominant portion of them. The specificity of human monoclonal antibodies promises to be at least as good as mouse antibodies. Whether the affinity of these antibodies is great enough, and the number of antigenic molecules they react with is large enough, to make them useful reagents both remain to be determined.

MEASUREMENT OF SERUM ANTIBODIES

An even more problematic area is role of monoclonal antibodies in the measurement of the serum antibody response to a tumor vaccine. Theoretically, an analogous sort of inhibition of the binding of a monoclonal antibody to its target epitope should be possible to detect serum antibodies. For example, if an unknown serum contained antibodies to the same epitope as the monoclonal antibody, preincubating target tumor cells bearing the appropriate antigens with the serum should competitively block the subsequent binding of peroxidase-labeled monoclonal antibody. However, only a small proportion of the serum antibodies (with a concentration probably measured in picograms/ml) might reasonably be expected to be directed against the single epitope against which a monoclonal antibody is directed. The use of a mixture of a panel of monoclonal antibodies to detect several different serum antibodies simultaneously might circumvent this difficulty. This is becoming much more of a possibility now that a variety of well-characterized monoclonals are available in several diseases, particularly melanoma and colon carcinoma. Thus far only routine, relatively insensitive assays for antibody such as mixed hemadsorption have been used with consistent success in man, in striking contrast to the highly sensitive and specific immunoassays we have indicated for measurement of antigens. A promising method that might be used to detect antibodies is frequently used for antigens, namely, immunoprecipitation with Staphylococcal protein A of immune complexes, after the incubation of the patient's serum with a selected, radiolabeled tumor cell lysate or extract of previously determined antigenic content. The presence of antibody and antigen in the (dissociated) immunoprecipitate could then be verified by standard physicochemical methods. Titration of the level of antibodies, such as by 2-fold serial dilutions, would also be possible with this method. Data in the literature, obtained with previously available serological methods, have suggested that most commonly the titer of human antitumor antibodies is very low: on the order of 1:32 or less.

GENERATION OF HUMAN MONOCLONAL ANTIBODIES FROM LYMPHOCYTES OF VACCINATED PATIENTS

Finally, it should be noted that, as Hanna and colleagues (13) have shown, human monoclonal antibodies can be generated by _in vivo_ education of human lymphocytes in patients given vaccines with therapeutic intent. They have successfully produced more than 30 antibodies to colon carcinoma by this means, harvesting peripheral blood lymphocytes 7 days after a vaccination. Since relatively few patients will be treated by vaccines in the immediate future, this is a relatively limited strategy by which to improve the yield of monoclonal antibodies. For those investigators who have access to patients treated with active immunotherapy, it does represent a potentially important way of boosting the number of antibody-producing peripheral blood B lymphocytes, and probably increasing the avidity of antibodies produced by them. Since the use of peripheral blood lymphocytes has been far less successful than that of lymph node cells, any methods of improving the situation beyond what is achievable with pokeweed mitogen stimulation are welcome.

CONCLUSION

The many intersections of active specific immunotherapy and monoclonal antibodies , some of which have been described here, thus make it highly appropriate to consider specific immunotherapy in the context of this conference on monoclonal antibodies.

REFERENCES

1. Kan-Mitchell J, Kempf RA, Knapp SH, Harper JR, Reisfeld RA, Mitchell MS (1985). Monoclonal antibodies in the development of active specific immunotherapy in melanoma. In Reisfeld, RA, Sell, S (eds): "Monoclonal antibodies and cancer therapy", New York: Alan R. Liss, p.

2. Mitchell MS, Oettgen HF (1982)(eds). "Hybridomas in Cancer Diagnosis and Treatment". New York: Raven.

3. Bast RC Jr, Klug TL, St. John E, Jenison E, Niloff JM, Lazarus H, Berkowitz RS, Leavitt T, Griffiths CT, Parker L, Zurawski VR Jr, Knapp RC (1983). A radioimmunoassay using a monoclonal antibody to monitor the course of epithelial ovarian cancer. New Engl J Med 309: 883.

4. Giacomini P, Ng AK, Kantor RR, Natali P.G., Ferrone S. (1983). Double determinant immunoassay to measure a human high-molecular weight melanoma-associated antigen. Cancer Res 43: 3586.

5. Herlyn M, Blaszczyk M, Sears HF, Verrill H, Lindgren J, Colcher D, Steplewski Z, Schlom J, Koprowski H (1983). Detection of carcinoembryonic antigen and related antigens in sera of patients with gastrointestinal tumors using monoclonal antibodies in double-determinant radioimmunoassays. Hybridoma 2:329.

6. Ross AH, Herlyn M, Ernst CS, Guerry D, Bennicelli J, Ghrist BFD, Atkinson B, Koprowski H (1984). Immunoassay for melanoma-associated proteoglycan in the sera of patients using monoclonal and polyclonal antibodies. Cancer Res 44: 4642.

7. Morgan AC Jr, Crane MM, Rossen RD (1984). Measurement of a monoclonal antibody-defined, melanoma-associated antigen in human sera: correlation of circulating antigen levels with tumor burden. J Natl Cancer Inst 72: 243.

8. Cote RJ, Morrisey DM, Houghton AN, Beattie FJ, Oettgen HF, Old LJ (1983).Generation of human monoclonal antibodies reactive with cellular antigens.   Proc. Natl Acad Sci USA   80: 2026.

9. Kan-Mitchell J, Imam A, Kempf, RA, Taylor CR, Mitchell MS (1984). Human monoclonal antibodies (MoAbs) with antimelanoma reactivities. Proc Amer Assoc Cancer Res 25:278.

10. Oettgen HF, Old LJ (1985). The humoral immune response to human cancer.   In Reif AE, Mitchell MS (eds): "Immunity to Cancer", Orlando: Academic, In Press.

11. LeGrue SJ, Kahan BD, Pellis NR (1980). Extraction of a murine tumor-specific transplantation antigen with l-butanol.   I. Partial purification by isoelectric focusing. J Natl Cancer Inst 65: 191.

12. Kahan BD, Pellis NR, LeGrue, SJ, Tanaka T (1982). Immunotherapeutic effects of tumor-specific transplantation antigens released by l-butanol. Cancer 49: 1168.

13. Haspel MV, Hoover HC Jr, McCabe RP, Pomato N, Hanna MG (1985). Human colorectal cancer: generation of human monoclonal antibodies.   Proc Amer Assoc Cancer Res 25: 236.

Monoclonal Antibodies and Cancer Therapy, pages 505–522
© 1985 Alan R. Liss, Inc.

HUMAN MONOCLONAL ANTIBODIES: GENERATION OF
TUMOR CELL REACTIVE MONOCLONAL ANTIBODIES USING
PERIPHERAL BLOOD LYMPHOCYTES FROM ACTIVELY
IMMUNIZED COLORECTAL CARCINOMA PATIENTS

Martin V. Haspel, Richard P. McCabe, Nicholas Pomato,
Herbert C. Hoover, Jr[*], Michael G. Hanna, Jr.

Litton Institute of Applied Biotechnology
1330 Piccard Drive
Rockville, Maryland 20850-4373

[*]Division of Surgical Oncology
Health Sciences Center
State University of New York at Stony Brook
Stony Brook, New York 11794

ABSTRACT   The use of human monoclonal antibodies
(MCA) in the detection and treatment of human cancer
has been limited by the apparent scarcity of MCA to
tumor cell surface antigens. Using peripheral blood
lymphocytes from autologous tumor-immunized patients,
we isolated 36 MCA that react to sections of colorectal carcinoma. Twenty of these human MCA were
directed against cell surface antigens. Two-thirds
of the human MCA-producing cell lines were diploid
human B-cells rather than human-mouse heterohybridomas. Direct antibody-binding assays performed
with the MCA indicated that they recognized antigenic determinants preferentially expressed on tumor
cells. Experiments with paired specimens of air-dried,
dissociated colon tumor cells and normal colonic
mucosa cells showed that the MCA bound significantly
more to the cell surfaces of tumor cells than to the
surfaces of normal colonic mucosa cells. Similarly,
tests with a panel of cryostat sections of paired
colon tumor and normal colonic mucosa showed that
MCA bound to the tumor cells and not to the normal
colonic mucosa. None of the MCA bound to cells from
frozen sections of normal breast, stomach, kidney,

liver, skeletal muscle or skin. Furthermore, the
human MCA did not react with carcinoembryonic antigen, human erythrocyte antigens or human lymphocyte
antigens as measured by various techniques. Our
data also demonstrated that these transformed B
cells and hybridomas were stable producers of human
MCA. Thus our studies show that these tumor-specific
human MCA may have the specificity and stability
necessary for in vivo evaluation of their use in the
detection and treatment of cancer.

INTRODUCTION

The usefulness of MCA for the detection, quantitation, and evaluation of the molecular structure of TAA
is well documented. The potential of MCA in the treatment of cancer has also been recognized particularly
because, unlike chemotherapy and radiation therapy, MCA
potentially can be directed specifically to tumor cells,
thus improving the therapeutic:toxicity ratio. Presently,
most MCA developed against human tumor cells are produced
by immunizing mice with human tumor cells or cell extracts.
While a great deal of progress has been made with murine
MCA generated against colon cancer (1-3) and reductions
in tumor load have been reported (4); it has been the
general experience that the epitopes recognized by murine
MCA are often not restricted to tumor cells but may be
present on CEA, blood group determinants and other normal
epithelial components (1,5). In addition, patients
treated with murine MCA often develop an antimouse immu-
nogloblulin response which neutralizes the effect of the
antitumor MCA (6,7). This is not surprising since the
presence of antibody to normal mouse antigens has been
detected by radioimmune precipitation procedures in the
majority of normal human sera (8).

A considerable effort has been made to develop human
hybridoma systems. Many hybridization techniques have
been developed, however, these procedures have been
severely limited by the rarity of antitumor B cell clones
in cancer patients, by technical problems and/or by instability of the clones, resulting in the loss of antibody
reactivity when the cells are grown in culture (9-12).
We have developed a strategy for producing human anti-
tumor MCA which uses circulating B cells from colorectal

patients actively immunized with autologous tumor cells
admixed with BCG. We recently reported results of a
randomized phase II active specific immunotherapy trial
that showed that immunization of colorectal patients with
autologous tumor cells admixed with BCG significantly
increased the delayed cutaneous hypersitivity responses of
the patients to autologous tumor cells, but not to autologous normal mucosa cells (13). Furthermore, no tumor-
specific delayed cutaneous hypersensitivity responses
against autologous tumor or mucosa cells were detected in
a group of nonimmunized control patients. The efficacy of
this tumor-specific cell-mediated immune response has been
manifested over 4 years in significantly decreased recurrence and mortality in immunized as compared with
nonimmunized patients (14). These observations suggested
that these patients may represent an ideal source of B
cells sensitized to TAA. We now report the isolation of
36 human MCA that react to colorectal adenocarcinoma cells
and tissues. Approximately half of these antibodies are
directed against cell surface antigens and are therefore
of potential value for cancer diagnosis and treatment. Of
particular interest is our finding that most of the MCA-
producing cell lines were not human-mouse heterohybridomas
but were diploid human B cells as determined by morpho-
logical and karotype analysis of the cells. Both the
hybridomas and human diploid B cells have the requisite
specificity and stability for the potential use of human
MCA for the diagnosis and treatment of human cancer.

MATERIALS AND METHODS

Cell Lines.

Human colonic adenocarcinoma cell lines HT-29, SW1463,
SW948, SW480, SW403, LoVo, and WiDr were obtained from the
American Type Culture Collection (Rockville, MD). Colon
adenocarcinoma cell line LS-174^t was obtained from Dr. J.
Schlom, (National Cancer Institute, Bethesda, MD).

Collection of PBL.

As previously reported (13), colorectal tumors, after
surgical resection, were minced, enzymatically dissociated
and cryopreserved by techniques that maintain cell viability (15). Patients in the experimental treatment group

received an intradermal vaccination each week for 2 weeks
of 10^7 irradiated autologous tumor cells and 10^7 BCG, and
a vaccination at the third week of 10^7 irradiated tumor
cells alone. Heparinized venous blood was collected one
week after the second immunization from 10 patients and
one week after the first immunization from 9 of the 10
patients. Blood samples were taken from 2 of the patients
before immunization and from 3 of the patients one week
after the third immunization.

Cell Fusion.

Mouse myeloma cells, NS-1, were used for fusion with
human PBL. The procedure has been previously described
(16).

Screening of Hybrids.

Paraffin sections of colorectal tumors fixed in 10%
formalin were deparaffinized and blocked with PBS 1% BSA
and 0.75 M L-lysine (16). In later experiments, air-dried
unfixed, nonpermeabilized, cytocentrifuged preparations,
as described below, of colon cancer cell lines HT-29, LS-
174^t and SW1463 were substituted for the cryostat sections.
The controls consisted of normal human immunoglobulin
matched in isotype and concentration to test MCA.
Air-dried Cytospin slide specimens of colon tumor
cell lines, colon tumor and normal mucosa were prepared
using a Cytospin II centrifuge (Shandon Instruments) as
previously described (16).

Staining of Cytospin Slides with Human MCA by use of an
Indirect Peroxidase Technique.

Cytospin slides, stored at -30°, were warmed to room
temperature. Cells were hydrated with PBS for 5 min
followed by a 5 min wash with 1% BSA-HBSS. Each MCA
supernatant fluid (0.1 ml) was incubated on the slides for
60 min at room temperature followed by a 4° overnight incubation. Each slide was washed in PBS, in 1% BSA-buffered
saline solution, and HBSS. The slides were then incubated
with goat antibody to human IgG, IgA, and IgM conjugated
to horseradish peroxidase and developed with diaminobenzidine as previously described (16). The cells were
counterstained with hematoxylin, and permanent slides
were prepared as described above.

Biotin-labeling of Human MCA.

Human MCA 6a3, 7a2, 7a4, 18-22 and 19b2 were purified from hybridoma culture medium by 60% ammonium sulfate salt fractionation and high pressure liquid chromatography. Each MCA at a concentration of 1.0 to 2.5 mg/ml in 0.01 M potassium phosphate buffer containing 0.15 molar KCl (pH 7.8) was allowed to react with biotin-N-hydroxysuccinimide (Calbiochem) at 4 to 8 mg/ml in dimethyl formamide to give a molar ratio of 120:1 (biotin:antibody). The reaction was gently mixed for 15 min at room temperature, terminated with 1.0 M NH_4Cl and dialyzed overnight against the 0.01 M potassium phosphate buffer.

Direct Staining of Cytospin Slides and Frozen Sections with Biotin-labeled Human MCA.

Cytospin slides, prepared as described, were incubated with a solution of 1.0 mg/ml human IgM in 0.05 M Tris (pH 8.0) containing 1% BSA to block sites of nonspecific binding of human IgM. Each biotin-labeled MCA was diluted 1:3 and 1:10 in the above blocking solution and 0.1 ml was added to each slide for 60 min at 37°. Biotin-labeled human IgM was included in each experiment at the same concentration as the biotin-labeled MCA as a nonspecificity control. After incubation, slides were washed twice, incubated 10 min at 37° with 0.1 ml ABC-horseradish peroxidase reagent (Vector Laboratories, Burlingame, CA). The slides were subsequently washed and stained as described above with diaminobenzidine, counterstained with hemotoxylin and mounted. Frozen sections were warmed to room temperature, and postfixed for 10 min. in 0.5% paraformaldahyde, 0.075 M L-lysine and 0.01 M sodium periodate. The slides were washed in Tris buffer for 10 min at room temperature, blocked with IgM-BSA-Tris, and allowed to react with the biotinylated MCA as described above.

RESULTS

Isolation of Human-mouse Heterohybridomas and Diploid B Cells That Synthesize MCA.

Twenty-two fusions were performed with PBL obtained from 10 tumor-immunized patients, and 2 fusions were done with PBL taken from patients before immunization (Table 1). The isolation of tissue-reactive MCA was not dependent upon the age of the patient, site of the primary tumor or the stage of the tumor (data not shown). Hybridomas were obtained in all 24 fusions performed with PBL obtained from preimmunized or tumor-immunized patients, with only 1 fusion not yielding immunoglobulin-producing cells. The least productive fusions, based on number of cultures with growth, the number of immunoglobulin-producing cell lines and the number of MCA reactive with cell surface tumor antigens, were fusions with PBL obtained before immunization or 1 week after the third immunization. The latter time point was the only immunization in which BCG was not used in the vaccine. More productive fusions were achieved with PBL obtained 1 week after the first or 1 week after the second immunization. PBL obtained 1 week after the second immunization were most productive overall. Evaluation of the fusions performed at weekly intervals after the first, second, and third immunizations indicated that of the 230 immunoglobulin-producing cell lines, 36 (15.7%) reacted with adenocarcinoma of the colon. Of these 36 tumor positive MCA, 20 (55.6%) reacted with tumor cell surface antigens. Most of the antibodies (25/36) were of the IgM isotype.

TABLE 1

ISOLATION OF HUMAN MCA REACTIVE WITH TUMOR CELL SURFACE ANTIGENS

Immunization	No. of fusions	No. of wells assayed / No. of wells seeded (%)	No. of Ig+ cell lines	No. tissue+ MCA	No. of Surface+ MCA / No. of Ig+ cell lines (%)	Isotype IgG	Isotype IgM	Culture pattern of cell lines Diploid	Culture pattern of cell lines Hybridoma
PRE	2	25/240 (10)	4	0	0				
1	9	441/1262 (35)	65	10	4/65 (6)	2	8	8	2
2	10	573/1688 (34)	154	25	16/154 (10)	9	16	16	9
3	3	112/494 (23)	11	1	0		1		1

The tissue-reactive human MCA were produced by two cells types distinctly different in morphology and growth pattern. Twelve of the 36 cell lines were morphologically indistinguishable from murine hybridomas and grew in a dispersed manner. Six representative cell lines were karyotyped and were found to contain both murine and human chromosomes. In contrast, most of the tissue-reactive MCA (24 out of 36) were produced by cells that were irregular

in shape and grew in large clusters typical of some human
lymphoblastoid cell lines. We isolated these cluster-
forming cells from 7 of 10 patients, a result that demonstrates that these cells can be readily isolated when PBL
from actively immunized patients are used. Eight cell
lines, representing 5 fusions from 4 patients, were karyotyped and were found to contain, on the average, 46
chromosomes. G banding of the chromosomes confirmed that
they were of human origin. Thus, the cell morphology
indicated that most of the tumor-reactive MCA-synthesizing
cell lines were not heterohybridomas, but were transformed
B cells. Eighteen representative cluster-forming cells
were screened for Epstein-Barr viral antigens. All but 1
of the cell lines were positive for EBNA and only 1 of the
EBNA-positive cell lines was positive for viral capsid
antigen.

Production of Human MCA.

    Human MCA were typically produced in the range of
5-20 µg/ml. No clear differences existed between diploid
and hybrid cells in the average quantities of immunoglobulin produced. No murine immunoglobulins were detected in
the supernatant fluids of any of the hybrid or diploid
cell lines.
    The diploid cell lines did not exhibit any of the in-
stability reported for lymphoblastoid cell lines obtained
by in vitro transformation by EBV. In fact, we observed
increases in antibody production with many of the diploid
lines during the course of long-term culture. We grew
these cells in continuous culture for almost a year without
any indication of a finite life span of antibody produc-
tivity. Using a single small (25 cc) hollow fiber car-
tridge, we have been able, over the course of two months,
to produce over 4 grams of human MCA 16-88. As expected,
the human-mouse heterohybridomas did have a finite but, in
most instances, a useful life span. Some of the hybrids,
as is the case with some mouse-mouse hybrids, were too
unstable to be cloned and are therefore not described in
this report. Most of the hybrids, however, do appear to
have sufficient stability to permit batch production of
clinically useful quantities of antibody. For example,
human-mouse heterohybridoma 7a2 was passaged for more than
20 generations from a recently cloned seed stock of 5×10^6
cells without a decrease in antibody production.

Immunohistochemical Reactivity Of Human MCA To Colorectal
Tumors.

The individual MCA usually reacted in a homogeneous
manner with individual tumors. Rarely did we find a
heterogeneous pattern of reactivity among tumor cells
either in paraffin or cryostat sections of an individual
tumor with any individual MCA.
The pattern of reactivity of 10 of the human MCA to
histological sections of colorectal adenocarcinomas from
15 patients is shown in Fig. 1. The matrix of reactivity
of the MCA tested indicates that individual antibodies
reacted to between 47 and 80% of the tumor specimens tested. No MCA reacted to all 15 tumors. In tissue sections
from individual patients, the range of reactivity varied
from tissues reactive to all 10 antibodies (e.g., patients
1, 8 and 11) to tissues reactive to as few as 1 or 2 MCA
(patients 2 and 9). All of the tissue specimens used for
determination of MCA reactivity were taken from patients
other than the 10 donors of B cells for the original
fusions.
We compared the pathologic stage of the tumors tested
to the percentage of reactivity with the group of MCA
tested, and found that the tumors with broadest reactivity
were moderately- to well-differentiated, adenocarcinomas;
the less common, poorly differentiated adenocarcinomas
(e.g., patient 9) were generally nonreactive. The antibodies typically reacted with metaştases (e.g., patient
4). No pattern of reactivity vis-a-vis site of the
primary tumor or Duke's stage was apparent.

Reactivity of Human MCA to Cell Surface Antigens of 8
Colon Carcinoma Cell Lines.

Thirty-six human MCA were assessed for reactivity
with tumor cell surface antigens against a panel of 8
human colon cancer cell lines prepared as air-dried cyto-
centrifuge specimens. Thirteen of 36 MCA recognized
antigens expressed on the surface of at least 2 human
colon carcinoma cell lines. All 13 surface-reactive MCA
were isotyped as IgM. These MCA were produced by both
heterohybridomas and diploid B-cell lines.
Experiments using murine MCA to structural cytoplasmic
antigens, such as actin, confirmed that cytoplasmic structures cannot be detected with properly prepared airdried
Cytospin cell preparations without prior permeabilization

of the cell membrane (data not shown). However, we confirmed the surface localization of the antigens recognized
on the Cytospin-prepared cells for most of the MCA by
direct immunofluorescence of live cells.

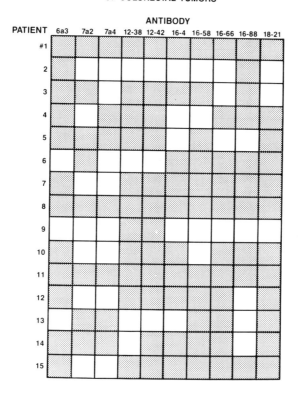

DISTRIBUTION OF ANTIGENS IN PARAFFIN SECTIONS
OF COLORECTAL TUMORS

FIGURE 1. Distribution of antigens in paraffin sections
of colorectal tumors. Shaded area indicates positive indirect immunoperoxidase staining of 15 tumors by 10 human
MCA.

Reactivity of Human MCA with Paraffin Sections of Paired
Colon Tumor and Normal Mucosa.

     Eight of the antibodies reacted with tumor cells and/
or cryostat sections but did not react with paraffin sections. The specificity of 22 of the 28 human MCA reactive

with paraffin sections was tested by indirect immunohisto-
chemistry against paired sections of colonic tumor and
autologous normal colonic mucosa from 5 patients (Table 2).
Eight of 25 MCA (44%) demonstrated no detectable reactivity with normal colonic mucosa in the 5 patients tested,
but all 8 reacted with tumor specimens. Fourteen of the
22 MCA, although reactive with the tumor specimens, also
reacted with normal colonic mucosa. Quantitatively in
these cases reactivity with normal colonic specimens was
less than with tumor specimens. Individual MCA reacted
with 1 to 4 of the normal colonic mucosa specimens tested.
Five of 14 of these crosssreactive MCA only reacted with
the normal colonic mucosa of 1 of the 5 patients. The
normal colonic mucosa of patient 8 reacted with 13 of the
23 antibodies that reacted with that patient's tumor.
Whether the normal colonic mucosa from this patient was
proximal or distal to the tumor is not known. Overall, in
the total paired colorectal tumor and normal colonic
mucosa specimens tested, approximately 30% crossreactivity
with normal colonic mucosa was seen, although the quantitative reactivity was significantly less than that observed
against the paired tumor specimen.

TABLE 2

**REACTIVITY OF HUMAN MCA ON PARAFFIN SECTIONS OF COLORECTAL
TUMORS (T) AND PAIRED NORMAL COLONIC MUCOSA (N)**

| | Patient Number | | | | | | | | | |
| | 2 | | 6 | | 7 | | 8 | | 10 | |
MCA	T	N	T	N	T	N	T	N	T	N
6a3	+	-	-		2+	-	2+	-	2+	-
7a2	-		3+	-	-		4+	-	-	
11B5	+	-	3+	-	3+	-	4+	2+	3+	+
12-38	-		-	-	2+	-	2+	-	3+	-
12-42	-		-		2+	-	3+	-	2+	-
12-47	+	-	-		+	-	2+	-	-	
12-53	-		3+	-	-		+	-	-	
15-24-2	-		3+	-	4+	2+	3+	+	-	
16-4	-		2+	-	+	-	3+	+	+	-
16-58	-		4+	+	4+	-	2+	+	-	
16-66	-		4+	-	+	+	3+	+	+	-
16-86	-		-		2+	-	+	-	+	-
16-88	+	-	2+	-	+	-	4+	+	+	-
18-15	+	-	2+	-	+	-	2+	+	+	-
18-21	-		3+	+	2+	+	3+	+	+	+
19b2	-		-		2+	+	4+	2+	-	
20A3	+	-	4+	+	+	-	2+	-	+	-
20A6	3+	-	2+	-	2+	-	2+	-	2+	+
20B7	3+	+	2+	-	+	-	3+	+	+	+
21B27	2+	+	2+	-	-		3+	+	+	-
23A4	-		2+	-	2+	-	2+	+	3+	-
27B1	2+	-	4+	+	3+	-	4+	2+	3+	+

Direct Binding of Biotin-labeled MCA to Frozen Tissue
Sections of Colon Tumor and Normal Colonic Mucosa.

Further direct characterization of the 5 biotin-
labeled MCA with regard to their specificity for tumor
versus normal cells was established with frozen tissue
sections of colon tumor and adjacent normal colonic mucosa
(Table 3). Absolute specificity was observed with 4 of
the MCA as shown by the fact that they strongly react
with at least 2 out of 5 colon tumors and did not reach
with any of the 4 matched normal colonic mucosa sections.
MCA 19b2 reacted strongly with 4 of 5 tumor sections and
showed a weak reaction with 1 of 4 normal colonic mucosa
sections.
Frozen tissue sections of normal breast, stomach,
kidney, liver, muscle and skin (Table 3) showed no staining by biotin-labeled human MCA except antibody 19b2
which exhibited a low level of binding to normal stomach
tissue. An overall background stain of connective tissue
components was observed. This background staining was
nonspecific and has been observed by others using biotin-
labeled MCA.

TABLE 3

REACTIVITY OF BIOTIN-LABELED MCA WITH FROZEN SECTIONS
OF COLON TUMORS (T) AND NORMAL TISSUES (N)

Source of Tissue	MCA									
	6a3		7a2		7a4		18-22		19b2	
	T	N	T	N	T	N	T	N	T	N
Colon	+	-	-	-	2+	-	+	-	2+	+
Colon	3+	-	2+	-	3+	-	+	-	2+	-
Colon	3+	-	+	-	3+	-	3+	-	3+	-
Colon	2+	-	+	-	-	-	-	-	-	-
Breast		-		-		-		-		-
Breast		-		-		-		-		-
Breast	-	-	-	-	-	-	-	-	-	-
Stomach		-		-		-		-		+
Kidney		-		-		-		-		-
Liver		-		-		-		-		-
Muscle		-		-		-		-		-
Skin		-		-		-		-		-
Skin		-		-		-		-		-

Reactivity of MCA with CEA, Erythrocyte and Leukocyte
Antigens.

To further establish the tumor specificity of the
MCA, we tested them for reactivity with CEA, human
erythrocyte antigens and human lymphocyte antigens by
various techiques. We found no evidence of reactivity
between these MCA and these antigens. Reactivity with
human erythrocyte antigens was measured by indirect
immunofluorescence and hemagglutination against an
erythrocyte panel representing all major and most minor
blood group systems. No reactivity was seen. ELISA,
cytotoxicity assays and direct immunofluorescence staining
of human lymphocytes showed no evidence of recognition of
human lymphocyte antigens by any of the MCA.

Functionality of Human MCA to Colorectal Cancer.

Specificity is a major consideration in the determination of the usefulness of these tumor-reactive MCA.
The lack of reactivity of some of the MCA with a certain
percentage of the tumor specimens tested is another factor
which must be considered. Thus is it unlikely, based upon
these data obtained with paraffin sections of tumors, dissociated primary tumor cells and tumor cell lines, that
any single MCA would react with all patient's tumors
making it an ideal MCA for universal therapeutic or
diagnostic applications.
The strategy of using immunized cancer patients has
provided a large number of clones from which certain sele-
tions can be made with regard to range of reactivities.
By selecting only 2 of the MCA that we have produced
which, based on their characteristics in a broad in vitro
screen, have the greatest amount of tumor reactivity with
the least amount of normal colonic mucosa reactivity, we
can propose and develop cocktails of antibodies that
together promise greater efficacy that any individual MCA.
As shown in Fig. 2, 2 monoclonal antibodies, 6a3-1 and 7a2
paired for their range of reactivity with both tissue
sections and dissociated tumor cells and selected based on
their relative lack of crossreactivity with normal colonic
mucosa, provide an antibody cocktail which will react with
14 of 15 tumor specimens and 9 of 9 dissociated tumor cell
specimens.

TWO MONOCLONAL ANTIBODIES REACT WITH MOST COLORECTAL TUMORS

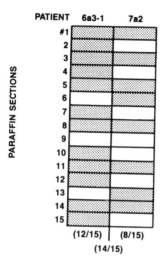

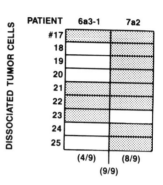

FIGURE 2.   Two MCA react with most colorectal tumors.
The reactivity of two monoclonal antibodies to paraffin
sections of 15 colorectal tumors and air-dried Cytospin
preparations of dissociated tumors from 9 patients are
compared.   Shaded area indicates positive indirect immunoperoxidase staining.

DISCUSSION

There are 3 important factors in the development and
production of human MCA for TAA.   These are strategy,
specificity, and stability.

Peripheral blood lymphocytes were obtained from
actively immunized patients that had been determined, by
delayed cutaneous hypersensitivity tests, to be immunologically responsive to their autologous tumor (13).   In
this prospectively randomized phase II protocol, this induced cell-mediated immune response has been associated
with an increase in the disease-free period and overall
survival rate for patients monitored for over 4 years (14).
We speculated that at some point during the course of immunization, which was developed primarily for stimulation of
a strong cellmediated immune response, there would be a
transient humoral immune response of some magnitude.   In

our studies the most productive fusions were obtained with
PBL taken 1 week after the first and 1 week afte the second
immunization. In these vaccines, 21 autologous tumor cells
cells were given admixed with BCG at a ratio of 10^7 viable
tumor cells to 10^7 viable BCG organisms. Less success in
terms of effective fusions was achieved with the PBL obtained 1 week after the third immunization, which used the
vaccine that consisted solely of tumor cells. No successful fusions with regard to demonstrated production of antibodies reactive with cell surface antigens were obtained
in fusions made from patients before immunization. We
speculate that the increase in fusion efficiency may be
associated with the active immunizations augmented by the
adjuvant BCG. BCG is known to influence the depletion of
bone marrow reserves and thereby to affect the presence of
progenitor B cells in circulation which normally would not
be present in peripheral blood of cancer patients or in
lymph nodes draining the sites of primary tumors.

Approximately 20% of the cultures tested produced
human immunoglobulin, with 15.6% of the MCA binding to
colon tumor cell antigens. MCA reactive with tumors were
isolated from 7 of the 10 immunized patients. Our results
demonstrated that human colon cancer is immunogenic, and
that the antigens recognized are not individually specific
but rather are expressed on tumors from various patients.
Antigenic diversity or complexity of antigen expression
has been reported to occur in carcinogen-induced experimental tumors (18). Most significant in our strategy is
the high proportion of MCA reactive with tumor cell surface
antigens. Results with our MCA suggest that colorectal
tumors similarly appear to express multiple TAA. None of
the MCA isolated thus far detected an antigen common to
all of the tumors. However, a cocktail of appropriately
complementary antibodies potentially could achieve the
broad reactivity necessary for in vivo diagnosis and
therapy. For example, 6a3-1 and 7a2 would react with 14
of 15 tumor specimens and 9 of 9 dissociated tumor cell
specimens. Other cocktails of this type can be developed;
however, clearly we must have a broad range of MCA to
selected from an extensive in vitro screen for testing a
large number of specimens in a variety of differentiation
states in order to utilize human MCA for therapeutic or
diagnostic purposes.

In the present study, one third of the cell lines
were mouse-human heterohybridomas based upon morphology

and karyotypic analysis. In contrast, most of the MCA-synthesizing cell lines were predominantly irregular in shape and grew in large aggregates. These large cluster-forming cells were isolated in 11 fusions performed with PBL from 7 of 10 patients. Thus, they appear to be quite common when our strategy of MCA development is used. Karyotype analysis demonstrated that these cells contain, on the average, 46 chromosomes. G banding of the chromosomes confirmed that they were of human origin. Thus based upon the criterion of cell morphology, it appears that most of the MCA-synthesizing cell lines are not hybridomas, but rather are transformed B cells.

An interesting and significant difference in the specific reactivity of these MCA as compared to many mouse MCA generated against human colon cancer is the absence of reactivity to well-known tissue components, particularly CEA, frequently recognized by mouse MCA (5). We found no reactivity of these human antibodies to CEA, blood group determinants or histocompatibility antigens, suggesting that the human MCA specificity is restricted to those structures recognized as immunogenic in the autologous host. It is not unreasonable to expect that when one immunizes mice with human tumor cells, there would be substantial antigenic competition resulting in the more abundant and more predominant tissue-type and differentiation antigens successfully competing with relatively minor TAA for immune responsiveness by the host. Thus, autologous immunization of man may result in the elicitation of antibodies against the group of antigens normally poorly immunogeneic in mice. This evidence suggests that humans and mice may respond to different TAA. Another apparent difference between human and mouse MCA is the patterns of labeling. Previous studies with mouse MCA have demonstrated that there is often a heterogenous labeling of cells within tumor sections. This pattern of reactivity has been attributed by some authors to antigenic heterogeneity of tumor cells (19,20). In contrast, the human MCA developed by our strategy were homogeneous in terms of their reactivity to tumors to which they did react.

Specificity aside, only MCA that can be produced in appropriate quantities can be considered clinically relevant. The diploid lymphoblastoid cells tend to produce increased rather than decreased amounts of MCA over time and have been kept in continuous culture almost a year. The human-mouse heterohybridomas, although less stable than the diploid lines, should be able, with frequent recloning, to produce sufficient quantities of monoclonal antibody for clinical use.

ACKNOWLEDGEMENT

The authors express appreciation to Ms. N. Janesch, J. Knowlton, L. Peters, M. Petalver, L. Petkofsky, M. C. Schneider and S. Berg for technical assistance and to Drs. R. Harty, A. B. Jenson and R. K. Oldham for valuable advice.

REFERENCES

1. Atkinson BF, Ernst CS, Herlyn M, Steplewski Z, Sears HF, Koprowski H (1982). Gastrointestinal cancer-associated antigen in immunoperoxidase assay. Cancer Res 42:4820.
2. Koprowski H, Steplewski Z, Mitchell K, Herlyn M, Herlyn D, Fuhrer P (1979). Colorectal carcinoma antigens detected by hybridoma antibodies. Somatic Cell Genet 5:957.
3. Moldofsky PJ, Sears HF, Mulhern CB, Hammond ND, Powe J, Gatenby RA, Steplewski Z, Koprowski H (1984). Detection of metastatic tumor in normal-sized retroperitoneal lymph nodes by monoclonal antibody imaging. New Eng J Med 311:106.
4. Sears HF, Herlyn D, Steplewski Z, Koprowski H (1984). Effects of monoclonal antibody immunotherapy on patients with gastrointestinal adenocarcinoma. J Biol Response Modifiers 3:138.
5. Herlyn M, Blasczyk M, Sears HF, Verrill H, Lindgren J, Colcher D, Steplewski Z, Schlom J, Koprowski H (1983). Detection of carcinoembryonic antigen and related antigens in sera of patients with gastrointestinal tumors using monoclonal antibodies in double-determinant radioimmunoassays. Hybridoma 2:329.
6. Levy R, Miller RA (1983). Tumor therapy with monoclonal antibodies. Fed Proc 42:2650.
7. Schroff RW, Foon KR, Beatty SM, Oldham RK, Morgan AC Jr (1985). Human anti-murine immunoglobulin response in patients receiving monoclonal antibody therapy. Cancer Res 45:879.
8. Hersh EM, Hanna MG Jr, Gutterman JU, Mavligit G, Yurconic M Jr, Gschwind CR (1974). Human immune response to active immunization with Rauscher leukemia virus. II. Humoral immunity. JNCI 53:327.

9. Cole SP, Campling BG, Louwman IH, Kozbor D, Roder JC (1984). A strategy for the production of human monoclonal antibodies reactive with lung tumor cell lines. Cancer Res 44:2750.

10. Cote RJ, Morrissey DM, Houghton AN, Beattie EJ Jr, Oettgen HF, Old LJ (1983). Generation of human monoclonal antibodies reactive with cellular antigens. Proc Natl Acad Sci USA 80:2026.

11. Iman A, Drushella MM, Taylor CR, Tökés Z (1985). Generation and immunohistological characterization of human monoclonal antibodies to mammary carcinoma cells. Cancer Res 45:263.

12. Schlom J, Wunderlich D, Teramoto UA (1980). Generation of human monoclonal antibodies reactive with human mammary carcinoma cells. Proc Natl Acad Sci USA 77:6841.

13. Hoover HC Jr, Surdyke M, Dangel R, Peters LC and Hanna MG Jr (1984). Delayed cutaneous hypersensitivity to autologous tumor cells in colorectal cancer patients immunized with an autologous tumor cell: bacillus Calmette-Guérin vaccine. Cancer Res 44:1671.

14. Hoover HC Jr, Surdyke MG, Dangel RB, Peters LC, Hanna MG Jr (1985). Prospectively randomized trial of adjuvant active specific immunotherapy for human colorectal cancer. Cancer 55:1236.

15. Peters LC, Brandhorst JS, Hanna MG Jr (1979). Preparation of immunotherapeutic autologous tumor cell vaccines from solid tumors. Cancer Res 39:1353.

16. Haspel MV, McCabe RP, Pomato N, Janesch NJ, Knowlton JV, Peters LC, Hoover HC Jr and Hanna MG Jr (1985). Generation of tumor cell reactive human monoclonal antibodies using peripheral blood lymphocytes from actively immunized colorectal carcinoma patients. Cancer Res (in press)

17. Knobler RL, Dubois-Dalcq M, Haspel MV, Claysmith AP, Lampert PW, Oldstone MBA (1981). Selective localization of wild-type and mutant mouse hepatitis virus (JHM strain) antigens in CNS tissue by fluorescence, light and electronmicroscopy. J Neuroimmunol 1:81.

18. Wortzel RD, Philipps C, Schreiber H (1983). Multiple tumour-specific antigens expressed on a single tumour cell. Nature 304:165.

19. Hand PH, Nuti M, Colcher D, Schlom J (1983). Defi-
     nition of antigenic heterogeneity and modulation among
     human mammary carcinoma cell populations using mono-
     clonal antibodies to tumor-associated antigens.
     Cancer Res 43:728.
20. Wright GL Jr, Beckett ML, Starling JJ, Schellhammer
     PF, Sieg SM, Ladaga LE, Poleskic S (1983). Immuno-
     histochemical localization of prostate carcinoma-
     associated antigens. Cancer Res 43:5509.

Monoclonal Antibodies and Cancer Therapy, pages 523–536
© 1985 Alan R. Liss, Inc.

MONOCLONAL ANTIBODIES IN THE DEVELOPMENT
OF ACTIVE SPECIFIC IMMUNOTHERAPY FOR MELANOMA[1]

June Kan-Mitchell, Raymond A. Kempf, Ashraf Imam,
Ralph A. Reisfeld and Malcolm S. Mitchell

Departments of Microbiology and Medicine
University of Southern California
School of Medicine
Los Angeles, California 90033
and
Department of Immunology
Scripps Clinic and Research Foundation
La Jolla, California 92037

ABSTRACT   We have attempted to design a trial of
active specific immunotherapy ("vaccination") in which
a more precise dose of tumor-associated antigens could
be administered.   Soluble extracts have been prepared
from surgical specimens. An estimate of the antigenic
contents of these extracts was made by a binding
inhibition assay with the mouse monoclonal antibody,
9.2.27, which detects the core protein p250 of the
noncartilage chondroitin sulfate proteoglycan present
on most human melanoma cells. Serial analysis of the
content of circulating p250 in the sera of vaccinated
patients on study was also performed with 9.2.27. To
identify melanoma-associated antigens immunogenic to
man, and therefore important to be included in tumor
vaccines, human monoclonal antibodies were produced by
the fusion of regional lymph node cells from melanoma
patients with a mouse myeloma line.   Six human

[1]This work was supported by grants from the National
Cancer Institute, CA 36233, the Concern Foundation, the
Eckstrom Trust, the Mirkin Foundation and the Lawrence D.
Lenihan Memorial Fund.

monoclonal antibodies, 4 IgGs and 2 IgMs, had reactivities against melanoma cells in tissue culture and fixed tissue sections. One antibody studied in greater detail bound to 23 of 23 skin melanomas, 2 ocular melanomas and 1 lentigo maligna. There was no reactivity to normal melanocytes in skin or pigmented cells in nonmalignant nevi, such as blue, compound, congenital, junctional, epithelioid (Spitz) and halo nevi. The only reactivity noted was against dysplastic nevi, which are premalignant lesions. Of most interest was that all of the human monoclonal antibodies identified cytoplasmic rather than surface antigens. These cytoplasmic antigens were distinct from carcinoembryonic antigen. A pool of butanol extracts from allogeneic melanoma was given subcutaneously (300 units of p250 per week for 6 weeks) without toxicity to 6 patients with Stage IV melanoma, either alone or preceded by low dose cyclophosphamide. Neither toxicity nor evidence of significant immunological effectiveness has thus far been observed in this early stage of our Phase I trial. Monoclonal antibodies will play a significant role in the quantitation of the immunogens administered in active specific immunotherapy, as well as the monitoring of its effectiveness on the host's immunity.

INTRODUCTION

Finding a consistent way to augment the immunological reactivity of cancer patients to their own tumor, thereby eradicating residual foci of tumor cells, has been the fond hope of tumor immunologists for decades. Hybridoma technology in particular has permitted a more precise identification of the antigens expressed on tumor cells and perhaps the determination of their importance as immunogens in man. It is towards these objectives that we have designed a trial of active specific immunotherapy in melanoma in which a more precise dose of tumor-associated antigens could be administered.

METHODS AND RESULTS

Preparation of Vaccines

Thirteen soluble extracts were prepared from human melanoma cells derived from fresh surgical specimens. The extraction was performed with 1-butanol, a method originally devised to selectively remove highly antigenic tumor-associated antigens but not histocompatibility antigens from methylcholanthrene-induced mouse sarcomas (1). The optimal conditions for extraction from human melanoma cells from tumor tissues were first determined with cultured melanoma cells. Incubation with 2.5% 1-butanol in Dulbecco's phosphate buffered saline for 5 min resulted in the maximal extraction of protein while still maintaining viability of the cells. Under these conditions, the cultured melanoma cells were shown to retain most of their HLA-A,B and HLA-DR antigens by an indirect binding radioimmunoassay with ^{125}I-labeled Staphylococcal Protein A .

Quantitation of Melanoma-Associated Antigens in Extracts

A binding inhibition assay was developed to measure the content of a particular antigen in our tumor vaccines with an appropriate monoclonal antibody. A predetermined quantity of the monoclonal antibody labeled with horseradish peroxidase (HPO) was first allowed to react with either the vaccine to be tested or a reference antigenic standard. If the antigen whose epitope is recognized by the monoclonal antibody is present in the extract, it preempts binding sites of the antibody. Thus, the degree of inhibition of binding of the monoclonal antibody to target melanoma cells bearing the corresponding epitope is a measurement of the specific content of the antigen in the vaccine. By referring to a standard curve of binding inhibition by serial dilutions of a reference antigenic extract, the relative number of antigenic units in the vaccine can be determined.

We have established a model assay with the 9.2.27 monoclonal antibody to detect and quantitate the core glycoprotein, p250, of melanoma-associated chondroitin sulfate proteoglycan (2). The reactivity of 9.2.27 has been shown to be highly restricted to melanoma cells and other

cells of neuroectodermal origin. To determine first the
appropriate amount of the 9.2.27-HPO conjugate to use in
these experiments, various dilutions were added to dried
melanoma cells in microtiter wells for 1 h at 37C. The
amount of antibody bound, as measured by the peroxidase
activity fixed to the cells, was proportional to the amount
of 9.2.27-HPO added. Under these conditions, 8 to 100ng of
antibody protein did not saturate all of the available
antigenic sites on the M21 cells. Thus, a non-saturating
amount of the antibody-HPO conjugate that gave a convenient
optical density was adopted for this binding inhibition
assay.

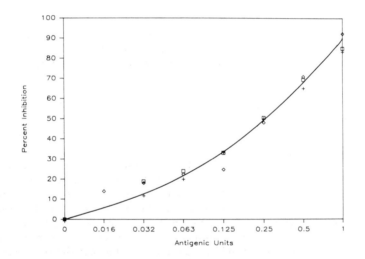

FIGURE 1.   Standard binding inhibition curve of
9.2.27-HPO by preincubation with serial dilutions of the
melanoma extract MA-17.   Three concentrations of 9.2.27-HPO
were used (◊ , 6.8 ug/ml; + , 8.5 ug/ml and □ , 10.2
ug/ml).

Figure 1 shows the percent inhibition of the binding of
9.2.27-HPO at 3 concentrations of antibody by various
dilutions of the antigenic extract MA-17, ranging from
undiluted (1.0) to 1/64 (0.016). The curve reproducibly
obtained was sigmoidal and appeared to be independent of
the concentration of 9.2.27-HPO used within this range

(6.8-10.2 ug/ml). Because MA-17 had a considerable concentration of p250, we used it as our standard to measure the relative amount of p250 in the other extracts. The amount of p250 antigenic activity in 10 ul of the MA-17 extract was defined as one antigenic unit.

TABLE 1

ANTIGENIC UNITS OF P250

IN 1-BUTANOL EXTRACTS OF TUMORS

Butanol Extract	% Inhibition of Binding	Antigenic Units/ml
MA-2	30	11.5
MA-3	46	22.0
MA-6	66	43.5
MA-7	35	15.0
MA-8	ND[a]	–
MA-10	44	21.0
MA-11	40	18.0
MA-12	74	60.0
MA-13	38	17.0
MA-14	ND	–
MA-15	ND	–
MA-16	22	6.5
MA-17	86	100.0
AML-1[b]	24	7.8
Lu-2[c]	20	5.6
Br-1[d]	26	9.2
Bl-1[e]	5	2.2

[a] not detectable
[b] acute myelocytic leukemia
[c] squamous lung carcinoma
[d] breast carcinoma
[e] bladder carcinoma.

By titrating MA-17 in parallel with an unknown preparation, the relative number of antigenic units of p250 in the new extract can be deduced from the standard curve. This approach enables us to give a standard dose of this antigen to each patient. Table 1 shows data on 13 melanoma extracts, 10 of which had detectable p250. The 3 preparations without p250 activity were from poorly preserved specimens. No appreciable p250 activity was found in the 4 control extracts, from acute myelocytic leukemia, lung carcinoma, breast carcinoma and bladder carcinoma.

Development of Human Monoclonal Antibodies for Use in Indicating Immunogenic Antigens

To identify melanoma antigens that are immunogenic to man, we developed human monoclonal antibodies by fusing human regional lymph node cells of melanoma patients with the mouse myeloma cell line M5, a subline of SP2/0Ag14 adapted to grow in agammaglobulinemic horse serum. Our method was based on that of Schlom and his colleagues to immortalize lymphocytes primed in vivo to antigens of breast carcinoma (3). Six human monoclonal antibodies were generated from a total of 9 fusions. The antibodies were derived from lymphocytes of 3 patients. Initial screening for reactivity against melanoma cultures by either fluorescein isothiocyanate (FITC)- or HPO-conjugated goat antihuman Ig was not sufficiently sensitive in our hands to demonstrate binding. The target antigens appeared to be present at concentrations much lower than other melanoma-associated antigens identified by mouse monoclonal antibodies. This problem was overcome by the use of the biotin-avidin-peroxidase amplification system. In this manner, all 6 antibodies were found to have reactivity against cytoplasmic antigens present in melanoma cells in short term cultures, fixed by a 3 minute exposure to formaldehyde. No binding was detected if the same concentration of normal polyclonal human Ig was used. Under these conditions, all 6 antibodies had little or no reactivity against a glioma cell culture and a lung squamous carcinoma cell culture.

To test the binding characteristics of these human antibodies efficiently against a variety of tissue types, we used formaldehyde-fixed, paraffin-embedded sections of human tissues, both normal and malignant. To circumvent the problem of background reactivity due to the endogeneous human immunoglobulins in specimens, we conjugated our purified monoclonal antibodies directly to biotin. Binding was demonstrated with the avidin-biotin-peroxidase complex without the use of a second antibody reactive against human immunoglobulins. Two of the 6 antibodies, 2-139-1 (2-139) and 6-26-3, were studied extensively with very similar results. For simplicity, we will present data only with 2-139 here.

2-139 was reactive against all melanoma tumor specimens tested, including 18 primary cutaneous lesions, 5 metastases and 2 ocular melanomas. One of 4 lentigo maligna, a low grade melanoma, was also reactive. No reactivity was detectable in 2 basal cell carcinomas and 2 squamous cell carcinomas (Table 2).

TABLE 2

REACTIVITY OF ANTIBODY 2-139 : HUMAN SKIN TUMORS

Diagnosis	+ve/Total	% Cells +ve (Intensity)[a]
Primary melanoma	18/18	60-70 (3+)
Metastatic melanoma	5/5	90 (3+)
Ocular melanoma	2/2	60 (2+)
Lentigo maligna	1/4	30 (2+)
Basal cell carcinoma	0/2	-
Squamous cell carcinoma	0/2	-

[a]Intensity of staining was scored on a arbitrary scale of 1 to 4+.

Melanocytes in normal skin and nonmalignant pigmented cells such as those found in many types of nevi were not stained by this antibody (Table 3) (4). The only nevi that were reactive with antibody 2-139 were 2 of the 5 dysplastic nevi. In this regard, it is interesting to note that dysplastic nevi are considered to be premalignant lesions.

TABLE 3
REACTIVITY OF ANTIBODY 2-139 : NEVI

Diagnosis	+ve/Total
Blue	0/2
Compound	0/3
Congenital	0/2
Junctional	0/1
Epithelioid (Spitz)	0/7
Halo	0/2
Dysplastic	2/5[a]

[a]40% cells positive; intensity 2+.

TABLE 4
ABSENCE OF REACTIVITY OF ANTIBODY 2-139
AGAINST VARIOUS TISSUES

Tissue	+ve/Total
Skin	0/3
Colon	0/2[a]
Liver	0/1
Lung	0/4
Kidney	0/6[b]
Pancreas	0/1[b]
Salivary gland	0/2[b]
Breast fibroadenoma	0/2
Benign prostatic hypertrophy	0/3
Lung small cell carcinoma	0/1
Lung adenocarcinoma	0/1

[a] Surface epithelium only positive
[b] Collecting tubules of kidney, ducts of
   pancreas, salivary gland positive.

Antibody 2-139 had no reactivity against a variety
of other tissues (Table 4).   Thus no reactivity was
observed against normal skin, liver and lung. The majority

of the tissue components of colon, kidney, pancreas and kidney were also not stained. However, binding was detected in the tip of the villi, that is the surface epithelium of the colon. The collecting tubules in the kidney were also stained, but this tissue is also (nonspecifically) reactive with many mouse monoclonal antibodies. The ducts of the pancreas and salivary gland were also stained by 2-139. Mammary fibroadenoma, benign prostate hypertrophy and small cell and adenocarcinoma of the lung were also not reactive.

In Table 5 is shown the reactivity of 2-139 against tumors other than melanoma (Table 5). The strongest reactivities were against colon and prostate carcinomas. Cross-reactivity was clearly not restricted to cells of neuroectodermal derivation, in contrast to the reactivities found with mouse monoclonal antibodies to melanoma cells.

TABLE 5
REACTIVITY OF ANTIBODY 2-139 WITH VARIOUS TUMORS

Diagnosis	+ve/Total	% Cells +ve	(Intensity)
Breast infiltrating ductal carcinoma	2/2	60	(1+)
Colon carcinoma	6/6	80	(3+)
Liver carcinoma	2/2	50	(2+)
Lung large cell carcinoma	1/1	20	(2+)
Lung squamous cell carcinoma	1/1	20	(2+)
Pancreatic carcinoma	1/2	50	(2+)
Prostate carcinoma	2/2	70	(4+)
Stomach carcinoma	1/1	70	(1+)

The human-mouse hybridomas isolated were relatively stable and retained their ability to produce and secrete monoclonal antibodies over at least 6 months. The relative stability may be due to the use of the mouse myeloma cell line M5, a derivative of SP2/OAg14. Previous human-mouse hybridizations have predominantly utilized mouse myelomas derived from the NS1 parent. Our fusions were performed within 2-4 hours after the lymph nodes were obtained, which may also have beneficially influenced our results. Another factor which appeared to be of importance was the lot of serum used. We have found several lots of horse serum to be toxic to the hybrid cells. Replacement with fetal calf sera always resulted in cessation of antibody secretion by our hybridomas.

Phase I Clinical Trial of Allogeneic Melanoma Vaccine: Preliminary Results

In order to test the toxicity and immunological effects of our allogeneic melanoma vaccine, we elected first to treat patients with metastatic melanoma, with at least a predicted 3-month survival. These individuals might be expected to have a relatively intact immune response, and might indicate to us the dose that could be administered to patients whose primary tumors had just been resected. This is the group that will ultimately be the subjects for an extensive Phase III clinical trial. A pooled preparation of 3 allogeneic melanoma extracts with the highest p250 activity was used to provide a uniform preparation for a group of 6 patients. We administered 300 units of antigen to 3 patients with absent skin test reactivity to the vaccine preparation (25 units, in 0.25 ml intradermally). The antigenic extracts were given in a total volume of 3.0 ml subcutaneously in the extremities. No adjuvant was used, to follow the procedures of Kahan et al (5) as closely as possible. The pooled antigens were given weekly for 6 weeks to the first 3 patients in the study, with repeat skin testing 1 week after the last dose to see whether delayed hypersensitivity to the extracts had developed. None of these patients in fact developed delayed hypersensitivity to the allogeneic vaccine. The next 3 patients were given 300 mg/m^2 of cyclophosphamide, to inhibit their suppressor T cells, before receiving the same dose of 300 units of vaccine antigens. These patients also did not develop skin test reactivity against the vaccine. All 6 patients with Stage IV melanoma had progression of their disease.

We are aware that the measurement of cytolytic T cells and specific serum antibodies directed against melanoma-associated antigens may be the best tests to monitor the efficacy of the vaccines. Serum antibodies, which we have sought to quantitate by a method based on blocking the binding of 9.2.27 to melanoma target cells, have not been consistently found in the patients after vaccination. One contributing factor may be that the concentration of an antibody reacting against the same epitope as 9.2.27 may be too low to detect. A panel of monoclonal antibodies to detect several antibodies in the serum at once may be more useful if such a competitive binding technique is to be applied to titrate specific antibody molecules. A procedure for quantitating cytolytic T cells is also under development.

Measurement of Serum Antigen with Monoclonal Antibody 9.2.27 to Monitor the Course of Disease

The amount of antigenic material given to the patients and the subcutaneous route both made it unlikely that the level of serum antigen p250 would be elevated by the vaccination procedure. Nevertheless, we were interested to determine whether measurement of levels of serum antigen might help to monitor the course of disease in the Phase I test population, all of whom had metastatic melanoma.

The assay we used was essentially that described for the determination of p250 activity in the vaccines. In pilot studies, we found that several human sera contained spurious reactivity against mouse immunoglobulins. We overcame this problem by the addition of 10 ug/ml of the mouse myeloma protein MOPC 21 to the reaction mixture. The lowest detectable level of p250 antigenic activity was 3-6 units/ml of serum. Analysis of variance of the assay allowed us to define a significant level of antigenic activity to be 8 units/ml or greater. We found no significant level of p250 activity in sera from 6 normal individuals, in 7 patients with benign diseases and in 40 patients with a variety of other cancers. The 13 patients with Stages I to III melanoma also had nondetectable levels of p250 in their sera. The situation is quite different in sera of patients with Stage IV melanoma. Seven of 26 patients (27%) had a significant level of p250 activity in their sera, ranging from 14 to 24 units/ml (Figure 2). While no statistical difference was observed among melanoma patients with different stages of disease (p=0.20), cluster analysis suggests that there is a subgroup of Stage IV patients with elevated serum p250 activity.

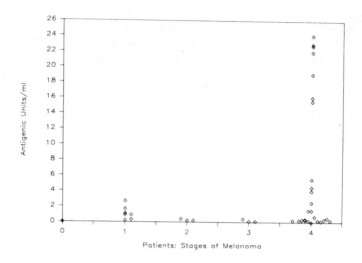

Figure 2.   Serum p250 activity in melanoma patients by
the stage of disease.   Each symbol represents an individual
patient.

From a total of 93 individuals studied, only 7 with
Stage IV melanoma, had high levels of circulating
p250activity.   To prove that this positive reactivity was
specific and not due to spurious inhibition by unusual
serum components, we analyzed by affinity chromatography 4
of the 7 serum samples from the Stage IV patients with high
p250 activity.   Two sera from cancer patients with
negligible activity (4 units/ml) were also analyzed as a
control. p250 activity was recovered from all of the highly
purified specific eluate of serum samples from the Stage IV
melanoma patients.   Three to 4 ml of each serum were first
passed through a column of Sepharose 4B beads conjugated to
MOPC 21 myeloma protein to adsorb nonspecifically-adherent
components.   The effluent was then passed over a 9.2.27-
conjugated Separose 4B column. After extensive washing, the
specifically bound molecules were eluted with 0.5M acetic
acid, pH 2.5, neutralized with Tris buffer and dialyzed to
remove excess salt. The specific effluents of the melanoma
sera were found to contain between 50 to 90% of the input
p250 antigenic activity.   No such activity was observed in
eluates from the 2 sera from other cancer patients.

The serum p250 activity of 6 patients receiving the allogeneic vaccine was followed serially over a course of 20 to 200 days. Only two individuals had elevated serum p250 activity of 16-19 units/ml, one of whom had a constant level and the other, a rise. The other 4 patients had no appreciable levels (2-8 units/ml) over a period of 50 to 200 days on as many as 10 determinations. Despite these differences, all the patients had evidence of slowly progressive disease and died 4 to 12 months after the study. From these results, it is apparent that some individuals never developed detectable serum p250 activity despite advancing disease. On the other hand, the significance of an elevation of p250 as a marker of progression of disease obviously requires far more study.

CONCLUSIONS

Since the human monoclonal antibodies have indicated that cytoplasmic antigens are most immunogenic in human beings, we have just embarked on the next phase of the vaccination study with a mechanical lysate of cultured melanoma cells rather than butanol extracts. It remains to be seen, in the Phase III trial, whether immunogenic can be equated with protective, because the importance of the cytoplasmic antigens in fostering eradication of the melanoma has not been formally tested in the past. The role of adjuvant materials will also be explored systematically, with the proviso that only alum and perhaps Bacillus Calmette-Guerin(BCG) are adjuvant materials with established safety for use in human beings.

With appropriate human or mouse monoclonal antibodies, it may be possible to design and monitor more rational trials of active specific immunotherapy than was previously possible.

REFERENCES

1. LeGrue, SJ, Kahan, BD, Pellis, NR (1980). Extraction of a murine tumor-specific transplantation antigen with l-butanol. I. Partial purification by isoelectric focusing. JNCI 65:191.

2. Bumol, TF, Reisfeld, RA (1982). A unique glycoprotein-proteoglycan complex defined by monoclonal antibody on human melanoma cells. Proc Natl Acad Sci USA 79:1245.
3. Schlom, J, Wunderlich, D, Teramoto, YA (1980). Generation of human monoclonal antibodies reactive with human mammary carcinoma cells. Proc Natl Acad Sci USA 77:6841.
4. Imam, A, Mitchell, MS, Modlin, RL, Taylor, CR, Kempf, RA, Kan-Mitchell, J (submitted). Human monoclonal antibodies that distinguish cutaneous malignant melanomas from benign nevi in fixed tissue sections.
5. Pellis, NR, Yamagishi, H, Macek, CM, Kahan, BD (1980). Specificity and biological activity of extracted murine tumor-specific transplantation antigens. Int J Cancer 26:443.

Monoclonal Antibodies and Cancer Therapy, pages 537–548
© 1985 Alan R. Liss, Inc.

APPROACHES TO AUGMENTING THE IMMUNOGENICITY OF

TUMOR ANTIGENS

Philip O. Livingston, L.J. Old, and H.F. Oettgen

Sloan-Kettering Institute, 1275 York Ave.,

New York, NY 10021

Supported by a Junior Faculty Award from the
American Cancer Society and grants from the Tortuga
Foundation, Pfizer Central Research and the National
Cancer Institute (CA-08748, CA-19267, CA-28461,
CA-28696).

INTRODUCTION

The treatment or prevention of cancer with
specific vaccines has been envisaged ever since the
first vaccines against infectious diseases were
developed. Although several thousand patients have
been injected with tumor cell preparations in this
country and elsewhere over the past 50-60 years (1),
the complexity of the studies has made an assessment of
the value of this approach to cancer therapy
impossible. Even under the most favorable clinical
circumstances, and with a most carefully designed
trial, the testing of human cancer cell vaccines is
fraught with difficulties arising from the uncertainty
of whether the vaccines contained in fact
tumor-specific antigens, and whether the patients
responded immunologically to these antigens. What is
required for the development of an immunogenic cancer
vaccine are methods to assess effectiveness that are

both rapid and objective and that can be used to guide
the process of vaccine testing step by step. With
regard to vaccines against infectious diseases,
serological responses to bacterial or viral antigens
have served this purpose. With the development of
serological typing systems for defining cell surface
antigens of melanoma and other cancers, we now have
serological tests of requisite sensitivity and
specificity that are comparable to those used for
monitoring vaccines against infectious diseases. This
is not to say that we think cell-mediated immunity is
less important in the host's defense against cancer, on
the contrary, just that at present serological
techniques are more precise and better suited to
screening approaches to vaccine construction. An
additional benefit from the serological approach to
monitoring vaccine trials is that it is likely to
indicate vaccines that are particularly effective in
activating B cells, B cells which can then be used for
hybridoma formation and monoclonal antibody production.

RESULTS AND DISCUSSION

Serologic Response of Melanoma Patients to Melanoma Vaccines

For several years, we have attempted to define
favorable conditions for active immunization against
melanoma antigens by investigating the immunogenicity
of a series of melanoma vaccines. These studies
originated in our serological analysis of cell surface
antigens of malignant melanomas by autologous typing.
We have shown that melanoma patients may have
antibodies in their serum that recognize i) unique
antigens, found only on the autologous melanoma and no
other cell, ii) shared antigens, which are highly
restricted differentiation antigens shared by melanomas
and other tumors of neural crest origin, as well as
melanocytes and brain tissue, and iii) widely
distributed antigens on malignant and normal tissues
(2). Two conclusions were derived from these studies.
First, the human immune system can in fact recognize
cell surface components of human malignant melanomas.
Second, only a small fraction of melanoma patients

produce antibodies against individually specific or shared melanoma antigens. Based on these findings, we have attempted to induce the production of antibodies against melanoma antigens by immunizing melanoma patients with vaccines expressing these antigens.

Vaccines we have used in earlier trials were i) cultured autologous melanoma cells, a possible source of unique melanoma antigens (3), ii) allogeneic melanoma cell lines expressing shared melanoma antigens (4,5), and iii) lysates of vesicular stomatitis virus (VSV)-infected autologous or allogeneic melanoma cell lines (6). While most patients produced antibodies against the HLA antigens expressed on allogeneic cell vaccines or VSV antigens present in the lysate vaccines, only exceptional patients produced antibodies against unique or shared melanoma cell surface antigens after administration of these vaccines. In an attempt to augment the immunogenicity of these antigens we have recently vaccinated 3 groups of Stage II melanoma patients with irradiated allogeneic melanoma cells (SK-MEL-93-2) that were modified by treatment with trypsin, neuraminidase or glutaraldehyde. Trypsin and neuraminidase were selected to remove or modify cell surface proteins or carbohydrates that might cover or block melanoma differentiation antigens. Glutaraldehyde was used to stabilize the cell membrane and to eliminate HLA antigenicity. The reactivity with cells treated in these ways using our typing sera against several shared tumor antigens was unchanged or slightly increased in tests on SK-MEL-93-2 cells treated in these 3 ways. The melanoma antigens that have been identified on SK-MEL-93-2 have been previously described (7-10). They include an individually specific antigen (DX) and several differentiation antigens expressed on melanomas and other tissues of neural crest origin (Mel 1 and the gangliosides GD2 and GD3). Reactivity of SK-MEL-93-2 with HLA antibodies, however, while unaffected by the first two treatments, was completely eliminated by glutaraldehyde treatment. The trypsin and neuraminidase treated cell trials are described and the serologic results summarized in Tables I and II.

Table I

SEROLOGIC RESPONSE OF MELANOMA PATIENTS VACCINATED WITH TRYPSIN-TREATED SK-MEL-93-2 MELANOMA CELLS *

Patient	No. of Vaccines	Peak Antibody Titers **	
		IA	PA
1	6	0	320
2	2	0	0
3	6	0	40
4	6	16	1280
5	6	0	640
6	6	8	8
7	6	8	1280
8	6	0	640
9	6	0	16
10	6	8	40
11	6	0	0
12	6	0	20

* SK-MEL-93-2 was grown in monolayer culture, detached by incubation with 0.1% trypsin (GIBCO, Grand Island, N.Y.) at 37° for 5 minutes, washed 3 times in PBS and irradiated with 5000 rads from Cobalt 60 source. The median number of viable melanoma cells per vaccine was 8×10^7. Before injection, the vaccine cells were mixed with 10^5 viable units of BCG (University of Illinois Medical Center) per vaccine. Vaccines were administered intradermally at weekly intervals.

** Immune adherence (IA) and protein (PA) assays were performed on unmodified SK-MEL-93-2 cells cultured in human serum. Patients showed no reactivity before vaccination.

Table II

SEROLOGIC RESPONSE OF MELANOMA PATIENTS VACCINATED WITH NEURAMINIDASE-TREATED SK-MEL-93-2 MELANOMA CELLS *

Patient	No. of Vaccines	Peak Antibody Titers **	
		IA	PA
1	5	0	0
2	5	0	1215
3	5	0	4096
4	5	0	15
5	5	0	1024
6	5	0	1245
7	5	0	21870

* SK-MEL-93-2 was grown in monolayer culture, suspended in an equal volume of Calbiochem Vibro Cholerae Neuraminidase (1 IU/ml), incubated at 37° for 1 hour, washed 3 times in PBS and irradiated with 5,000 rads from a Cobalt 60 source. The median number of viable cells per vaccine was 1.1×10^7. Before injection, the vaccine cells were mixed with 10^5 viable units of BCG (University of Illinois Medical Center) per vaccine. Vaccines were administered intradermally at weekly intervals.

** Immune adherence (IA) and protein (PA) assays were performed on unmodified SK-MEL-93-2 cells cultured in human serum. Patients showed no reactivity before vaccination.

Positive sera were absorbed with EBV transformed B cells from patient DX (the donor of SK-MEL-93-2) as previously described (4). All reactivity was removed by absorption with the companion B cells, indicating that only HLA related antigens were detected. Of interest is that no such reactivity developed in the third trial despite the use of 2×10^8 cells per vaccine and 8 vaccines, confirming the destruction of HLA related antigens by glutaraldehyde treatment. Once again, however, increased serologic reactivity against individually specific or shared melanoma antigens was not detected. Table III summarizes the serologic results of all our vaccine trials.

Table III

COMPLETED MELANOMA VACCINE TRIALS

VACCINE	ADJUVANT	NUMBER OF PATIENTS	SEROLOGICAL RESPONSE MELANOMA ANTIGENS	HLA (or VSV)
UNMODIFIED CELLS				
Autologous Melanoma	BCG	13	2	
Allogeneic Melanoma				
SK-MEL-13	BCG	20	1	20
SK-MEL-29, 33, 37	BCG or C parvum	17	0	17
MODIFIED CELLS				
VSV Lysates				
Autologous Melanoma	—	13	1	(12)
SK-MEL-13 (AH)	—	11	0	11
Trypsin-Treated				
SK-MEL-93-2	BCG	12	0	11
Neuraminidase-Treated				
SK-MEL-93-2	BCG	6	0	5
Glutaraldehyde Treated				
SK-MEL-93-2	BCG	6	0	0

Thus though we have selected our vaccine cells on the basis of expression of individually specific or shared melanoma antigens and though these antigens are clearly immunogenic in some nonvaccinated melanoma patients and normal donors as indicated by the presence of antibodies in their serum, very few of our vaccinated patients have made antibody as a consequence of vaccination. We turned, therefore, to experimental tumors in the mouse to test a wider range of approaches to augmenting the immunogenicity of serologically defined individually specific and shared melanoma antigens.

Serologic Response of Mice to Whole Cell Vaccines

Previous attempts at augmenting the immunogenicity of tumor cells in experimental animals have relied on transplantation studies. Three general approaches have been widely used: immunization with irradiated tumor cells mixed with adjuvants, immunization with irradiated tumor cells modified by treatment with chemicals or viruses and recently, administration of tumor cell vaccines in conjunction with reagents such as cyclophosphamide which are assumed to decrease suppressor cell activity . However, these studies have not provided information regarding the relative efficacy of the approaches used. In our initial study we tested the effectiveness of more than 20 of these approaches in inducing antibody responses to the serologically defined (11) individually specific cell surface antigen of the chemically induced sarcoma Meth A (12). Our results showed: 1) antibodies against the Meth A antigens were not induced by fewer than 15 vaccinations using irradiated Meth A cells alone, 2) several of the adjuvants and cell surface modifiers induced serologic responses after four to six vaccinations, and 3) pretreatment of the host with cyclophosphamide (Cy) followed by vaccination with irradiated tumor cells resulted in high titer serologic responses after only one or two vaccinations. In a subsequent study it was determined that additional

augmentation of the serological response to sarcoma
Meth A could be obtained by using pretreatment with Cy
in conjunction with certain adjuvants such as
monophosphoryl lipid A (MPLA) (13). The results of
these experiments are summarized in Table IV.

Table IV

REQUIREMENTS FOR INDUCING A
SEROLOGIC RESPONSE AGAINST THE METH A ANTIGEN

Vaccine	No. of Vaccinations	Type Antibody Produced
5×10^6 cells alone	>20	IgM
5×10^6 cells + adjuvant	>4	IgM
5×10^6 cells + Cy pretreatment	1	IgM
1×10^5 cells + Adjuvant + Cy	1	IgM

Antibodies against the Meth A antigen are induced in
most mice pretreated with Cy by one vaccination with as
few Meth A cells as 10^5 mixed with MPLA. The
combination of Cy and MPLA was also shown to be
effective in augmenting the serological response
against 2 other chemically induced BALB/c sarcomas
which are known to be less immunogenic than Meth A,
CMS4 and CMS5, (13), and against the C57BL/6 melanoma
JB-RH. While the antigens defined on CMS4 and CMS5 are
individually specific tumor antigens, JBRH is of
particular interest because it expresses, and the
induced antibodies recognize, the ganglioside GM2 which
is a shared melanoma antigen also expressed by some
human melanomas. One peculiarity in these results is

that the antibodies induced by vaccines against these 4 tumors were all of the IgM class. No significant switch to IgG has resulted even after multiple vaccinations administered I.V., I.P. or subcutaneously and with or without Cy or various adjuvants. It appears, therefore, that the use of Cy and irradiated tumor cells plus MPLA is applicable to stimulating IgM serological responses against a variety to tumor cell surface antigens. We are currently testing the effect of this approach on transplantation immunity in the mouse and on serologic reactivity to Class 1 and 2 melanoma antigens in man.

Serologic Response of Mice to Purified Ganglioside Vaccines

In the past, vaccine studies with purified tumor antigens have been limited by the quantity of antigen available. Two shared melanoma antigens are now available in purified form in quantities sufficient for vaccine studies, the gangliosides GD2 (also termed the AH antigen and OFA-I-2) (9,14) and GM2 (OFA-I-1) (15). Both antigens are expressed predominantly on subsets of cells of neuroectodermal lineage and both are known to be potentially immunogenic in man as they have been identified by a variety of human sera (7,9,16). We have, however, been unable to develop consistently immunogenic vaccines in man using whole cells or cell lysates expressing these gangliosides. Consequently, we have begun to explore the effect of purified GM2 and GD2 vaccines in the mouse as a prelude to similar trials in man. While our results are preliminary, they have confirmed that these gangliosides administered alone are rarely immunogenic, in C57BL/6 mice, and have identified several approaches capable of greatly augmenting their immunogenicity. A summary of these experiments and the results obtained is presented in Table V.

Table V

SEROLOGICAL RESPONSE TO G_{M2} VACCINES *

VACCINE	CYCLOPHOSPHAMIDE PRETREATMENT	NO. MICE VACCINATED	NO. MAKING ANTIBODIES	MEAN TITER ON JB-RH
G_{M2} PLUS:				
-	-	10	1	40
-	+	10	0	0
CFA	-	3	0	0
CFA	+	3	0	0
DETOX	+	10	0	0
LIPOSOMES	+	5	0	0
LIPOSOMES + MDP	+	5	1	64
LIPOSOMES + MPLA	+	10	6	4,000
SALMONELLA	+	10	6	80

* G_{M2} was prepared from G_{M1} (Supelco) by treatment with beta-galactosidase as previously described (14). Fifty micrograms of G_{M2} were used per vaccine and all mice (C57BL/6) were vaccinated subcutaneously twice at a 3-4 week interval.

Abbreviations: CFA, complete Freund adjuvant (Difco Laboratories);DETOX, monophosphoryl Lipid A plus BCG cell wall skeletons (Ribi Immunochem Research); MDP, muramyl dipeptide (Ciba-Geigy); MPLA, monophosphoryl Lipid A (Ribi Immunochem Research); and the liposomes are prepared from sphingomyelin, cholesterol and dicetylphosphate at molar ratios of 2:1.5:0.22 by sonication.

Serologic titer was determined by IA (detecting predominantly IgM) and PA (detecting IgG) assays on cultured JB-RH melanoma cells. JB-RH was selected because it contained more GM2 by thin layer chromatography and by direct tests with anti GM2 monoclonal antibody than the other 4 murine melanomas tested. GM2 alone or mixed with CFA or DETOX, or incorporated into liposomes or liposomes plus MDP was poorly immunogenic. However, when GM2 was presented on heat killed Salmonella (17) or in liposomes containing MPLA, serologic reactivity developed in 6 of 10 mice after one or two vaccinations (including 4 with high titer IgG antibodies). The success of these murine trials has encouraged us to proceed with similar trials in melanoma patients.

CONCLUSIONS

We have conducted a series of whole melanoma cell and cell lysate vaccine trials in small numbers of melanoma patients with the intent of producing a vaccine that could consistently raise antibodies against individually specific (Class 1) or shared (Class 2) melanoma antigens, a vaccine that could then be used in larger clinical trials. Only occasional responses have been seen, so we have initiated studies with experimental tumors in the mouse to test a broader range of immunization procedures. Whole cell vaccines against individually specific or shared tumor antigens on a variety of tumors were found to be optimal when irradiated tumor cells were mixed with adjuvants such as monophosphoryl lipid A (MPLA) and injected several days after administration of a low dose of cyclophosphamide. We have also investigated the use of purified antigen vaccines. Two shared melanoma antigens, the gangliosides GM2 and GD2, can now be produced biochemically and so are available in quantities sufficient for immunization experiments. In ongoing studies we have found that vaccines containing GM2 attached to Salmonella minnesota or in liposomes with MPLA were significantly more immunogenic than GM2 alone and resulted in serologic responses, both IgM and IgG, in the majority of mice. Based on these results in the mouse, similar vaccines are planned for testing in melanoma patients. These include vaccines containing irradiated cultured autologous melanoma cells (as potential sources of Class 1 and 2 melanoma antigens) plus MPLA in cyclophosphamide pretreated patients, and vaccines containing GM2 and GD2 (Class 2 melanoma antigens) attached to Salmonella minnesota or in liposomes with MPLA.

REFERENCES

1.   Livingston PO, Oettgen HF, and Old LJ:
     Specific active immunotherapy in cancer therapy,
     IN: Immunological aspects of cancer theapeutics,
     Dr. Enrico Mihich (ed), John Wiley and Sons,
     Inc. Publ., 363-404, 1982.

2.   Old, LJ: Cancer immunology: The search for
     specificity-GHA Clowes Memorial Lecture.
     Cancer Research 41: 361-375,1981.

3.   Livingston PO, Watanabe T, Shiku H, Houghton AN,
     Albino A, Takahashi T, Resnick A, Michitsch R,
     Pinsky CM, Oettgen HF, and Old LJ: Serological
     response of melanoma patients receiving melanoma
     cell vaccines, I. Autologous cultured melanoma cells.
     Int J Cancer 30: 413-422, 1982.

4.   Livingston PO, Takeyama H, Pollack MS, Houghton
     AN, Albino A, Pinsky CM, Oettgen HF and Old LJ:
     Serological responses of melanoma patients to
     vaccines derived from allogeneic cultured
     melanoma cells. Int J Ca 31: 567-575, 1983.

5.   Livingston PO, Kaelin E, Pinsky CM, Oettgen HF
     and Old LJ: IV. Serological response in Stage II
     melanoma patients receiving allogeneic melanoma
     cell vaccines. Cancer, (In press).

6.   Livingston PO, Albino AP, Chung TJC, Real FX,
     Houghton AN, Oettgen HF and Old LJ: Serological
     response of melanoma patients to vaccines prepared
     from VSV lysates of autologous and allogeneic cultured
     melanoma cells. Cancer Vol 55: 713-720, 1985.

7.   Houghton AN, Taormina MC, Ikeda H, Watanabe T,
     Oettgen HF, and Old LJ. Serological survey of
     normal humans for natural antibody to cell surface
     antigens of melanoma. Proc Natl Acad Sci USA, 77:
     4260-4264, 1980.

8.   Albino AP, Lloyd KO, Houghton AN, Oettgen HF and
     Old LJ. Heterogeneity in surface antigen
     expression and glycoprotein expression of cell lines
     derived from different metastases of the same patient:
     implications for the study of tumor antigens. J Exp
     Med 154-1764, 1981.

9.   Watanabe T, Pukel CS, Takeyama H, Lloyd KO,
     Shiku H, Li LTC, Travassos LR, Oettgen HF,
     and Old LJ. Human melanoma antigen AH is
     an autoantigenic ganglioside related to GD2.

J Exp Med 156:1884, 1982.

10. Pukel CS, Lloyd KO, Travassos LR, Dippold WG, Oettgen HF, Old LJ. GD3, a prominent ganglioside of human melanoma. Detection and characterization by mouse monoclonal antibody. J Exp Med 155:1133, 1982.

11. DeLeo AB, Shiku H, Takahashi T, Old LJ. Serological definition of cell surface antigens of chemically induced sarcomas of inbred mice. In: R.W. Ruddon (ed.). Biological markers of neoplasia: Basic and applied aspects. New York: Elsevier/North-Holland Publishing Corp, pp 25-34, 1978.

-12. Livingston PO, DeLeo AB, Jones M, Oettgen HF, Old LJ. Comparison of approaches for augmenting the serological response to the Meth A antigen. Pre-treatment with Cyclophosphamide is most effective. J of Immunology 131: 2601, 1983.

13. Livingston PO, Jones M, Oettgen HF, Old LJ. Augmentation of the serological response to Meth A antigen by cyclophosphamide and endotoxin. Proc Amer Assoc Cancer Res 25:279, 1984.

14. Cahan LD, Irie RF, Singh R, Cassidenti A, Paulson JC. Identification of a human neuroectodermal tumor antigen (OFA-I-2) as ganglioside GD2. Proc Natl Acad Sci USA 79:7629-7633, 1982.

15. Tai T, Paulson JC, Cahan LD, Irie RF. Ganglioside GM2 as a human tumor antigen (OFA-I-1). Proc Natl Acad Sci USA 80:5392-5396, 1983.

16. Irie RF, Irie K, Morton DL. A membrane antigen common to human cancer and fetal brain tissues. Can Res 36:3510-3517, 1976.

17. Galanos C, Luderitz O, Wetphal O. Preparation and properties of Antisera against the lipid-A component of bacterial lipopolysaccharides. Euro J Biochem 24:110, 1971.

XI. MONOCLONAL ANTIBODIES TO ONCOGENE PRODUCTS

Monoclonal Antibodies and Cancer Therapy, pages 551–564
© 1985 Alan R. Liss, Inc.

USE OF MONOCLONAL ANTIBODIES TO PROBE THE
FUNCTIONAL ACTIVITY OF THE CELLULAR SRC
GENE PRODUCT IN POLYOMA VIRUS TRANSFORMED CELLS

Wes Yonemoto, Joseph Bolen[*], Mark Israel[*],
Leah Lipsich, and Joan S. Brugge

Department of Microbiology
State University of New York
Stony Brook, New York 11794

[*]Pediatric Branch
Carcinogenesis Branch
National Institutes of Health
Bethesda, Md. 20205

ABSTRACT

The transforming protein of polyomavirus, middle T antigen, associates in a complex with $pp60^{c-src}$, the cellular homolog of the Rous sarcoma virus transforming protein, in polyoma virus-infected and -transformed cells. The tyrosine kinase activity associated with $pp60^{c-src}$: middle T antigen complexes is enhanced 30- to 50-fold compared to unbound $pp60^{c-src}$ molecules, and the $pp60^{c-src}$ protein associated with middle T antigen displays a novel pattern of tyrosine phosphorylation. These results suggest that transformation by polyomavirus involves an alteration in the functional activity of the cellular src gene product which is mediated by the formation of a protein complex between T antigen and $pp60^{c-src}$.

INTRODUCTION

Investigations of oncogenic transformation by tumor-inducing retroviruses has led to the identification of a group of genes, denoted oncogenes, which are responsible for the development of virus-induced neoplasias (review, 1). These viral genes are all homologous to highly conserved cellular genes, denoted proto-oncogenes. It is likely that retroviruses acquired these genes by recombination between viral structural genes and cellular chromosomal genes. Transformation by some retroviruses which do not encode oncogenes is mediated by retrovirus-induced alterations in the expression of cellular proto-oncogenes as a result of integration of the viral genome into the host cell chromosome. In the past few years, it has become evident that alterations in the expression of these cellular proto-oncogenes are involved in the genesis of human neoplasias (review,2). Thus, investigations of these cellular oncogene products may yield important information on the mechanism of human tumorigenesis.

The protein products of one class of oncogenes (shown in Table 1) have been found to share a considerable degree of amino acid homology and to possess a common enzymatic activity. The proteins encoded by all of these oncogenes possess protein kinase activity and show a strict specificity for the phosphorylation of tyrosine residues. There are several lines of evidence which suggest that phosphorylation of tyrosine residues on cellular proteins is involved in oncogenic transformation.

Table 1. Retrovirus encoded oncogenes which possess tyrosine-specific protein kinase activity

Oncogene	Virus
src	Rous sarcoma virus
abl	Abelson leukemia virus
fps	Fuginami sarcoma virus PRC II sarcoma virus
fes	Synder-Theilen feline sarcoma virus Gardner-Arnstein feline sarcoma virus
yes	Yamaguchi 73 sarcoma virus
ros	UR-2 sarcoma virus
fgr	Gardner-Rasheed feline sarcoma virus
erb-b	Avian erythroblastosis virus

1) Eight different oncogenes associated with tumor-inducing retroviruses encode tyrosine-specific protein kinases (1).

2) Elevated levels of tyrosine phosphorylation are detected in cells transformed by viruses which encode tyrosine kinases, and the loss of kinase activity in mutant oncogene products correlates with a loss of transforming activity (review, 3).

3) The chromosomal translocation responsible for generating the Philadelphia chromosome in patients with chronic myologenous leukemia involves a rearrangement in the c-abl oncogene (4). The protein product of this gene shows significantly enhanced levels of tyrosine kinase activity compared to its non-rearranged homolog (5,6).

4) Rat neuroblastomas induced by nitrosurea have been found to possess an oncogene whose product is highly related to the erb-b protein and possesses tyrosine-specific protein kinase activity (7).

Rous sarcoma virus (RSV) has served as a model system for investigations of transformation mediated by tyrosine-specific protein kinases. The oncogene which is associated with RSV, v-src, encodes a 60,000 d. phosphoprotein (8,9) which is associated with the cytoplasmic face of the plasma membrane of RSV-transformed cells (review,10). The protein encoded by the cellular homolog of this gene, denoted c-src, is also associated with the plasma-membrane and possesses tyrosine kinase activity (1). Recent evidence indicates that tyrosyl kinase activity of the v-src gene product, $pp60^{v-src}$, is 50 to 100-fold greater than actvity associated with the cellular src gene product, $pp60^{c-src}$ (Iba, Cross and Hanafusa; Coussens and Shalloway; personal communications). Hanafusa and coworkers (personal communication) have shown that mutations which activate the oncogenic potential of the c-src gene correlate with a 30 to 100-fold increase in the activity of the c-src protein in in vitro kinase assays. This activation of the tyrosyl kinase activity of the c-src gene is analogous to the elevation of kinase activity associated with the rearranged protein product of the c-abl gene detected in patients with chromic myelogenous leukemia (5,6). Thus, these two systems provide evidence that oncogenic activation of cellular proto-oncogenes which encode tyrosine kinases

involves mutagenic alterations which result in enhancement
of the enzymatic activity of the protein products of these
genes.

We have developed monoclonal antibodies which
recognize the viral and cellular src protein as well as
other tyrosine-kinase transforming proteins (11). These
antibodies do not interfere with the enzymatic activity of
these enzymes, and provide the means to analyze the
tyrosine kinase activity of these oncogenes in a rapid,
immune-complex-bound assay. Thus, these antibodies can be
used to probe the functional activity of tyrosine kinases
in naturally occuring tumors and in experimental tumors
induced by carcinogenesis or other types of tumor viruses.
In this report, we will provide evidence that oncogenic
transformation by polyoma virus, a DNA-containing tumor
virus, is at least partially mediated by an enchancement in
the tyrosine kinase activity of the cellular src protein.

RESULTS

Polyoma virus (Py) encodes three tumor antigens which
cooperate to induce the production of tumors in rodents
(review,12). One antigen, designated middle tumor antigen
or MTAg, is believed to play a control role in Py-induced
tranformation since it is capable of transforming
immortalized cells in culture (13). It was previously
reported that immunoprecipitates containing MTAg possess an
associated tyrosine kinase activity (14-16). Current
evidence indicates that this activity is not intrinsic to
MTAg, and that MTAg is associated in a complex with the
cellular src protein in Py-transformed and -infected cells
(17-19). This evidence raises the question of whether Py
recruits the the c-src protein kinase to mediate crucial
aspects of transformation; and if so, how does MTAg
influence the functional activity of pp60^{c-src}?

To address these questions, we examined the protein
kinase activity of the c-src protein in Py-transformed
cells. The immune-complex protein kinase procedure used to
assay pp60^{c-src}-specific protein kinase activity is shown
in Figure 1. In these assays, we monitored either the
phosphorylation of the c-src and MTAg, or the
phosphorylation of an exogenous substrate, like casein.

Immune-Complex Protein Kinase Assay

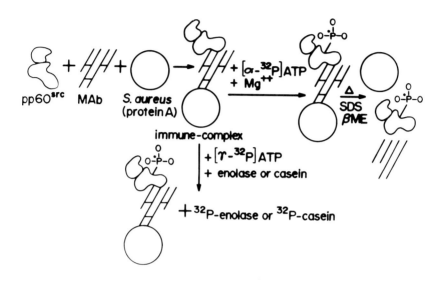

Figure 1.   Immune complex protein kinase activity

Lysates are prepared by disruption of cells with a detergent lysis buffer (RIPA) and clarification at 49,000 xg as described previously (11). The lysate is then incubated with antibody directed against the protein of interest. The antigen:antibody complexes are collected by adsorption to formalin fixed <u>Staphlyococcus</u> <u>aureus</u> bacteria, and the immune-complexes are washed with the detergent buffer. After a final wash with 10 mM Tris-HCl, pH 7.2, 100 mM NaCl, 5 mM $MgCl_2$, the immunoprecipitated proteins are incubated with 5 μCi [γ-^{32}P-ATP], 5 μM ATP, 10 mM Tris-HCL, pH 7.2, and 5 mM $MgCl_2$ for 15 min. at 22°C. To assay the phosphorylation of an exogenous substrate, 2 μg of casein or enolase are added to the kinase reaction mix. The proteins are then eluted from the immune-complex with electrophoresis sample buffer and electrophoresed on 7.5% SDS-polyacrylamide gel. The radiolabeled protein are detected by autoradiography.

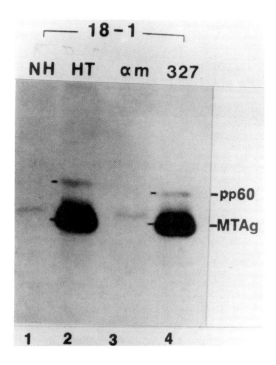

Figure 2. Phosphorylation of of pp60^{c-src} and MTAg after immunoprecipitation from cells transformed by MTAg.

Lysates prepared from 18-1 cells were incubated with normal hamster serum (lane 1), HT serum (lane 2), anti-mouse immunoglobulin (lane 3), and MAb-src #327 (lane 4). The washed immunoprecipitates were assayed for endogenous protein phosphorylation as described in the legend to Figure 1.
In the experiment shown in Figure 2, pp60 and MTAg were immunoprecipitated with either monoclonal antibody to pp60^{c-src} (MAb-src) or antibodies to Py tumor antigens from polyclonal antiserum (HT serum) obtained from hamsters bearing Py induced tumors. After isolation of the immune complexes, the phosphorylation of casein was assayed. In the MAb-src immunoprecipitates from lysates of normal Fisher rat 3T3 cells, casein phosphorylation was not detectable above the background levels found in the control immunoprecipitates formed with normal hamster serum or

rabbit antiserum to mouse immunoglobulins. In contrast, 5- to 10-fold higher levels of casein phosphorylation were detected in MAb-src or HT serum immunoprecipitates from Fisher rat cells transformed by MTAg. Elevated levels of c-src phosphorylation were also detected in the immunoprecipitates. We have found that the steady state levels of pp60^{c-src} are identical in the FR-3T3 and MTAg-transformed FR-3T3 cells, indicating that the elevated levels of casein phosphorylation are not a consequence of elevated synthesis of the c-src protein in Py-transformed cells. We have also found that only a small percentage of the c-src protein is associated with MTAg; and, vice versa, only a small proportion of MTAg molecules are bound to pp60^{c-src} (19). When lysates from Py-transformed cells were successively preincubated with antibody to MTAg to remove the pp60^{c-src}:MTAg complexes from cell lysates, the casein phosphorylating activity in MAb-src immunoprecipitates was reduced to background levels. This result indicates that enhancement of the c-src protein kinase activity requires an association between MTAg and pp60^{c-src}. Since the 10-15% of pp60^{c-src} molecules which are bound to MTAg are responsible for the 5 to 10-fold increase in the total levels of casein phosphorylating activity, this suggests that the actual increase in the specific activity of the c-src protein is 30 to 100-fold.

This evidence suggests the possibility that at least one aspect of Py-induced celluar transformation is induced by the enhancement of pp60^{c-src} phosphorylating activity which results from MTAg binding to the c-src protein. This system provides an example of a novel mechanism for the activation of a cellular proto-oncogene; namely that the activation results from a protein-protein interaction, rather than by mutation of the genes encoding the cellular proto-oncogene.

In light of these results, it was of interest to determine whether the "activated" c-src protein which was bound to MTAg could be distinguished in any way from the unbound molecules of pp60^{c-src} in Py transformed cells.

Figure 3 shows that the pp60^{c-src} protein which was phosphorylated in immunoprecipitates formed using antibody directed against MTAg displayed a slightly slower electrophoretic mobility than the c-src molecules phosphorylated in MAb-327 immunoprecipitates.   Peptide and

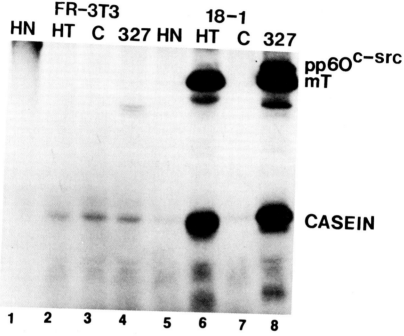

Figure 3.   Phosphorylation of casein in immunoprecipitates from normal and MTAg transformed FR-3T3 cells.

Lysates containing five hundred micrograms of protein extracted from normal Fisher rat 3T3 (FR-3T3) cells and 18-1 cells [MTAg transformed FR3T3 cells (19)] were immunoprecipitated with normal hamster serum (lanes 1,5), HT serum (lanes 2,6), anti-mouse immunoglobulin (lane 3,7), or anti-mouse immunoglobulin and MAb-src #327 (11) (lanes 4,8).   The phosphorylation of casein was assayed as described in the legend to figure 1.

phosphoaminoacid analysis of the pp60^{c-src} protein phosphorylated in these reactions indicated that the pp60^{c-src} protein phosphorylated in the anti-MTAg immunoprecipitates was phosphorylated on a tyrosine residue within the aminoterminal 18,000 d. of pp60^{c-src} (20). This contrasts the typical pattern of phosphorylation of pp60^{c-src} found in immune complexes where the single site of phosphorylation is tyrosine residue #416, which is within the carboxylterminal-half of the c-src protein molecule. These results indicate that MTAg binding to pp60^{c-src} causes a change in pattern of pp60^{c-src} phosphorylation. The detection of a novel phosphorylation site in the c-src molcules bound to MTAg raises the question of whether aminoterminal tyrosine phosphorylation of the c-src molecule is responsible for the activation of c-src protein kinase activity, or merely a reflection of an alteration in pp60^{c-src} caused by MTAg binding.

Recently, several lines of evidence have suggested the possibility that alterations within the aminoterminal region of the c-src protein might influence the kinase activity of the catalytic domain which is present within the carboxylterminal-half of pp60^{c-src}.

1) The COOH-terminal-half of the v-src protein molecule can be separated from the aminoterminal portion of the molecule by mild protease treatment (21,22). This protease-resistant fragment of pp60^{v-src} possesses 30 to 50-fold higher levels of tyrosine kinase actvity than the intact pp60^{v-src} molecule (22). This evidence suggests that the aminoterminal sequences of pp60^{v-src} might restrict the kinase activity of the catalytic domain.

2) Collett and coworkers have provided evidence suggesting that the kinase activity of partially purified pp60^{v-src} is enhanced by tyrosine phosphorylation on sites within the aminoterminal-half of the molecule (23-25).

3) The pp60^{c-src} protein expressed in rat central nervous system neurons contains a modification within the aminoterminal 18,000 d. of the molecule. The presence of this modification correlates with a 6- to 12-fold increase in the specific activity of pp60^{c-src} in immune-complex kinase reactions (Cotton, P.C. Ph.D. Dissertation, State University of New York at Stony Brook, Stony Brook, N.Y., and Brugge, Cotton, Queral, Donner, Barrett, and Keane, unpublished results).

4) The pp60^{c-src} protein expressed in several human neuroblastoma cell lines is phosphorylated on a tyrosine(s) within the aminoterminal portion of the molecule (Bolen, Rosen, and Israel, unpublished results). This form of the c-src protein displays enhanced levels of tyrosine kinase activity.

5) Ralston and coworkers have reported that treatment of mouse 3T3 cells with platelet-derived growth factor (PDGF) causes a retardation in the electrophoretic mogility of pp60^{c-src} (Ralston and Bishop, personal communication). Tyrosine phosphorylation within the aminoterminal 16,000 d. of pp60^{c-src} was shown to correlate with this electrophoretic alteration, and a slight increase in the kinase activity of pp60^{c-src} was detected in lysates the treated cells.

In order to access the significance of the aminoterminal tyrosine phosphorylation on the activation of pp60^{c-src} in Py transformed cells, we have examined the phosphorylation of the c-src protein in vivo in Py-transformed cells. Figure 4 shows that the variant of pp60^{c-src} which displayed a retarded electrophoretic mobility is not detectble in Py-transformed cells labeled in vivo with ^{32}P-orthophosphate. Phosphoamionoacid analysis of the pp60^{c-src} protein immunoprecipitated with either MAB-src or anti-MTAg (HT serum) did not reveal the presence of phosphotyrosine within the aminoterminal portion of pp60^{c-src} (Yonemoto and Brugge, unpublished results). These results suggest that the "activated" form of pp60^{c-src} isolated from Py transformed cells is not phosphorylated on tyrosine residues within the aminoterminal-half of the molecule, and thus provide evidence that this modification may not be involved in the activation of pp60^{c-src} following MTAg binding.

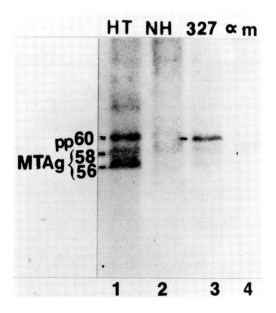

Figure 4. ^{32}P-labeled proteins immunoprecipitated from Py-transformed mouse cells

Py transformed mouse cells (Py6 cells) were incubated for 20 hours with ^{32}P-orthophosphate (1mC/ml), lysed in RIPA buffer and the clarified lysate incubated with normal hamster serum (lane 1), HT serum (lane 2), anti-mouse immunoglobulin and MAb-src #327 (lane 3), and anti-mouse immunoglobulin alone (lane 4). The immunoprecipitates were adsorbed to formalin-fixed <u>Staphylococcus aureus</u> bacteria and washed as described previously (11). The proteins were eluted from the immunoprecipitates and electrophoresed as described in the legend to Figure 1.

DISCUSSION

Elucidation of the ultimate importance of MTAg-induced activation of pp60^{c-src} awaits demonstration of the consequences of this enhancement of tyrosine kinase activity <u>in vivo</u>. Elevated levels of tyrosine phosphorylation of cellular proteins have not been detected in Py transformed cells, as in RSV transformed cells. However, it is possible that the activation of $pp60^{c-src}$ by MTAg involves the phosphorylation of a single, or limited number, of substrates which are essential for eliciting the phenotypic changes induced by MTAg in Py-infected cells. Identification of such substrates is crucial to elucidation of the mechanism of transformation induced by Py, and will have obvious importance to the understanding of transformation induced by other viruses carrying tyrosine-specific protein kinases. Investigation of the $pp60^{c-src}$-specific tyrosine kinase activity in human tumors should also indicate whether human tumorigenesis involves similar mechanisms of transformation.

ACKNOWLEDGMENTS

The authors would like to acknowledge the technical assistance of Maureen Jarvis-Morar and Ana Queral in many of the experiments described in this report, and the secretarial assistance of Kathleen Donnelly. This work was supported by grants from the National Cancer Institute and the American Cancer Society.

REFERENCES

1. Bishop JM, Varmus H (1982). Functions and Origins of Retroviral Transforming Genes. In Weiss R, Teich N, Varmus H, Coffin J (eds): "RNA Tumor Viruses," Cold Spring Harbor: Cold Spring Harbor Press, p999.

2. VandeWoude G, Levine AJ, Topp WC, Watson JD (1984). "Cancer Cells 2: Oncogenes and Viral Genes," Cold Spring Harbor: Cold Spring Harbor Press.

3. Weber M (1984). Malignant transformation by Rous sarcoma virus: From phosphorylation to phenotype. Adv Viral Oncology, in press.

4. Groffein J, Stephenson JR, Heisterkamp JR, deKlein A, Bartiam CR, Grosfeld G (1984). Philadelphia chromosomal breakpoints are clustered within a limited region, bcr, on chromosome 22. Cell 36:93.

5. Konopka J, Watanabe S, Witte OW (1984). An alteration of the human c-abl protein in K562 leukemia cells unmasks associated tyrosine kinase activity. Cell 37:1035.

6.   Davis RL, Konopka JB, Witte OW (1985). Activation of the c-abl oncogene by viral transduction or chromosomal translocation generates altered c-abl proteins with similar in vitro kinase properties. Mol Cell Biol 5:204.

7.   Schechter AL, Stern DF, Vaidyanathan L, Decker SJ, Drebin JA, Green GI, Weinberg RA (1984). The nev oncogene: an erb-b-related gene encoding a 185,000-M_r tumor antigen. Nature 312:513.

8. Brugge JS and Erikson RL (1977).   Identification of a transformation-specific antigen induced by an avian sarcoma virus. Nature 269:348.

9. Purchio AF, Erikson E, Brugge JS, Erikson RL (1978). Identification of a polypeptide encoded by the avian sarcoma virus src gene. Proc Natl Acad Sci USA 75:1567.

10. Krueger JG, Garber EA, Goldberg AR (1983). Subcellular localization of pp60^{src} in RSV-transformed cells. Curr Top Microbiol Immunol 107:51.

11.   Lipsich LA, Lewis AJ, Brugge JS (1983). Isolation of monoclonal antibodies which recognize the transforming proteins of avian sarcoma viruses. J Virol 48:352.

12.   Tooze J, (1980) "DNA Tumor Viruses." Cold Spring Harbor Laboratory.

13.   Rassoulzadegan M, Cowie A, Carr A, Glaichenhaus N, Kamen R, Cuzin F (1982). The roles of individual polyoma virus early proteins in oncogenic transformation. Nature (London) 300:713.

14. Eckhart W, Hutchinson MA, Hunter T (1979). An activity phosphorylating tyrosine in polyoma T antigen immunoprecipitates. Cell 18:925.

15. Schaffhausen B, Benjamin TL (1979). Phosphorylation of polyoma T antigen. Cell 18:935.

16. Smith A, Smith R, Griffin B, Fried M (1979). Protein kinase activity associated with polyoma middle T antigen in vitro. Cell 18:915.

17. Courtneidge S and Smith AE (1983). Polyoma virus transforming protein associates with the product of the c-src cellular gene. Nature 303:435.

18. Lipsich LA, Yonemoto W, Bolen JB, Israel MA, Brugge JS (1983). Structural and functional studies of Rous sarcoma virus transforming protein pp60^{c-src}. In Van de Woude GF, Levine AJ, Topp WC, Watson JD (eds): "Cancer Cell II: Oncogenes and Viral Genes," Cold Spring Harbor Laboratory, p 43.

19. Bolen JB, Thiele, CJ, Israel MA, Yonemoto W, Lipsich LA, Brugge JS (1984). Enhancement of cellular src gene-product associated tyrosyl-kinase activity following polyoma virus infection and transformation. Cell 38:767.

20. Yonemoto W, Jarvis-Morar M, Brugge JS, Bolen J, Israel M (1985). Novel tyrosine phosphorylation within the aminoterminal domain of pp60^{c-src} molecules associated with polyoma virus middle tumor antigen. Proc. Natl. Acad. Sci. USA, in press.

21. Levinson AD, Courtneidge SA, Bishop JM (1981). Structural and functional domains of the Rous sarcoma virus-transforming protein (pp60^{src}). Proc Natl Acad Sci USA 78:1624.

22. Brugge JS, Darrow D (1984). Analysis of the catalytic domain of phosphotransferase activity of two avian sarcoma virus-transforming proteins. J Biol Chem 259:4550.

23. Collett MS, Belzer SK, Purchio AF (1984). Structurally and functionally modified forms of pp60^{v-src} in Rous sarcoma virus-transformed cell lysates. Mol Cell Biol 4:1213.

24. Purchio AF, Wells SK, Collett MS (1984). Increase in the phosphotransferase activity of purified Rous sarcoma virus, pp60^{v-src} protein after incubation with ATP plus Mg^{+}. Mol Cell Biol 4:1589.

25. Collett M, Wells S, Purchio A (1983). Physical modification of purified Rous sarcoma virus pp60^{v-src} protein after incubation with ATP/Mg^{2+}. Virology 128:285.

Monoclonal Antibodies and Cancer Therapy, pages 565–572
© 1985 Alan R. Liss, Inc.

A MONOCLONAL ANTIBODY RAISED AGAINST A RAS RELATED SYNTHETIC PEPTIDE SHOWS IMMUNOREACTIVITY WITH HUMAN CARCINOMAS

Walter P. Carney[1], H.J. Wolfe[2], D. Petit[1], L. Bator[2], R. DeLellis[2], A.S. Tischler[2], Y. Dayal[2], P. Hamer[1], G. Cooper[3] and H. Rabin[1]

ABSTRACT A murine monoclonal antibody, DWP, was raised against a synthetic dodecapeptide representing amino acid residues 5–16 of the mutated ras protein (P21) expressed in the T24 bladder carcinoma cells. DWP reacted specifically in competition assays with peptides containing valine or cysteine at position 12 but was unreactive with peptides containing glycine, arginine, serine, alanine, aspartic or glutamic acid at position 12. DWP reacted immunocytochemically with formalin-fixed, paraffin embedded NIH3T3 cells transformed with activated human ras genes but was not reactive with NIH3T3 cells or NIH3T3 cells transformed by overexpression of the normal Harvey ras P21. Western blot analysis of cells expressing either glycine or valine at position 12 demonstrated that DWP reacted specifically with the mutated protein of approximately 21 kilodaltons but not with normal Harvey ras P21. Initial immunohistochemical analysis of formalin-fixed, paraffin-embedded tumor tissues demonstrated DWP reactivity on greater than 60% of a variety of human carcinomas but not on a panel of normal human tissues.

1. E.I. DuPont deNemours, Biomedical Products Dept., 331 Treble Cove Road, North Billerica, Mass. 01862
2. Department of Pathology, Tufts New England Medical Center 171 Harrison Avenue, Boston, Mass.
3. Department of Pathology, Dana Farber Cancer Institute Boston, Mass.

INTRODUCTION

Transfection experiments using the mouse NIH3T3 cell line
as recipients of human tumor cell DNA have led to the
identification of a family of human transforming genes
homologous to the oncogenes described in the Harvey (1) and
Kirsten (2) retroviruses. Activated ras oncogenes have
been described in a variety of human tumors and have been
shown to encode a 21,000 dalton protein (P21) with amino
acid changes at position 12 and 61 (3,4,5). The cellular
Harvey ras (C-Ha-ras) gene isolated and cloned from the T24
bladder carcinoma has been shown to transform NIH3T3 cells
and to encode a P21 protein that contains valine at
position 12 instead of the normal amino acid glycine (6).
A monoclonal antibody that could detect specific amino acid
alterations at positions 12 and 61 of the ras P21 would
provide an important tool in evaluating the presence of
altered ras gene expression in human tumors. The use of
synthetic peptides to generate antibodies of predefined
specificity has been important in the study of a variety of
biologically important proteins (7,8). We utilized this
approach to raise monoclonal antibodies to synthetic
peptides representing regions of the P21 encompassing
position 12 or 61 containing specific amino acid
substitutions. This report describes a monoclonal antibody
(MOAb), DWP, which recognizes peptides having valine or
cysteine at position 12 but which fails to recognize
peptides having the normal constituent, glycine at this
position.

MATERIALS AND METHODS

Peptides and Mouse Immunizations

Dodecapeptides used for mouse immunization and hybridoma
screening were obtained from Peninsula Laboratories,
Belmont, Cal. The peptide Lys-Leu-Val-Val-Val-Gly-Ala-
Val-Gly-Val-Gly-Lys was conjugated to carrier proteins
bovine thyroglobulin (BTg) or Keyhole Limpet Hemocyanin
(KLH) using 1-ethyl-3-(3 dimethyl amino propyl)
carbodiimide hydrochloride coupling reagent (9).
Peptide-BTg conjugates were inoculated intraperitoneally
(i.p.) at approximately 2 week intervals with complete
Freund's adjuvant. On day 59, a final i.p. inoculation of
peptide-BTg conjugate was given and 3 days later the mouse
was sacrificed for fusion.

Hybridoma Selection

Cell hybridization was carried out by methods previously
described (10). Mouse sera and hybridoma supernatants were
evaluated on microtiter wells coated with peptides
conjugated to KLH by enzyme linked immunosorbent assay
(ELISA) using a goat anti-mouse horseradish peroxidase and
0-phenylene-diamine system (DuPont-NEN Products, Boston,
Mass.). Hybridomas were doubly cloned by limiting
dilution, inoculated into Pristane-primed mice for ascites
production and MOAb DWP purified from ascites fluid by
ammonium sulfate precipitation followed by sequential
chromatography on DEAE Affigel blue and Sephadex G150. DWP
was determined to be an IgG2b kappa molecule by ELISA using
rabbit antibodies against the various classes of mouse
immunoglobulins.

Western Blot and Immunoperoxidase Analysis

Biochemical evaluation of cell lines transformed with
activated human ras genes for reactivity with DWP was
carried out by Western blot procedures (11,12).
Immunocytochemical analysis on cell lines and human tumor
tissue utilized the avidin-Biotin complex immunoperoxidase
assay (13) on formalin-fixed paraffin-embedded materials.
In all cases, a negative class matched myeloma protein,
MOPC 141, (Litton Bionetics, Rockville, MD) was used at a
similar protein concentration to DWP.

Cell Lines

Untransformed NIH3T3 mouse fibroblasts and NIH3T3 cell
lines transformed with the T24 bladder carcinoma DNA or DNA
from the lung carcinoma cell line, Calu 1, were maintained
in DMEM-high glucose medium supplemented with 10% fetal
calf serum. The PSV 13 cell line which overexpresses the
normal C Ha-ras P21 protein was produced by transforming
the NIH3T3 cell line with a molecular construct containing
the cloned C-Ha-ras gene and an SV40 promoter linked to the
gene for neomycin resistance. The PSV LM (EJ) cell line
was produced in a similar fashion except that the C Ha-ras
gene contained a mutation in the position 12 codon leading
to the expression of a P21 containing valine at position
12. The PSV LM (EJ) also overexpresses the mutated P21.

Results

Ten Balb/c X C57Bl/6 mice were immunized with the
dodecapeptide Lys-Leu-Val-Val-Val-Gly-Ala-Val-Gly-
Val-Gly-Lys conjugated to BTg representing the primary
amino acid structure of positions 5-16 of the ras P21
expressed in T24 bladder carcinomas cells which have valine
at position 12. Mouse sera were evaluated periodically for
the presence of anti-peptide antibodies, and mice were
selected for fusion based on anti-peptide antibody titers.
Immune spleen cells were fused with Sp2/0 cells and 2 to 3
weeks later culture supernatants were evaluated by ELISA
and immunoglobulins reactive with peptides (conjugated to
KLH) containing valine at position 12 but not reactive with
peptides containing glycine at position 12 were selected
for further analysis. The hybridoma secreting the antibody
of desired reactivity was evaluated for binding with
peptides conjugated to KLH, with unconjugated peptides, or
with BTg and KLH carrier proteins. Assays evaluating two
fold serial dilutions of DWP on valine containing peptides
conjugated to KLH showed strong positive reactivity at
dilutions greater than one to fifty million. DWP also
showed strong reactivity on unconjugated valine containing
peptides. In contrast, DWP was unreactive on conjugated
and unconjugated glycine-containing peptides as well as on
carrier proteins BTg and KLH.

To define MOAb DWP specificity further, a competition assay
was performed in which a series of peptides containing
various amino acid substitutions at position 12 were tested
for the ability to bind DWP and inhibit its binding to
valine containing peptides conjugated to KLH. Results
indicated that peptides containing glycine, alanine,
serine, arginine, aspartic or glutamic acid at position 12
were unreactive with MOAb DWP thereby allowing maximum
binding of the DWP MOAb to the peptide-KLH conjugate. In
contrast, the valine and to a lesser extent the cysteine
containing peptides bound DWP, thereby making it
unavailable for binding to the peptide (val at 12)-KLH
conjugate. These results demonstrate specificity of DWP
for dodecapeptides containing valine and cysteine at
position 12.

In the next series of experiments DWP immunoreactivity was evaluated on cell lines expressing glycine, valine or cysteine at position 12 of the ras P21 protein. Cell lines overexpressing the normal and mutated P21 proteins were also included in this study. Results demonstrated that cell lines containing glycine at position 12 were unreactive with DWP whereas cell lines containing altered P21s with valine or cysteine showed positive immunoperoxidase reactivity. Cell lines incubated with class matched, affinity purified MOPC 141 immunoglobulin were unreactive in all cases.

Several attempts at immunoprecipitating ras P21 from cell lines using DWP were unsuccessful. Western blot analysis was then utilized to study the PSV-LM-EJ and PSV-13 cell lines for DWP immunoreactivity. Ras P21 was concentrated from these cell lines with rat MOAb 259 (14) prior to SDS-polyacrylamide gel electrophoresis and transfer to nitrocellulose paper. Results showed that DWP detected a 21K dalton protein from the PSV-LM-EJ cells but not from PSV-13 cells. These results closely resembled those seen in the PSV-LM-EJ immunoblotting studies with the 259 control antibody. Control studies employing normal rat serum or murine MOPC 141 antibodies showed no reactivity with P21.

In the final series of experiments paraffin embedded human tissues were examined for DWP immunoreactivity using the avidin-biotin immunoperoxidase technique. DWP was found to be reactive with approximately 60% of lung colon, breast and ovarian carcinomas studied whereas all carcinomas tested with the negative control MOPC 141 were not reactive. In most carcinomas examined in this study, heterogeneity in the number of tumor cells reactive with MOAb DWP was consistently observed. Epithelial fibroblastic, and lymphoid elements of normal lung, colon, spleen, heart, liver and stomach were unreactive with both the MOPC 141 control and DWP. However, some smooth muscle in normal colon, lung and stomach tissues showed positive reactivity with DWP.

Discussion

MOAb DWP was reactive with conjugated and unconjugated dodecapeptides containing valine or cysteine at position 12 but not reactive with peptides containing a variety of

other amino acid changes. MOAb DWP was reactive by
immunoperoxidase and Western blot analysis on cell lines
expressing valine or cysteine at position 12 of the ras P21
but not reactive with a cell line transformed by
overexpression of normal P21. Analysis of formalin fixed
paraffin-embedded human tissues indicated that DWP reacted
with both primary and metastatic human carcinomas but was
not reactive on a series of normal tissues with the
exception of smooth muscle.

To our knowledge, DWP represents the first monoclonal
antibody which is capable of distinguishing altered P21
from normal P21. Previous reports have described a rat
monoclonal antibody 259 which is reactive with normal and
mutated ras P21 proteins found in both mammalian (15) and
yeast cells (16). Another series of anti-ras MOAbs,
designated RAP antibodies, were raised against synthetic
peptides corresponding to positions 10-17 of the ras P21.
These antibodies are reactive with both normal and altered
cellular P21 proteins as well as 97% of colon carcinomas
and 90% of intraductal carcinomas of the breast by the
avidin biotin immunoperoxidase procedure (17,18).

The observation that DWP reacts with greater than 60% of
the carcinomas tested is interesting in light of published
reports which describe activated ras genes in 10-20% of
human tumors. While DWP has shown immunological
specificity in vitro its reactivity with human carcinomas
should be interpreted with caution. It will be necessary
to determine the biochemical basis for its immunoreactivity
with these tissues before a claim can be made that DWP is
specifically detecting altered ras gene products in these
cells.

MOAb DWP may prove valuable in identification and
classification of human tumors. Secondly, this antibody
may provide a useful tool in studying the role of ras P21
in cellular transformation and the interaction of P21 with
other cellular proteins.

REFERENCES

1. Harvey JJ (1964) An unidentified virus which causes the rapid production of tumours in mice. Nature 204.1104

2. Kirsten WH, Mayer LA (1967) Morphologic responses to a murine erythroblastosis virus. JNCI 39.311

3. Der CJ Kroniris TG, Cooper GM (1982) Transforming genes of human bladder and lung carcinoma cell lines are homologous to the ras genes of Harvey and Kirsten sarcoma viruses. PNAS USA 79.3637.

4. Eva A, Trowick SR, Gol RA, Pierce JH, Aaronson SA (1983) Transforming genes of human hematopoietic tumors. Frequent detection of ras related oncogenes whose activation appears to be independent of tumor phenotype. PNAS 80.4926.

5. Der, CJ, Cooper, GM (1983) Altered gene products are associated with activation of cellular ras K genes in human lung and colon carcinomas. Cell 32.201

6. Taparowsky E, Suard Y, Fascino O. Shimizu K, Goldfarb M, Wigler M (1982) Activation of the T24 bladder carcinoma transforming gene is linked to a single amino acid change   Nature 300.762.

7. Niman HL, Houghten RA. Walker LE, Reisfeld RA. Wilson IA, Hogle JM, Lerner RA (1983) Generation of protein-reactive antibodies by short peptides is an event of high frequency. Implications for the structural basis of immune recognition. PNAS USA 80.4949.

8. Niman, HL (1984) Antisera to a synthetic peptide of the sis viral oncogene product recognize human platelet-derived growth factor. Nature 307.180.

9. Goodfriend TL. Levine L, Fasman GD (1964) Antibodies to Bradykinin and Angiotensin a use of carbodiimides in immunology. Science 144:1344

10. Galfre G, Milstein C, Wright B (1979) Rat X rat hybrid myeloma and a monoclonal anti-Fc portion of mouse IgG. Nature 277:131.

11. Towbin H, Staehelm T, Gordon J (1979) Electrophoretic transfer of proteins from polyacrylamide gels to nitrocellulose sheets. Procedure and some applications PNAS USA 76.4350.

12. Burnette WN (1981) "Western Blotting". Electrophoretic transfer of proteins from sodium dodecyl sulfate-polyacrylamide gels to unmodified nitrocellulose and radiographic detection with antibody and radioiodinated protein A. Analytical Biochemistry 112:195.

13. Hsu SM, Raine L, Fanger H (1981) A comparative study of the peroxidase anti-peroxidase method and avidin-biotin complex method for staining polypeptide hormones with RIA antibodies. Am. J Clin. Path. 75.734

14. Furth ME, Davis LJ, Fleurdelys B, Scolnick EM (1982) Monoclonal antibodies to the P21 products of the transforming gene or Harvey murine sarcoma virus and of the cellular ras gene family. J. Virol. 43.294

15. Ellis RW, DeFeo D, Papageorge A Scolnick EM (1983) Expression of endogenous P21 ras genes. In Oncogenes and Retroviruses. Evaluation of Basic Findings and Clinical Potential 67-77.

16. Tamanoi F Walsh M, Kataoka T Wigler M. (1984) A product of yeast RAS 2 gene is a guanine nucleotide binding protein PNAS 81.6924.

17. Horan P, Thor A, Wunderlich D, Muraro R, Caruso A, Schlom J. (1984) Monoclonal antibodies of predefined specificity detect activated ras gene expression in human mammary and colon carcinomas. PNAS 81:5227.

18. Thor A, Hand PH, Wunderlich D, Caruso A, Muraro R, Schlom J (1984) Monoclonal antibodies define differential ras gene expression in malignant and benign colonic diseases. Nature 311:562.

Monoclonal Antibodies and Cancer Therapy, pages 573–585
© 1985 Alan R. Liss, Inc.

BIOLOGIC CONSIDERATIONS FOR THE DEVELOPMENT
OF ANIMAL MODELS TO STUDY TREATMENT
OF METASTATIC HUMAN NEOPLASMS.

Isaiah J. Fidler and Raffaella Giavazzi

Department of Cell Biology, The University of Texas
M. D. Anderson Hospital and Tumor Institute
at Houston, Houston, Texas 77030

ABSTRACT   Human and rodent neoplasms are heterogeneous and contain many subpopulations of cells with
different biologic properties that include metastatic
potential.   Young athymic nude mice can be used to
ascertain the metastatic potential of tumor cells and
for selection of metastatic subpopulations of cells
from both mouse and human neoplasms.   The metastatic
potential of mouse or human cells varies with the
site of initial implantation. Thus, both tumor cell
properties and host factors must be taken into consideration in the design of studies dealing with the
biology and therapy of human cancer metastasis in the
athymic nude mouse.

INTRODUCTION

The growth of metastases depends on both tumor cell
properties and host factors, and the relative contributions of these factors can vary from one tumor system to
another (1-5).   It is imperative that, at this stage in
the development of monoclonal antibodies for the diagnosis and treatment of cancer, the main objective of this
work not be obscure: In the main, the challenge to the
clinical oncologist is the eradication of metastases that
occur in the primary host.   Therefore, to develop and
evaluate new therapeutic modalities for disseminated
cancer such as monoclonal antibodies, it is necessary to
test them in meaningful model systems.

The design of effective therapeutic modalities, including the use of monoclonal antibodies for treatment of metastases, must be based upon considerations of the biology of cancer metastasis.

The pathogenesis of metastasis involves a series of sequential steps wherein tumor cells must first invade tissues surrounding the primary neoplasm, thereby gaining entrance into blood vessels or lymphatics. Some tumor cells can detach and disseminate to reach capillary beds of distant organs. After some cells extravasate into the organ parenchyma, new lesions can develop. The process of metastasis is highly selective, and the final outgrowth of tumors in various distant organs represents the end point of many destructive events that not every tumor cell can survive (5-7). Only a few tumor cells of a primary tumor can invade blood vessels, and of those cells that enter the circulation, less than 0.1% survive transport (5). Similarily, not all malignant cells that survive transport can arrest in the microcirculation, undergo extravasation into organ parenchyma, escape systemic and local host defense mechanisms, respond to local or systemic growth stimuli, and proliferate into metastases (5). In turn it is important to remember that the response to therapeutic agents of tumor cells that survive to become metastases is influenced by both the tumor cell properties and host factors such as organ environment, local and systemic defense mechanisms, and the presence of growth-modifying factors.

The Origin and Development of Biologic Heterogeneity in Metastases

The major obstacle to the effective treatment of metastases is the fact that cells populating both primary and secondary neoplasms are not uniform. By the time of diagnosis, and certainly in clinically advanced lesions, malignant neoplasms contain multiple populations of cells with infinite biological heterogeneity (1-7). Cells obtained from individual tumors can exhibit different cell surface properties, antigenicity, immunogenicity, growth rate, karyotype, sensitivity to various cytotoxic drugs, and potential for invasion and metastasis (3,8). Biologic heterogeneity is not confined to cells in primary tumors and is even more prominent among cells populating metastases (5,8). In general, metastases do not result from the random survival of tumor cells detaching from the primary tumor, but from the selective growth of specialized cells that preexist in a heterogeneous neoplasm (9). Metastases, like primary tumors, may have a unicellular or a multicellular origin. Studies from our laboratory (10) and others (11) have recently shown that some metastases can be clonal in origin, and that different metatases can originate from different progenitor cells (10). Such data provide a partial explanation for the clinical observation that different metastases can react differently to cytotoxic drugs or to identification with monoclonal antibodies (8). However, the issue of biologic heterogeneity in metastases is more complex. Even within a single metastasis of clonal origin, biologic diversity develops rapidly (12-15). Thus by the time of diagnosis, when metastases are large (>8 mm), they contain multiple subpopulations of cells. This process of evolution and progression of metastases probably results from the phenotypic instability associated with clonal populations of cells (12,15) and from the high rate of spontaneous mutation unique to highly metastatic cells (15-17).

The corollary of these findings is that the genesis of cellular diversity within tumors is a powerful mechanism for increasing the ability of a tumor to survive a diverse array of destructive selection pressures. Moreover, the continuous emergence of new clonal subpopulations of tumor cells with diverse phenotypes increases the probability that one or more subpopulations will survive natural or iatrogenic selection pressures.

Host Factors and the Pathogenesis and Treatment of Metastases

Whether experimental tumor systems are valid models for therapeutic modalities for human cancer, or indeed whether specific therapeutic modalities shown to be effective in one animal tumor system can be applied to another system, is debatable (18). Animal models for human disease can provide answers only for carefully defined questions. For example, if the major objective of an investigation is to determine whether the systemic administration of a monoclonal antibody can lead to destruction of melanoma metastases, the model must not use nonmetastatic cells growing in irrelevant anatomical sites. Rather, the model must employ metastatic melanoma cells proliferating in organs where malignant melanoma metastases usually occur, i.e. lungs, lymph nodes, and brain.

To better use animal models in therapy studies, some obvious rules must be routinely followed. All animals must be of a precise age, sex, strain, and health status. Even conditions considered trivial by some may have profound influence on the outcome of experiments. For example, rodents infested with endoparasites, e.g. pin worms, or ectoparasites, e.g. lice, do not react to tumor challenge in the same way as animals that are parasite free. Similarly, rodents infected with pathogenic bacteria or viruses cannot be used in immunological studies. The use of such animals assures peculiar results and lack of reproducibility (18).

Ideally, all experimental animals should be given identical environmental conditions and care. The lack of uniformity in housing, diet, and so on has been shown to bring about discrepancies in experimental results (18). Sometimes, however, totally unsuspected factors can influence the outcome of otherwise well-planned experiments. Our own experience with the adverse effects of hyperchlorinated drinking water on mice is an appropriate example (19). Historically, hyperchlorinated drinking water has been given to experimental animals to avoid the so-called "early death syndrome" in lethally irradiated animals due to pathogenic enteric bacteria such as Pseudomonas. The recommended level of hyperchlorination has been 12-16 parts per million (ppm). Owing to the unusually high incidence of Pseudomonas sp. within certain breeding units of our experimental animal facilities, we temporarily increased the hyperchlorination of the drinking water to 25-30 ppm. Within several weeks, abnormalities in the mice were noticeable. Weight-gain problems developed, and the number of macrophages fell drastically. Thus, a routine procedure used in animal husbandry heretofore considered safe and of little consequence to the outcome of investigations affected the pathogenesis of experimental metastasis (19).

The Use of Young Nude Mice to Study Heterogeneous Metastatic Human Neoplasms.

Since the first report by Rygaard and Povlsen that xenogeneic human tumors can grow in athymic nude mice (20), there have been numerous studies using his animal model for the propagation and expansion of human neoplasms (review 21,22). Successful growth of xenogeneic tumors in nude mice is contingent upon both tumor cell properties and host factors. Tumor-related properties, such as the origin and type of tumor and the route of inoculation appear important. For example, human melanomas, carcinomas of soft tissues, and sarcomas are easily transplanted (23). In contrast, carcinomas of the breast, prostate, and stomach are more difficult to grow in nude mice (24). To successfully grow leukemias and lymphomas, the recipient nude mouse must be further immunocompromised or receive intracranial tumor injections or both (25). Many host-related factors such as age, strain, state of health, and housing conditions influence the growth of rodent or human tumors in the athymic nude mouse (26,27). For example, three-week-old mice develop significantly more lung metastases than do six- to eight-week-old mice similarly challenged with tumor cells (27). Nude mice infected with mouse hepatitis virus strongly resist transplanted xenogeneic human tumors (26), and nude mice maintained in specific pathogen-free conditions are consistently more receptive to transplanted human neoplasms than animals maintained under conventional conditions (28).

The nude mouse is not deficient in natural defense mechanisms. Indeed, both natural killer (NK) cell and macrophages of nude mice play a prominent role in the rejection of transplanted neoplasms. Moreover, results from our laboratory and many others suggest that NK cells are particularly efficient in destroying circulating tumor emboli (review 29).

The observation that three-week-old nude mice, in which the NK cell system is not yet fully activated, can be used for the quantitation of the metastatic potential of neoplasms allowed us to use this mouse to select metastatic subpopulations of cells from two allogeneic hetrogeneous melanomas, the B16 melanoma syngeneic to the C57BL/6 mouse (30,31) and the K-1735 melanoma syngeneic to the C3H/HEN mouse (30,31), and from a xenogeneic human

melanoma, the A-375 line (21,31). Three-week-old
BALB/cAn nude mice received intravenous injections of
viable cells of the B16 melanoma, the K-1735 melanoma, or
the human A-375 melanoma. Four to five weeks later, the
mice were sacrificed, and solitary lung tumor colonies
were harvested from different mice and transplanted via
trocar into the subcutis of new, young nude mice (1
metastasis/mouse) to expand the populations. Suspensions
of single viable tumor cells were prepared from each
individual subcutaneous tumor by collagenase dissociation. The metastatic potential of the parent tumor and
of the established metastases was determined by the
injection of portions of the cell suspensions into the
tail vein of unanesthetized immunocompetent syngeneic
(B16, K-1735) or three-week-old allogeneic nude mice
(B16, K-1735, A-375). Four weeks later, the mice were
sacrificed, the lungs were placed in Bouin's fluid, and
peripheral lung tumor colonies were counted with use of
the dissecting microscope. Results were recorded as the
median and range of lung tumor counts. Differences in
metastatic incidence among the groups were further
analyzed by the Mann-Whitney U-test. In all tumor
systems, cells isolated from the lung tumor colonies
produced a significantly higher incidence of metastases
(P<0.001) than did cells of the unselected parent tumor
(Tables 1 and 2). This enhanced metastatic potential was
expressed in both the allogeneic nude mice and, for the
mouse tumors, in normal syngeneic recipients (30,31).

More recently, we examined the metastatic behavior
of seven human tumor lines grown in three-week-old nude
mice. Two cell lines were derived from melanomas, two
from prostate adenocarcinomas, two from renal adenocarcinomas, and one from a colon carcinoma. The incidence of
metastasis produced by these cells subsequent to intravenous (experimental metastasis), subcutaneous (spontaneous
metastasis), or intrasplenic (experimental/spontaneous
metastasis), implantation was primarily dependent on the
biological characteristics of the individual tumor cells.
However, manipulation of such host factors as natural
killer-cell activity by chronic administration of 17 β-
estradiol or site of tumor cell implantation increased
the metastatic potential of the cells (22).

Table 1. <u>In vivo</u> selection for tumor cells with increased metastatic potential from the B16 melanoma and the K-1735 melanoma growing in athymic nude mice[1]

Mouse Strain	Source of Cells[2]	Median Number (Range) Pulmonary Metastases[3]	
		Nude Mice (3-wk-old)	Syngeneic Mice (6-wk-old)
C57BL/6	B16 Parent	0.5 (0-7)	1.0 (0-11)
	Lung Met-1	9.5 (1-39)	8.0 (1-16)
	Lung Met-2	40.0 (3-101)	27.0 (7-40)
	Lung Met-3	87.0 (37-298)	68.0 (2-98)
	Lung Met-4	25.0 (4-56)	11.0 (3-23)
C3H/HeN	K-1735 Parent	19 (3-56)	44 (10-148)
	Lung Met-1	>500 (all >500)	>500 (all >500)
	Lung Met-2	406 (184->500)	>500 (all >500)
	Lung Met-3	>500 (all >500)	>500 (all >500)
	Lung Met-4	124 (57-186)	200 (134-245)

[1] From Pollack and Fidler (30)

[2] B16 melanoma cells; 10,000 cells/dose/mouse. K-1735 cells; 25,000 cells/dose/nude mouse; and 50,000 cells/dose/syngeneic mouse.

[3] Ten mice/group. Median number of lung tumor colonies differed significantly between groups injected with cells isolated from metastases or from parent tumor ($P<0.001$).

Table 2. The isolation of cells with enhanced metastatic potential from the A-375 human melanoma line growing in athymic nude mice.[1]

Source of Cells	Dose Injected Intravenously	Median Number (Range) Pulmonary Metastases[2]
A375 Parent	10^5	0 (0)
	8×10^5	3 (0-21)
Lung Met-1	10^5	all >250
Lung Met-2	10^5	all >250
Lung Met-3	10^5	>250 (63->250)
Lung Met-4	10^5	138 (16-182)
Lung Met-5	10^5	131 (6-160)
Lung Met-6	10^5	84 (65-115)
Lung Met-7	10^5	71 (12-93)

[1] From Fidler, Pollack and Hanna (31).

[2] Ten mice/group. Differences in incidence of metastasis produced by cells harvested from metastases and those of parent tumor were highly significant (P<0.001).

We were particularly impressed with how important the implantation of tumor cells into a relevant organ site was to the outcome of metastasis. Tumor cells of colon carcinoma, renal carcinoma, and prostatic carcinoma injected into the spleen produced metastases in the liver, lungs, and lymph nodes, whereas the same tumor cells implanted subcutaneously formed only local neoplasms (Table 3). All the tumor lines isolated in our laboratory have been routinely examined by karyotypic and isozyme analyses to verify their human origin, ruling out artefacts (32).

CONCLUSIONS

The pathogenesis of a metastasis is complex, and the growth of secondary lesions represents the end point of many destructive events that few tumor cells can survive. The heterogeneity of neoplasms for metastatic properties, however it originates, has important implications for the study and treatment of cancer metastases. A model for such studies must therefore use a relevant cell populations (metastatic cells) implanted into a relevant organ environment. These are demanding criteria for setting up models for therapy. Nonetheless, the complex problem of treating metastasis may demand the abandoning of simple and admittedly easier models, which may provide answers of little clinical relevance.

Table 3. The production of metastasis by human tumor lines injected into athymic nude mice[1]

Cell Line	Implantation Site	Number of Animals with Metastasis[2]
A-375 melanoma parent line	i.v.	1/5
	s.c. (thorax)	0/10
	s.c. (hind footpad)	0/20
A375 melanoma metastatic line[3]	i.v.	5/5
	s.c. (thorax)	9/10
	s.c. (hind footpad)	19/20
Prostatic Ca parent line	i.v.	0
	s.c. (thorax)	1/10
	s.c. (hind footpad)	2/10
	intrasplenic	16/20
Prostatic Ca metastatic line[3]	i.v.	13/15
	s.c. (thorax)	8/10
	s.c. (hind footpad)	3/10
	intrasplenic	20/20

[1] From Kozlowski et al. (21,22).

[2] Lung, liver, and lymph nodes of nude mice were examined histologically to confirm the presence of growing metastases.

[3] Metastatic lines were isolated from rare metastases produced by parental tumors.

REFERENCES

1. Fidler IJ, Poste G (1982). The heterogeneity of metastatic properties in malignant tumor cells and regulation of the metastatic phenotype. In Owens A (ed): "Tumor Cell Heterogeneity," New York: Academic Press, p 127.
2. Nicolson GL, Poste G (1982). Tumor cell diversity and host responses in cancer metastasis. Curr Prob Cancer 7:4.
3. Fidler IJ, Hart IR (1982). Biological diversity in metastatic neoplasms: Origins and implications. Science 217:998.
4. Heppner G (1984). Tumor heterogeneity. Cancer Res 214:2259.
5. Fidler IJ (1984). The evolution of biological heterogeneity in metastatic neoplasms. In Nicolson GL, Milas L (eds): "Cancer Invasion and Metastasis: Biologic and Therapeutic Aspects," New York: Raven Press, p 5.
6. Fidler IJ, Gersten DM, Hart IR (1978). The biology of cancer invasion and metastasis. Adv Cancer Res 28:149.
7. Poste G, Fidler IJ (1980). The pathogenesis of cancer metastasis. Nature 283:139.
8. Hart IR, Fidler IJ (1981). The implications of tumor heterogeneity for studies on the biology and therapy of cancer metastasis. Biochim Biophys Acta 651:37.
9. Fidler IJ, Kripke ML (1977). Metastasis results from preexisting variant cells within a malignant tumor. Science 197:893.
10. Talmadge JE, Wolman SR, Fidler IJ (1982). Evidence for the clonal origin of spontaneous metastases. Science 217:361.
11. Poste G, Greig R, Tzeng J, Koestler T, Corwin S (1984). Interactions between tumor cell subpopulations in malignant tumors. In Nicolson GL, Milas L (eds): "Cancer Invasion and Metastasis: Biologic and Therapeutic Aspects," New York: Raven Press, p. 223.
12. Poste G, Doll J, Fidler IJ (1981). Interactions between clonal subpopulations affect the stability of the metastatic phenotype in polyclonal populations of the B16 melanoma cells. Proc Natl Acad Sci USA 78:6226.

13. Poste G, Tzeng J, Doll J, Greig R, Reiman D, Zeidman I (1982). Evolution of tumor cell heterogeneity during progressive growth of individual lung metastases. Proc Natl Acad Sci USA 79:6574.

14. Talmadge JE, Benedict K, Madsen J, Fidler IJ (1984). The development of biological diversity and susceptibility to chemotherapy in cancer metastases. Cancer Res 44:3801.

15. Cifone MA, Fidler IJ (1982). Increasing metastatic potential is associated with increasing genetic instability of clones isolated from murine neoplasms. Proc Natl Acad Sci USA 78:6949.

16. Bosslet K, Schirrmacher V (1982). High frequency generation of new immunoresistant tumor variants during metastasis of a cloned murine tumor line (ESb). Int J Cancer 29:195.

17. Harris JF, Chambers AF, Hill RP, Ling V (1982). Metastatic variants are generated spontaneously at a high rate in mouse KHT tumor. Proc Natl Acad Sci USA 79:5547.

18. Fidler IJ (1982). The role of host factors and tumor heterogeneity in the testing of therapeutic agents. In Fidler IJ, White RJ (eds): "Design of Models for Testing Cancer Therapeutic Agents," New York: Van Nostrand Reinhold, p. 239.

19. Fidler IJ (1977): Depression of macrophage in mice drinking hyperchlorinated water. Nature 270:735.

20. Rygaard J, Povlsen CO (1969). Heterotransplantation of human malignant tumor to nude mice. Acta Pathol Microbiol Scand (A) 77:758.

21. Kozlowski JM, Hart IR, Fidler IJ, Hanna N (1984). A human melanoma line heterogeneous with respect to metastatic capacity in athymic nude mice. JNCI 72(4):913.

22. Kozlowski JM, Fidler IJ, Campbell D, Xu Z, Kaighn ME, Hart IR (1984). Metastatic behavior of human tumor cell lines grown in the nude mouse. Cancer Res 44:3522.

23. Giovanella BC, Stehlin JS, Williams LJ Jr (1974). Heterotransplantation of human malignant tumors in nude thymusless mice. II. Malignant tumors induced by injection of cell cultures derived from human solid tumors. JNCI 52:921.

24. Reid LC, Shin SI (1978). Transplantation of hetero-logous endocrine tumor cells in nude mice. In Fogh JE, Giovanella BC (eds) "The Nude Mouse in Experimental and Clinical Research," New York: Academic Press, p. 313.

25. Epstein AL, Herman MM, Kim H, Dorfman RF, Kaplan HS (1976). Biology of the human malignant lymphomas, III. Intracranial heterotransplantation in the nude, athymic mouse. Cancer 37:2158.

26. Kyriazis A, DiPersio L, Michael JG, Pesce AJ (1979). Influence of the mouse hepatitis virus (MHV) infection on the growth of human tumors in the athymic mouse. Int J Cancer 23:402.

27. Hanna N (1980). Expression of metastatic potential of tumor cells in young nude mice is correlated with low levels of natural killer cell-mediated cytotoxicity. Int J Cancer 26:675.

28. Hanna N, Davis TW, Fidler IJ (1982). Environmental and genetic factors determine the level of NK activity of nude mice and affect their suitability as models for experimental metastasis. Int J Cancer 30:371.

29. Hanna N (1982). Role of natural killer cells in control of cancer metastasis. Cancer Met Rev 1:45.

30. Pollack VA, Fidler IJ (1982). Use of young nude mice for selection of subpopulations of cells with increased metastatic potential from nonsyngeneic neoplasms. JNCI 69:137.

31. Fidler IJ, Pollack VA, Hanna N (1984). The use of nude mice for studies of cancer metastasis. In Sordat B (ed) "Immune Deficient Animals," Basel: Karger A.G., p. 388.

32. Goldenberg D, Pavia R (1981). Malignant potential of murine stromal cell after transplantation of human tumors into nude mice. Science 212:65.

Index